Essential Benefits
The Power of Essential Oils

Contents

Chapter 1

Introduction to the Essential Oils

1.1 Essential oil

For the Midnight Oil album, see Essential Oils (album).

An **essential oil** is a concentrated hydrophobic liquid containing volatile aroma compounds from plants. Essential oils are also known as **volatile oils**, **ethereal oils**, **aetherolea**, or simply as the **oil of the plant** from which they were extracted, such as oil of clove. An oil is "essential" in the sense that it contains the "essence of" the plant's fragrance—the characteristic fragrance of the plant from which it is derived.[1] The term essential used here does not mean indispensable as with the terms essential amino acid or essential fatty acid which are so-called since they are nutritionally required by a given living organism.[2] Rather, it has been suggested by aromatherapists that "essential oil" is a contraction of "quintessential oil," from the Aristotelian theory of matter. [3]

Essential oils are generally extracted by distillation, often by using steam. Other processes include expression, solvent extraction, absolute oil extraction, resin tapping, and cold pressing. They are used in perfumes, cosmetics, soaps and other products, for flavoring food and drink, and for adding scents to incense and household cleaning products.

Essential oils have been used medicinally in history. Medical applications proposed by those who sell medicinal oils range from skin treatments to remedies for cancer and often are based solely on historical accounts of use of essential oils for these purposes. Claims for the efficacy of medical treatments, and treatment of cancers in particular, are now subject to regulation in most countries.

As the use of essential oils has declined in evidence-based medicine, one must consult older textbooks for much information on their use.[4][5] Modern works are less inclined to generalize; rather than refer to "essential oils" as a class at all, they prefer to discuss specific compounds, such as methyl salicylate, rather than "oil of wintergreen".[6][7]

Interest in essential oils has revived in recent decades with the popularity of aromatherapy, a branch of alternative medicine that claims that essential oils and other aromatic compounds have curative effects. Oils are volatilized or diluted in a carrier oil and used in massage, diffused in the air by a nebulizer, heated over a candle flame, or burned as incense.

The earliest recorded mention of the techniques and methods used to produce essential oils is believed to be that of Ibn al-Baitar (1188–1248), an Andalusian physician, pharmacist and chemist.[8]

1.1.1 Production

Main article: Extraction (fragrance)

Distillation

See also: Distillation

Today, most common essential oils — such as lavender, peppermint, tea tree oil and eucalyptus — are distilled. Raw plant material, consisting of the flowers, leaves, wood, bark, roots, seeds, or peel, is put into an alembic (distillation apparatus) over water. As the water is heated, the steam passes through the plant material, vaporizing the volatile compounds. The vapors flow through a coil, where they condense back to liquid, which is then collected in the receiving vessel.

Most oils are distilled in a single process. One exception is *ylang-ylang* (*Cananga odorata*), which takes 22 hours to complete through a fractional distillation.

The recondensed water is referred to as a hydrosol, hydrolat, herbal distillate or plant water essence, which may be sold as another fragrant product. Popular hydrosols include rose water, lavender water, lemon balm, clary sage and orange blossom water. The use of herbal distillates in cosmetics is increasing. Some plant hydrosols have unpleasant smells and are therefore not sold.

Expression

Most citrus peel oils are expressed mechanically or cold-pressed (similar to olive oil extraction). Due to the relatively large quantities of oil in citrus peel and low cost to grow and harvest the raw materials, citrus-fruit oils are cheaper than most other essential oils. Lemon or sweet orange oils that are obtained as byproducts of the citrus industry are even cheaper.

Before the discovery of distillation, all essential oils were extracted by pressing.

Solvent extraction

Most flowers contain too little volatile oil to undergo expression; their chemical components are too delicate and easily denatured by the high heat used in steam distillation. Instead, a solvent such as hexane or supercritical carbon dioxide is used to extract the oils. Extracts from hexane and other hydrophobic solvents are called *concretes*, which are a mixture of essential oil, waxes, resins, and other lipophilic (oil-soluble) plant material.

Although highly fragrant, concretes contain large quantities of nonfragrant waxes and resins. Often, another solvent, such as ethyl alcohol, which is more polar in nature, is used to extract the fragrant oil from the concrete. The alcohol solution is chilled to −18C/0F for more than 48 hour which causes the waxes and lipids to precipitate out. The precipitates are then filtered out and the ethanol is removed from the remaining solution by evaporation, vacuum purge, or both, leaving behind the *absolute*.

Supercritical carbon dioxide is used as a solvent in supercritical fluid extraction. This method has many benefits including avoiding petrochemical residues in the product and the loss of some "top notes" when steam distillation is used. It does not yield an absolute directly. The supercritical carbon dioxide will extract both the waxes and the essential oils that make up the concrete. Subsequent processing with liquid carbon dioxide, achieved in the same extractor by merely lowering the extraction temperature, will separate the waxes from the essential oils. This lower temperature process prevents the decomposition and denaturing of compounds. When the extraction is complete, the pressure is reduced to ambient and the carbon dioxide reverts to a gas, leaving no residue.

Supercritical carbon dioxide is also used for making decaffeinated coffee. Although it uses the same basic principles, it is a different process because of the difference in scale.

Florasols extraction

Florasol (R134a), a refrigerant, was developed to replace Freon. Although Florasol is an "ozone-friendly" product, it is still a fluorochemical (1,1,1,2-Tetrafluoroethane) and it poses significant danger to the environment due to its global warming potential (GWP; 100-yr GWP = 1430).[9] The European Union has banned its use, with a phase-out process beginning in 2011, to be completed in 2017 [10] One advantage is that the extraction of essential oils occurs at or below room temperature so degradation through high temperature extremes does not occur. The essential oils are mostly pure and contain little to no foreign substances.

Production quantities

Estimates of total production of essential oils are difficult to obtain. One estimate, compiled from data in 1989, 1990 and 1994 from various sources, gives the following total production, in tonnes, of essential oils for which more than 1,000 tonnes were produced.[11]

For a video on smaller-scale domestic use production and extraction, see The Essential Series: Essential Concoction. <EupterraFoundation.com>

1.1.2 Pharmacology

Although medicinal use of essential oils is seen as pseudoscience in the healthcare community,[12] essential oils retain considerable popular use among advocates of alternative medicine. Therefore, it is difficult to obtain reliable references concerning their pharmacological merits.

Studies have shown that certain essential oils may have the ability to prevent the transmission of some drug-resistant strains of pathogen, specifically Staphylococcus, Streptococcus and Candida.[13]

Taken by mouth, many essential oils can be dangerous in high concentrations. Typical effects begin with a burning feeling, followed by salivation. In the stomach, the effect is carminative, relaxing the gastric sphincter and encouraging eructation (belching). Further down the gut, the effect typically is antispasmodic.[4]

Typical ingredients for such applications include eucalyptus oils, menthol, capsaicin, anise and camphor. Other essential oils work well in these applications, but it is notable that others offer no significant benefit. This illustrates the fact that different essential oils may have drastically different pharmacology. Those that do work well for upper respiratory tract and bronchial problems act variously as mild expectorants and decongestants. Some act as locally anaesthetic counterirritants and, thereby, exert an antitussive effect.[4][14]

Some essential oils, such as those of juniper and agathosma, are valued for their diuretic effects.[15] With relatively recent concerns about the overuse of antibacterial agents,[16] many essential oils have seen a resurgence in off-label use for such properties and are being examined for this use clinically.[17]

Many essential oils affect the skin and mucous membranes in ways that are valuable or harmful. Many essential oils, particularly tea tree oil, may cause a contact dermatitis.[18][19][20][21] They are used in antiseptics and liniments in particular. Typically, they produce rubefacient irritation at first and then counterirritant numbness. Turpentine oil and camphor are two typical examples of oils that cause such effects. Menthol and some others produce a feeling of cold followed by a sense of burning. This is caused by its effect on heat-sensing nerve endings. Some essential oils, such as clove oil or eugenol, were popular for many hundred years in dentistry as antiseptics and local anaesthetics. Thymol is well known for its antiseptic effects.

1.1.3 Use in aromatherapy

Main article: Aromatherapy

Aromatherapy is a form of alternative medicine in which healing effects are ascribed to the aromatic compounds in essential oils and other plant extracts. Some essential oils are claimed to have an uplifting effect on the mind. Such claims, if meaningful, are not necessarily false but are difficult to quantify in the light of the sheer variability of materials used in the practice.

1.1.4 Dilution

Essential oils are usually lipophilic (literally: *"oil-loving"*) compounds that usually are not miscible with water. They can be diluted in solvents like pure ethanol and polyethylene glycol.

1.1.5 Raw materials

Main article: List of essential oils

Essential oils are derived from sections of plants. Some plants, like the bitter orange, are sources of several types of essential oil.

Eucalyptus oil

Main article: Eucalyptus oil

Most Eucalyptus oil on the market is produced from the leaves of *Eucalyptus globulus*. Steam-distilled eucalyptus oil is used throughout Asia, Africa, Latin America and South America as a primary cleaning/disinfecting agent added to soaped mop and countertop cleaning solutions; it also possesses insect and limited vermin control properties. Note, however, there are hundreds of species of eucalyptus, and perhaps some dozens are used to various extents as sources of essential oils. Not only do the products of different species differ greatly in characteristics and effects, but also the products of the very same tree can vary grossly.[5]

Rose oil

Main article: Rose oil

Rose oil is produced from the petals of *Rosa damascena* and *Rosa centifolia*. Steam-distilled rose oil is known as "rose otto", while the solvent extracted product is known as "rose absolute".

Lavender essential oil

Lavender essential oil has long been used in the production of perfume [22] However, it can be estrogenic and antiandrogenic, causing problems for prepubescent boys and pregnant women, in particular.[23] Lavender essential oil is also used as an insect repellent.[24]

Balsam of Peru

Balsam of Peru, an essential oil derived from the *Myroxylon*, is used in food and drink for flavoring, in perfumes and toiletries for fragrance, and in medicine and pharmaceutical items for healing properties.[25] However, a number of national and international surveys have identified Balsam of Peru as being in the "top five" allergens most commonly causing patch test allergic reactions in people referred to dermatology clinics.[26][27][28]

1.1.6 Dangers

The potential danger of an essential oil is generally relative to its level or grade of purity. Many essential oils are designed exclusively for their aroma-therapeutic quality; these essential oils generally should not be applied directly to the skin in their undiluted or "neat" form. Some can cause severe irritation, provoke an allergic reaction and, over time, prove hepatotoxic.

Essential oils should not be used with animals, as they possess extreme hepatotoxicity and dermal toxicity for animals. Some essential oils, including many of the citrus peel oils, are photosensitizers, increasing the skin's vulnerability to sunlight.[29]

Industrial users of essential oils should consult the safety data sheets (SDS) to determine the hazards and handling requirements of particular oils. Even certain therapeutic grade oils can pose potential threats to individuals with epilepsy or pregnant women.

Handling

Exposure to essential oils may cause a contact dermatitis.[30][31][32] Essential oils can be aggressive toward rubbers and plastics, so care must be taken in choosing the correct handling equipment. Glass syringes are often used, but have coarse volumetric graduations. Chemistry syringes are ideal, as they resist essential oils, are long enough to enter deep vessels, and have fine graduations, facilitating quality control. Unlike traditional pipettes, which have difficulty handling viscous fluids, the chemistry syringe has a seal and piston arrangement which slides inside the pipette, wiping the essential oil off the pipette wall.

Pregnancy

The use of essential oils in pregnancy is not recommended due to inadequate published evidence to demonstrate evidence of safety. Pregnant women often report an abnormal sensitivity to smells and taste,[33] essential oils can cause irritation and nausea.

Gynecomastia

Estrogenic and antiandrogenic activity have been reported by *in vitro* study of tea tree oil and lavender essential oils. Case reports suggest the oils may be implicated in some cases of gynecomastia, an abnormal breast tissue growth, in prepubescent boys.[34][35] However, these claims have been challenged [36] and the European Commission's Scientific Committee on Consumer Safety has dismissed the claims saying "Since the hormonal active ingredients of Tea Tree Oil were shown not to penetrate the skin, the hypothesized correlation of the finding of 3 cases of gynecomastia to the topical use of Tea Tree Oil is considered implausible." [37]

Pesticide residues

There is some concern about pesticide residues in essential oils, particularly those used therapeutically. For this reason, many practitioners of aromatherapy buy organically produced oils. Not only are pesticides present in trace quantities, but also the oils themselves are used in tiny quantities and usually in high dilutions. Where there is a concern about pesticide residues in food essential oils, such as mint or orange oils, the proper criterion is not whether the material is alleged to be organically produced, but whether it meets the government standards based on actual analysis of its pesticide content.[38]

Ingestion

Essential oils are used extensively as GRAS flavoring agents in foods, beverages and confectioneries according to strict Good Manufacturing Practice (GMP) and flavorist standards. Therapeutic grade essential oils are generally safe for human consumption in small amounts. Pharmacopoeia standards for medicinal oils should be heeded. Some oils can be toxic to some domestic animals, cats in particular.[39] The internal use of essential oils can pose hazards to pregnant women, as some can be abortifacients in dose 0.5–10 ml, and thus should not be used during pregnancy.

Flammability

The flash point of each essential oil is different. Many of the common essential oils, such as tea tree, lavender, and citrus oils, are classed as a Class 3 Flammable Liquid, as they have a flash point of 50–60 °C.

Toxicology

The following table lists the LD_{50} or median lethal dose for common oils; this is the dose required to kill half the members of a tested population. LD_{50} is intended as a guideline only, and reported values can vary widely due to differences in tested species and testing conditions.[40]

It is important to understand that the foregoing figures are far less relevant in everyday life than far smaller, often localized levels of exposure. For example, a dose of many an essential oil that would do no harm if swallowed in diluted solution or emulsion, could do serious damage to eyes or lungs in a higher concentration.[4][41]

1.1.7 Standardization of its derived products

In 2002, ISO published ISO 4720 in which the botanical names of the relevant plants are standardized.[42] The rest of the standards with regards to this topic can be found in the section of ICS 71.100.60 [43]

Further information: British Pharmacopoeia and United States Pharmacopoeia

1.1.8 See also

- Aroma lamp
- Enfleurage
- Fragrance oil
- Herb farm
- List of essential oils
- List of vegetable oils
- Volatility

1.1.9 Notes

[1] "essential oil". *Oxford English Dictionary* (online American English ed.). Retrieved 2014-07-21.

[2] Reeds, Peter J (2000). "Dispensable and Indispensable Amino Acids for Humans" (PDF). *Journal of Nutrition* **130**: 1835S-1840S. Retrieved 9 August 2015.

[3] "What are Essential Oils?". National Association for Holistic Aromatherapy. Retrieved 9 August 2015.

[4] Sapeika, Norman (1963). *Actions and Uses of Drugs*. A.A. Balkema.

[5] *Thorpe's Dictionary of Applied Chemistry* **8** (4th ed.). Longmans Green. 1947.

[6] Gilman, A. G.; Rall, T. W.; Nies, Alan S.; Taylor, Palmer, eds. (1990). *Goodman & Gilman's The Pharmacological Basis of Therapeutics* (8th ed.). New York: Pergamon. ISBN 0-08-040296-8.

[7] Klaassen, Curtis D.; Amdur, Mary O.; Casarett, Louis J.; Doull, John (1991). *Casarett and Doull's Toxicology: The Basic Science of Poisons*. New York: McGraw-Hill. ISBN 0071052399.

[8] Houtsma, M.Th. (1993). *E. J. Brill's First Encyclopaedia of Islam, 1913–1936* 4. Brill. pp. 1011–. ISBN 9004097902.

[9] Forster, P; et al. (2007). "Changes in Atmospheric Constituents and in Radiative Forcing" (PDF). In Solomon, S; et al. *Climate Change 2007: The Physical Science Basis. Contribution of Working Group I to the Fourth Assessment Report of the Intergovernmental Panel on Climate Change*. Cambridge University Press.

[10] *Refrigerant 1234YF's Potential Impact in Automotive Applications*.

[11] "ISO TC 54 Business Plan — Essential oils" (PDF). Retrieved 2006-09-14. It is unclear from the source what period of time the quoted figures include.

[12] Carroll, Robert Todd. "Aromatherapy". *The Skeptic's Dictionary* (online ed.). Retrieved 6 February 2013.

[13] Warnke, PH; Becker, ST; Podschun, R; Sivananthan, S; et al. (2009). "The battle against multi-resistant strains: Renaissance of antimicrobial essential oils as a promising force to fight hospital-acquired infections". *Journal of Cranio-Maxillofacial Surgery* **37** (7): 392–7. doi:10.1016/j.jcms.2009.03.017. PMID 19473851.

[14] Haneke, Karen E (February 2002), *Turpentine (Turpentine Oil, Wood Turpentine, Sulfate Turpentine, Sulfite Turpentine) [8006-64-2]: Review of Toxicological Literature* (PDF) (Contract No. N01-ES-65402), National Institute of Environmental Health Sciences

[15] Watt, John Mitchell; Breyer-Brandwijk, Maria Gerdina (1962). *The Medicinal and Poisonous Plants of Southern and Eastern Africa* (2nd ed.). Edinburgh: E & S Livingstone.

[16] Levy, SB (June 2001). "Antibacterial household products: Cause for concern" (PDF). *Emerging Infectious Diseases* (conference presentation) **7** (3 Suppl.): 512–5.

[17] Singh, G; Kapoor, IPS; Pandey, SK; Singh, UK; et al. (2002). "Studies on essential oils: Part 10; Antibacterial activity of volatile oils of some spices". *Phytotherapy Research* **16** (7): 680–2. doi:10.1002/ptr.951. PMID 12410554.

[18] "Tea tree oil.". *Dermatitis*. doi:10.1097/DER.0b013e31823e202d. PMID 22653070.

[19] "Occupational contact dermatitis due to essential oils.". *Contact Dermatitis*. doi:10.1111/j.1600-0536.2007.01275.x. PMID 18416758.

[20] "Allergic contact dermatitis following exposure to essential oils.". *Australas J Dermatol*. PMID 12121401.

[21] "Occupational allergic contact dermatitis in two aromatherapists.". *Contact Dermatitis*. PMID 10902596.

[22] N. Groom. New Perfume Handbook. Springer Science & Business Media, 1997 ISBN 9780751404036, pp. 184-186

[23] Henley, DV; Lipson, N; Korach, KS; Bloch, CA (2007). "Prepubertal gynecomastia linked to lavender and tea tree oils". *New England Journal of Medicine* **356** (5) 479–85. doi:10.1056/NEJMoa064725. PMID 17267908.

[24] Debboun, Mustapha; Frances, Stephen P.; Strickman, Daniel, eds. (2014). *Insect Repellents Handbook* (2nd ed.). CRC Press. p. 362. ISBN 1466553553.

[25] "Balsam, Peru". *www.hippylife.co.uk*. Hippylife. Retrieved 2006-08-17.

[26] Arenholt-Bindslev, D; Jolanki, R; Kanerva, L (2008). "Diagnosis of Side Effects of Dental Materials, with Special Emphasis on Delayed and Immediate Allergic Reactions". In Schmalz, Gottfried; Arenholt-Bindslev, Dorthe. *Biocompatibility of Dental Materials*. Springer. p. 352. doi:10.1007/978-3-540-77782-3_14. ISBN 9783540777823. Retrieved March 5, 2014.

[27] Habif, Thomas P. (2009). *Clinical Dermatology*. Elsevier Health Sciences. ISBN 9780323080378. Retrieved March 6, 2014.

[28] Yiannias, JA (2013). "Contact Dermatitis". In Bope, Edward T.; Kellerman, Rick D. *Conn's Current Therapy 2014: Expert Consult*. Elsevier Health Sciences. ISBN 9780323225724. Retrieved March 6, 2014.

[29] Kaddu, S; Kerl, H; Wolf, P (2001). "Accidental bullous phototoxic reactions to bergamot aromatherapy oil". *Journal of the American Academy of Dermatology* 45 (3): 458–61. doi:10.1067/mjd.2001.116226. PMID 11511848.

[30] "Occupational contact dermatitis due to essential oils.". *Contact Dermatitis*. doi:10.1111/j.1600-0536.2007.01275.x. PMID 18416758.

[31] "Allergic contact dermatitis following exposure to essential oils.". *Australas J Dermatol*. PMID 12121401.

[32] "Occupational allergic contact dermatitis in two aromatherapists.". *Contact Dermatitis*. PMID 10902596.

[33] Nordin, S; Broman, DA; Olofsson, JK; Wulff, M (2004). "A longitudinal descriptive study of self-reported abnormal smell and taste perception in pregnant women". *Chemical Senses* 29 (5): 391–402. doi:10.1093/chemse/bjh040. PMID 15201206.

[34] Henley, DV; Lipson, N; Korach, KS; Bloch, CA (2007). "Prepubertal gynecomastia linked to lavender and tea tree oils". *New England Journal of Medicine* 356 (5): 479–85. doi:10.1056/NEJMoa064725. PMID 17267908.

[35] "Oils make male breasts develop". *BBC News*. February 1, 2007. Retrieved September 9, 2007.

[36] Carson, CF; Tisserand, R; Larkman, T (April 2014). "Lack of evidence that essential oils affect puberty". *Reproductive Toxicology* (letter to the editor) 44: 50–1. doi:10.1016/j.reprotox.2013.09.010. PMID 24556344.

[37] Scientific Committee on Consumer Products (December 16, 2008), *Opinion on tea tree oil* (PDF) (Report No. SCCP/1155/08), Directorate-General for Health and Consumers: European Commission: European Union

[38] Menary, RC (2008). *Minimising pesticide residues in essential oils*. Rural Industries Research and Development Corporation. ISBN 9781741517095.

[39] Bischoff, K; Guale, F (April 1998). "Australian tea tree (Melaleuca alternifolia) oil poisoning in three pure-bred cats". *J. Vet. Diagn. Invest.* 10 (2): 208–10. doi:10.1177/104063879801000223. PMID 9576358.

[40] Dweck, AC (September 2009). "Toxicology of essential oils reviewed" (PDF). *Personal Care*.

[41] "Essential Oils 101". *taoessentialoils*. Retrieved 21 October 2015.

[42] International Organization for Standardization. "ISO 4720:2002 Essential oils — Nomenclature". Retrieved April 23, 2009.

[43] International Organization for Standardization. "71.100.60: Essential oils". Retrieved June 14, 2009.

1.1.10 References

- Kurt Schnaubelt (1999). *Advanced Aromatherapy: The Science of Essential Oil Therapy*. Healing Arts Press. ISBN 0-89281-743-7.

- Wanda Sellar (2001). *The Directory of Essential Oils* (Reprint ed.). Essex: The C.W. Daniel Company, Ltd. ISBN 0-85207-346-1.

- Robert Tisserand (1995). *Essential Oil Safety: A Guide for Health Care Professionals*. Churchill Livingstone. ISBN 0-443-05260-3.

- K.H.C. Baser and G. Buchbauer (2010). *Handbook of Essential Oils: Science, Technology and Applications*. CRC Press, Boca Raton, London, New York. ISBN 978-1-4200-6315-8.

Chapter 2

Related Essential Oil Topics

2.1 Anethole

Anethole (anise camphor) is an organic compound that is widely used as a flavoring substance. It is a derivative of phenylpropene, a type of aromatic compound that occurs widely in nature, in essential oils. It contributes a large component of the odor and flavor of anise and fennel (both in the botanical family Apiaceae), anise myrtle (Myrtaceae), liquorice (Fabaceae), camphor, magnolia blossoms, and star anise (Illiciaceae). Closely related to anethole is its isomer estragole, abundant in tarragon (Asteraceae) and basil (Lamiaceae), that has a flavor reminiscent of anise. It is a colorless, fragrant, mildly volatile liquid.[1] Anethole is only slightly soluble in water but exhibits high solubility in ethanol. This difference causes certain anise-flavored liqueurs to become opaque when diluted with water, the ouzo effect.

2.1.1 Structure and production

Anethole is an aromatic, unsaturated ether related to lignols. It exists as both *cis-trans* isomers (see also *E-Z* notation), involving the double bond outside the ring. The more abundant isomer, and the one preferred for use, is the *trans* or *E* isomer.

Like related compounds, anethole is poorly soluble in water. Historically, this property was used to detect adulteration in samples.[2]

Most anethole is obtained from terpentine-like extracts from trees.[1][3] Also of only minor commercial significance, anethole can be isolated from essential oils.[4][5]

It is also readily prepared from anisole and propionic acid via the intermediacy of 4-methoxypropiophenone.[1]

2.1.2 Uses

Flavoring

It is distinctly sweet, measuring 13 times sweeter than sugar. It is perceived as being pleasant to the taste even at higher concentrations. It is used in alcoholic drinks ouzo , ((rakı)) and Pernod. It is also used in seasoning and confectionery applications, oral hygiene products, and in small quantities in natural berry flavors.[5]

Precursor to other compounds

Because they metabolize anethole into several aromatic chemical compounds, some bacteria are candidates for use in commercial bioconversion of anethole to more valuable materials.[6] Bacterial strains capable of using trans-anethole as the sole carbon source include JYR-1 (*Pseudomonas putida*)[7] and TA13 (*Arthrobacter aurescens*).[6]

2.1.3 Research

Antimicrobial and antifungal activity

Anethole has potent antimicrobial properties, against bacteria, yeast, and fungi.[8] Reported antibacterial properties include both bacteriostatic and bactericidal action against *Salmonella enterica*[9] but not when used against *Salmonella* via a fumigation method.[10] Antifungal activity includes increasing the effectiveness of some other phytochemicals (e.g. polygodial) against *Saccharomyces cerevisiae* and *Candida albicans*;[11] *In vitro*, anethole has antihelmintic action on eggs and larvae of the sheep gastrointestinal nematode *Haemonchus contortus*.[12] Anethole also has nematicidal activity against the plant nematode *Meloidogyne javanica* in vitro and in pots of cucumber seedlings.[13]

Insecticidal activity

Anethole also is a promising insecticide. Several essential oils consisting mostly of anethole have insecticidal action against larvae of the mosquitos *Ochlerotatus caspius*[14] and Aedes aegypti.[15][16] In similar manner, anethole itself is effective against the fungus gnat *Lycoriella ingenua* (Sciaridae)[17] and the mold mite *Tyrophagus putrescentiae*.[18] Against the mite, anethole is a slightly more effective pesticide than DEET, but anisaldehyde, a related natural compound that occurs with anethole in many essential oils, is 14 times more effective.[18] The insecticidal action of anethole is greater as a fumigant than as a contact agent. (E)-anethole is highly effective as a fumigant against the cockroach *Blattella germanica*[19] and against adults of the weevils *Sitophilus oryzae*, *Callosobruchus chinensis* and beetle *Lasioderma serricorne*.[20]

As well as an insect pesticide, anethole is an effective insect repellent against mosquitos.[21]

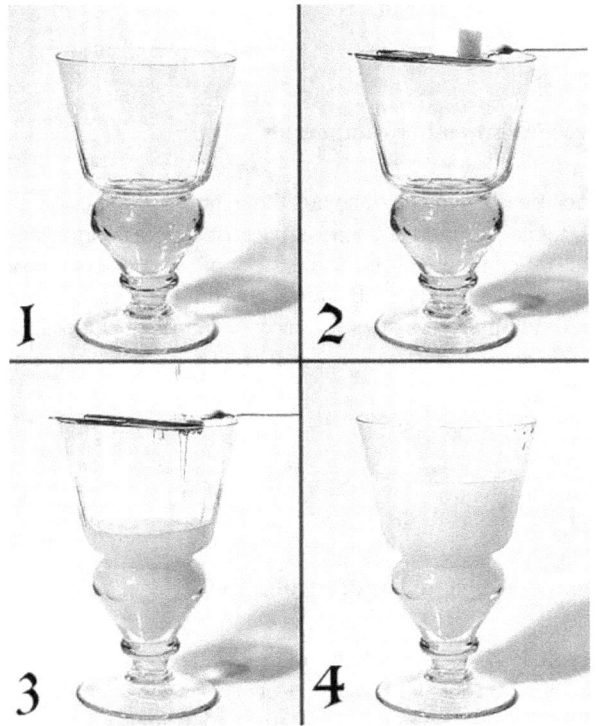

Diluting absinthe with water produces a spontaneous microemulsion (ouzo effect)

Anethole is responsible for the "ouzo effect", the spontaneous formation of a microemulsion[22][23] that gives many alcoholic beverages containing anethole and water their cloudy appearance. Such a spontaneous microemulsion has many potential commercial applications in the food and pharmaceutical industries.[24]

Precursor to illicit drugs

Anethole is an inexpensive chemical precursor for paramethoxyamphetamine (PMA),[25] and is used in its clandestine manufacture.[26] Anethole is present in the essential oil from guarana, which is alleged to have a psychoactive effect. The absence of PMA or any other known psychoactive derivative of anethole in human urine after ingestion of guarana leads to the conclusion that any purported psychoactive effect of guarana is not due to aminated anethole metabolites.[27] Anethole is also present in absinthe, a liquor with a reputation for psychoactive effects; these effects however are attributed to ethanol.[28] (See also thujone, anethole dithione (ADT), and anethole trithione (ATT)).

2.1.4 Safety

Formerly generally recognized as safe (GRAS), after a hiatus anethole was reaffirmed by Flavor and Extract Manufacturers Association (FEMA) as GRAS.[29] The hiatus was due to concerns about liver toxicity and possible carcinogenic activity, reported in rats.[30] Anethole is associated with a slight increase in liver cancer in rats,[30] although the evidence is scant and generally regarded as evidence that anethole is *not* a carcinogen.[30][31] An evaluation of anethole by the Joint FAO/WHO Expert Committee on Food Additives (JECFA) found its notable pharmacologic properties to be reduction in motor activity, lowering of body temperature, and hypnotic, analgesic, and anticonvulsant effects.[32] A subsequent evaluation by JECFA found some reason for concern regarding carcinogenicity, but there is currently insufficient data to support this.[33] At this time, the JECFA summary of these evaluations is that anethole has *no safety concern at current levels of intake when used as a flavoring agent.*[34]

In large quantities, anethole is slightly toxic and may act as an irritant.[35]

2.1.5 See also

- Category:Anise liqueurs and spirits

- List of liqueurs#Anise-flavored liqueurs

- Chavicol

- Safrole

- Fenchone

2.1.6 References

[1] Karl-Georg Fahlbusch, Franz-Josef Hammerschmidt, Johannes Panten, Wilhelm Pickenhagen, Dietmar Schatkowski, Kurt Bauer, Dorothea Garbe, Horst Surburg "Flavors and Fragrances" in *Ullmann's Encyclopedia of Industrial Chemistry*, Wiley-VCH, Weinheim: 2002. Published online: 15 January 2003; doi:10.1002/14356007.a11_141.

[2] S. Waldbott (1920). "Essential oils". *Chemical Abstracts* **14** (17): 3753–3755.

[3] Davis, Curry B. (February 20, 1990). "United States Patent 4902850: Purification of anethole by crystallization". Free Patents Online.

[4] Ram Nath Chopra and I. C. Chopra and K. L. Handa and L. D. Kapur (1958). *Chopra's Indigenous Drugs of India* (2nd ed.). Academic Publishers. pp. 178–179. ISBN 978-81-85086-80-4.

[5] Philip R. Ashurst (1999). *Food Flavorings*. Springer. p. 460. ISBN 978-0-8342-1621-1.

[6] Shimoni E, Baasov T, Ravid U, Shoham Y (2002). "The trans-anethole degradation pathway in an *Arthrobacter* sp". *J. Biol. Chem.* **277** (14): 11866–72. doi:10.1074/jbc.M109593200. PMID 11805095.

[7] Ryu J, Seo J, Lee Y, Lim Y, Ahn JH, Hur HG (July 2005). "Identification of syn- and anti-anethole-2,3-epoxides in the metabolism of trans-anethole by the newly isolated bacterium *Pseudomonas putida* JYR-1". *J. Agric. Food Chem.* **53** (15): 5954–8. doi:10.1021/jf040445x. PMID 16028980.

[8] De M, De AK, Sen P, Banerjee AB (February 2002). "Antimicrobial properties of star anise (*Illicium verum* Hook f)". *Phytother Res* **16** (1): 94–5. doi:10.1002/ptr.989. PMID 11807977.

[9] Kubo I, Fujita K (December 2001). "Naturally occurring anti-Salmonella agents". *J. Agric. Food Chem.* **49** (12): 5750–4. doi:10.1021/jf010728e. PMID 11743758.

[10] Weissinger WR, McWatters KH, Beuchat LR (April 2001). "Evaluation of volatile chemical treatments for lethality to *Salmonella* on alfalfa seeds and sprouts". *J. Food Prot.* **64** (4): 442–50. PMID 11307877.

[11] Fujita K, Fujita T, Kubo I (January 2007). "Anethole, a potential antimicrobial synergist, converts a fungistatic dodecanol to a fungicidal agent". *Phytother Res* **21** (1): 47–51. doi:10.1002/ptr.2016. PMID 17078111.

[12] Camurça-Vasconcelos AL, Bevilaqua CM, Morais SM, Maciel MV, Costa CT, Macedo IT, Oliveira LM, Braga RR, Silva RA, Vieira LS (2007). "Anthelmintic activity of Croton zehntneri and Lippia sidoides essential oils". *Vet. Parasitol.* **148** (3–4): 288–94. doi:10.1016/j.vetpar.2007.06.012. PMID 17629623.

[13] Oka Y, Nacar S, Putievsky E, Ravid U, Yaniv Z, Spiegel Y (July 2000). "Nematicidal activity of essential oils and their components against the root-knot nematode". *Phytopathology* **90** (7): 710–5. doi:10.1094/PHYTO.2000.90.7.710. PMID 18944489.

[14] Knio KM, Usta J, Dagher S, Zournajian H, Kreydiyyeh S (2008). "Larvicidal activity of essential oils extracted from commonly used herbs in Lebanon against the seaside mosquito, *Ochlerotatus caspius*". *Bioresour. Technol.* **99** (4): 763–8. doi:10.1016/j.biortech.2007.01.026. PMID 17368893.

[15] Cheng SS, Liu JY, Tsai KH, Chen WJ, Chang ST (July 2004). "Chemical composition and mosquito larvicidal activity of essential oils from leaves of different *Cinnamomum osmophloeum* provenances". *J. Agric. Food Chem.* **52** (14): 4395–400. doi:10.1021/jf0497152. PMID 15237942.

[16] Morais SM, Cavalcanti ES, Bertini LM, Oliveira CL, Rodrigues JR, Cardoso JH (2006). "Larvicidal activity of essential oils from Brazilian *Croton* species against *Aedes aegypti* L". *J. Am. Mosq. Control Assoc.* **22** (1): 161–4. doi:10.2987/8756-971X(2005)22[161:LAOEOF]2.0.CO;2. PMID 16646345.

[17] Park IK, Choi KS, Kim DH, Choi IH, Kim LS, Bak WC, Choi JW, Shin SC (August 2006). "Fumigant activity of plant essential oils and components from horseradish (*Armoracia rusticana*), anise (*Pimpinella anisum*) and garlic (*Allium sativum*) oils against *Lycoriella ingenua* (Diptera: Sciaridae)". *Pest Manag. Sci.* **62** (8): 723–8. doi:10.1002/ps.1228. PMID 16786497.

[18] Lee HS (June 2005). "Food protective effect of acaricidal components isolated from anise seeds against the stored food mite, *Tyrophagus putrescentiae* (Schrank)". *J. Food Prot.* **68** (6): 1208–10. PMID 15954709.

[19] Chang KS, Ahn YJ (February 2002). "Fumigant activity of (E)-anethole identified in *Illicium verum* fruit against *Blattella germanica*". *Pest Manag. Sci.* **58** (2): 161–6. doi:10.1002/ps.435. PMID 11852640.

[20] Kim DH, Ahn YJ (March 2001). "Contact and fumigant activities of constituents of *Foeniculum vulgare* fruit against three coleopteran stored-product insects". *Pest Manag. Sci.* **57** (3): 301–6. doi:10.1002/ps.274. PMID 11455661

[21] Padilha de Paula J, Gomes-Carneiro MR, Paumgartten FJ (2003). "Chemical composition, toxicity and mosquito repellency of *Ocimum selloi* oil". *J Ethnopharmacol* **88** (2–3): 253–60. doi:10.1016/s0378-8741(03)00233-2. PMID 12963152.

[22] Sitnikova, Natalia L.; Rudolf Sprik, Gerard Wegdam and Erika Eiser (2005). "Spontaneously Formed trans-Anethol/Water/Alcohol Emulsions: Mechanism of Formation and Stability" (PDF). *Langmuir* **21** (16): 7083–7089. doi:10.1021/la046816l. PMID 16042427. Archived (PDF) from the original on 18 March 2009. Retrieved 2009-03-15.

[23] David Carteau, Dario Bassani, and Isabelle Pianet (April–May 2008). "The "Ouzo effect": Following the spontaneous emulsification of trans-anethole in water by NMR". *Comptes Rendus Chimie* **11** (4–5): 493–498. doi:10.1016/j.crci.2007.11.003.

[24] Spernath A, Aserin A (2006). "Microemulsions as carriers for drugs and nutraceuticals". *Adv Colloid Interface Sci.* 128–130: 47–64. doi:10.1016/j.cis.2006.11.016. PMID 17229398.

[25] Waumans D, Bruneel N, Tytgat J (2003). "Anise oil as para-methoxyamphetamine (PMA) precursor". *Forensic Sci. Int.* **133** (1–2): 159–70. doi:10.1016/S0379-0738(03)00063-X. PMID 12742705.

[26] Waumans D, Hermans B, Bruneel N, Tytgat J (2004). "A neolignan-type impurity arising from the peracid oxidation reaction of anethole in the surreptitious synthesis of 4-methoxyamphetamine (PMA)". *Forensic Sci. Int.* **143** (2–3): 133–9. doi:10.1016/j.forsciint.2004.02.033. PMID 15240033.

[27] Benoni H, Dallakian P, Taraz K (1996). "Studies on the essential oil from guarana". *Z Lebensm Unters Forsch* **203** (1): 95–8. doi:10.1007/BF01267777. PMID 8765992.

[28] Lachenmeier DW (March 2008). "[Thujone-attributable effects of absinthe are only an urban legend—toxicology uncovers alcohol as real cause of absinthism]". *Med Monatsschr Pharm* (in German) **31** (3): 101–6. PMID 18429531.

[29] Newberne P, Smith RL, Doull J, Goodman JI, Munro IC, Portoghese PS, Wagner BM, Weil CS, Woods LA, Adams TB, Lucas CD, Ford RA (1999). "The FEMA GRAS assessment of trans-anethole used as a flavouring substance. Flavour and Extract Manufacturer's Association". *Food Chem. Toxicol.* **37** (7): 789–811. doi:10.1016/S0278-6915(99)00037-X. PMID 10496381.

[30] Newberne PM, Carlton WW, Brown WR (1989). "Histopathological evaluation of proliferative liver lesions in rats fed trans-anethole in chronic studies". *Food Chem. Toxicol.* **27** (1): 21–6. doi:10.1016/0278-6915(89)90087-2. PMID 2467866.

[31] Waddell WJ (2002). "Thresholds of carcinogenicity of flavors". *Toxicol. Sci.* **68** (2): 275–9. doi:10.1093/toxsci/68.2.275. PMID 12151622.

[32] "Trans-anethole". WHO Food Additives Series **14** (466). International Program on Chemical Safety (IPCS).

[33] "Trans-anethole". WHO Food Additives Series **28** (717). International Program on Chemical Safety (IPCS). 1998.

[34] "Summary of Evaluations Performed by the Joint FAO/WHO Expert Committee on Food Additives: Trans-anethole". International Program on Chemical Safety (IPCS). November 12, 2001. Archived from the original on 11 March 2009. Retrieved March 10, 2009.

[35] "Safety data for anethole". Physical & Theoretical Chemistry Laboratory Safety, Oxford University. Retrieved March 10, 2009.

2.2 Aroma lamp

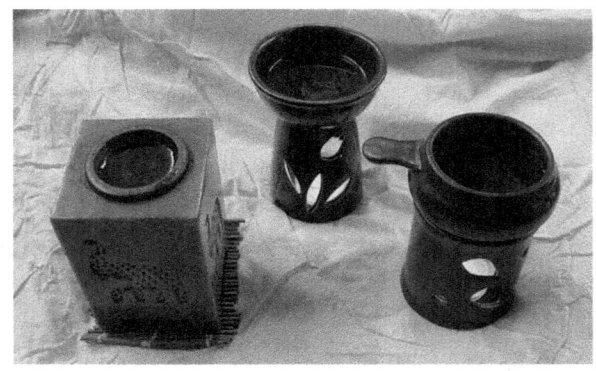

Various aroma lamps

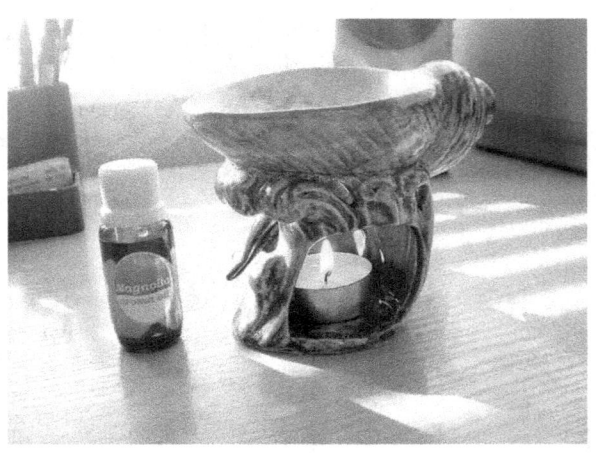

Aroma lamp with essential oil

Aroma lamps are used to diffuse essential oils in Aromatherapy, Esoterics or just in order to feel good. There are two different types of aroma lamps:

- Candle driven lamps use a small candle under a bowl to vaporize a mixture of water and oil.

- Electrical lamps use a combination of electrical and mechanical principles to vaporize the essence.

Certain plug-in nightlight units made by companies such as Air Wick are used in combination with glass bulbs of scented oil, filling a room with fragrance and light.

2.2.1 See also

- Censer

2.2.2 Links

- US patent describing the construction of an aroma lamp

2.3 Aromatherapy

Aromatherapy uses plant materials and aromatic plant oils, including essential oils, and other aromatic compounds for the purpose of altering one's mood, cognitive, psychological or physical well-being.[1]

It can be offered as a complementary therapy or, more controversially, as form of alternative medicine. Complementary therapy can be offered alongside standard treatment,[2] with alternative medicine offered 'instead of conventional treatments', conventional treatments being often scientifically proven.[3]

Aromatherapists, who specialise in the practice of aromatherapy, utilise blends of therapeutic essential oils that can be issued through topical application, massage, inhalation or water immersion to stimulate a desired response.

Some essential oils such as tea tree[4] have demonstrated anti-microbial effects, but there is still a lack of clinical evidence demonstrating efficacy against bacterial, fungal, or viral infections. Evidence for the efficacy of aromatherapy in treating medical conditions remains poor, with a particular lack of studies employing rigorous methodology.[5][6]

2.3.1 History

The use of essential oils for therapeutic, spiritual, hygienic and ritualistic purposes goes back to a number of ancient civilizations including the Chinese, Indians, Egyptians, Greeks, and Romans who used them in cosmetics, perfumes and drugs.[7]

Oils are described by Dioscorides, along with beliefs of the time regarding their healing properties, in his *De Materia Medica*, written in the first century.[8] Distilled essential oils have been employed as medicines since the invention of distillation in the eleventh century,[9] when Avicenna isolated essential oils using steam distillation.[10]

The concept of aromatherapy was first mooted by a small number of European scientists and doctors, in about 1907. In 1937, the word first appeared in print in a French book

on the subject: *Aromathérapie: Les Huiles Essentielles, Hormones Végétales* by René-Maurice Gattefossé, a chemist. An English version was published in 1993.[11] In 1910, Gattefossé burned a hand very badly and later claimed he treated it effectively with lavender oil.[12]

A French surgeon, Jean Valnet, pioneered the medicinal uses of essential oils, which he used as antiseptics in the treatment of wounded soldiers during World War II.[13]

2.3.2 Modes of application

The modes of application of aromatherapy include:

- *Aerial diffusion*: for environmental fragrancing or aerial disinfection
- *Direct inhalation*: for respiratory disinfection, decongestion, expectoration as well as psychological effects
- *Topical applications*: for general massage, baths, compresses, therapeutic skin care[14]

2.3.3 Materials

Some of the materials employed include:

- *Essential oils*: Fragrant oils extracted from plants chiefly through steam distillation (e.g., eucalyptus oil) or expression (grapefruit oil). However, the term is also occasionally used to describe fragrant oils extracted from plant material by any solvent extraction. This material includes incense reed diffusers.
- *Absolutes*: Fragrant oils extracted primarily from flowers or delicate plant tissues through solvent or supercritical fluid extraction (e.g., rose absolute). The term is also used to describe oils extracted from fragrant butters, concretes, and enfleurage pommades using ethanol.
- *Carrier oils*: Typically oily plant base triacylglycerides that dilute essential oils for use on the skin (e.g., sweet almond oil).
- *Herbal distillates* or hydrosols: The aqueous by-products of the distillation process (e.g., rosewater). There are many herbs that make herbal distillates and they have culinary uses, medicinal uses and skin care uses. Common herbal distillates are chamomile, rose, and lemon balm.
- *Infusions*: Aqueous extracts of various plant material (e.g., infusion of chamomile).

- *Phytoncides*: Various volatile organic compounds from plants that kill microbes. Many terpene-based fragrant oils and sulfuric compounds from plants in the genus "*Allium*" are phytoncides, though the latter are likely less commonly used in aromatherapy due to their disagreeable odors.

- *Vaporizer (Volatized) raw herbs*: Typically higher oil content plant based materials dried, crushed, and heated to extract and inhale the aromatic oil vapors in a direct inhalation modality.

2.3.4 Theory

Aromatherapy is the treatment or prevention of disease by use of essential oils. Other stated uses include pain and anxiety reduction, enhancement of energy and short-term memory, relaxation, hair loss prevention, and reduction of eczema-induced itching.[15][16]

Two basic mechanisms are offered to explain the purported effects. One is the influence of aroma on the brain, especially the limbic system through the olfactory system.[17] The other is the direct pharmacological effects of the essential oils.[18]

In the English-speaking world, practitioners tend to emphasize the use of oils in massage . Aromatherapy tends to be regarded as a complementary modality at best and a pseudoscientific fraud at worst.[19]

2.3.5 Choice and purchase

Oils with standardized content of components (marked FCC, for Food Chemical Codex) are required to contain a specified amount of certain aroma chemicals that normally occur in the oil. There is no law that the chemicals cannot be added in synthetic form to meet the criteria established by the FCC for that oil. For instance, lemongrass essential oil must contain 75% aldehyde to meet the FCC profile for that oil, but that aldehyde can come from a chemical refinery instead of from lemongrass. To say that FCC oils are "food grade" makes them seem natural when they are not necessarily so.

Undiluted essential oils suitable for aromatherapy are termed 'therapeutic grade', but there are no established and agreed standards for this category. The market for essential oils is dominated by the food, perfume, cosmetics and pharmaceutical industries, so aromatherapists have little choice but to buy the best of whatever oils are available.

Analysis using gas liquid chromatography (GLC) and mass spectrometry (MS) establishes the quality of essential oils. These techniques are able to measure the levels of compo-nents to a few parts per billion. This does not make it possible to determine whether each component is natural or whether a poor oil has been 'improved' by the addition of synthetic aromachemicals, but the latter is often signaled by the minor impurities present. For example, linalool made in plants will be accompanied by a small amount of hydro-linalool, whilst synthetic linalool has traces of dihydro-linalool.

2.3.6 Popular uses

- Lemon oil is said to be uplifting and to relieve stress. In a Japanese study, lemon essential oil in vapour form has been found to reduce stress in mice.[20] Research at The Ohio State University indicates that lemon oil aroma may enhance one's mood, and help with relaxation.[21]

- Thyme oil[22]

- Sage oil has been suggested to boost short-term memory performance in many using it as a dietary supplement.[23]

2.3.7 Efficacy

Some benefits that have been linked to aromatherapy, such as relaxation and clarity of mind, may arise from the placebo effect rather than from any actual physiological effect.[24] The consensus among most medical professionals is that while some aromas have demonstrated effects on mood and relaxation and may have related benefits for patients, there is currently insufficient evidence to support the claims made for aromatherapy.[25] Scientific research on the cause and effects of aromatherapy is limited, although in vitro testing has revealed some antibacterial and antiviral effects.[26][27] There is no evidence of any long-term results from an aromatherapy massage other than the pleasure achieved from a pleasant-smelling massage.[28] A few double blind studies in the field of clinical psychology relating to the treatment of severe dementia have been published.[29][30] Essential oils have a demonstrated efficacy in dental mouthwash products.[31]

Aromatherapy has been also promoted for its ability to fight cancer; however, according to the American Cancer Society, "available scientific evidence does not support claims that aromatherapy is effective in preventing or treating cancer".[25]

2.3.8 Safety concerns

Further information: Alternative medicine § Criticism

Aromatherapy carries a risk of a number of adverse effects and this consideration, combined with the lack of evidence of its therapeutic benefit, makes the practice of questionable worth.[32]

Because essential oils are highly concentrated they can irritate the skin when used in undiluted form.[33] Therefore, they are normally diluted with a carrier oil for topical application, such as jojoba oil, olive oil, or coconut oil. Phototoxic reactions may occur with citrus peel oils such as lemon or lime.[34] Also, many essential oils have chemical components that are sensitisers (meaning that they will, after a number of uses, cause reactions on the skin, and more so in the rest of the body). Some of the chemical allergies could even be caused by pesticides, if the original plants are cultivated.[35][36] Some oils can be toxic to some domestic animals, with cats being particularly prone.[37][38]

Two common oils, lavender and tea tree, have been implicated in causing gynaecomastia, an abnormal breast tissue growth, in prepubescent boys, although the report which cites this potential issue is based on observations of only three boys, and two of those boys were significantly above average in weight for their age, thus already prone to gynaecomastia.[39] A child hormone specialist at the University of Cambridge claimed "... these oils can mimic estrogens" and "people should be a little bit careful about using these products."[40] The Aromatherapy Trade Council of the UK has issued a rebuttal.[41] The Australian Tea Tree Association, a group that promotes the interests of Australian tea tree oil producers, exporters and manufacturers issued a letter that questioned the study and called on the *New England Journal of Medicine* for a retraction.[42] The *New England Journal of Medicine* has so far not replied and has not retracted the study.

As with any bioactive substance, an essential oil that may be safe for the general public could still pose hazards for pregnant and lactating women.

While some advocate the ingestion of essential oils for therapeutic purposes, licensed aromatherapy professionals do not recommend self-prescription due the highly toxic nature of some essential oils. Some very common oils like eucalyptus are extremely toxic when taken internally. Doses as low as one teaspoon have been reported to cause clinically significant symptoms and severe poisoning can occur after ingestion of 4 to 5 ml.[43] A few reported cases of toxic reactions like liver damage and seizures have occurred after ingestion of sage, hyssop, thuja, and cedar.[44] Accidental ingestion may happen when oils are not kept out of reach of children.

Oils both ingested and applied to the skin can potentially have negative interactions with conventional medicine. For example, the topical use of methylsalicylate-heavy oils like sweet birch and wintergreen may cause hemorrhaging in

users taking the anticoagulant warfarin.

Adulterated oils may also pose problems depending on the type of substance used.

2.3.9 See also

- Aromachologist

- List of ineffective cancer treatments

2.3.10 References

[1] "Aromatherapy". *Better Health Channel*. Retrieved 2014-08-14.

[2] http://www.hindawi.com/journals/ecam/2005/270901/abs/

[3] http://www.macmillan.org.uk/Cancerinformation/Cancertreatment/Complementarytherapies/Alternativetherapies/Alternativetherapies.aspx

[4] Carson, C. F.; Hammer, K. A.; Riley, T. V. (2006). "Melaleuca alternifolia (Tea Tree) Oil: A Review of Antimicrobial and Other Medicinal Properties". *Clinical Microbiology Reviews* **19** (1): 50–62. doi:10.1128/CMR.19.1.50-62.2006. PMC 1360273. PMID 16418522.

[5] van der Watt, Gillian; Janca, Aleksandar (August 2008). "Aromatherapy in nursing and mental health care". *Contemporary Nurse* **30** (1): 69–75. doi:10.5555/conu.673.30.1.69 (inactive 2015-01-09). PMID 19072192.

[6] Edris, Amr E. (2007). "Pharmaceutical and therapeutic Potentials of essential oils and their individual volatile constituents: A review". *Phytotherapy Research* **21** (4): 308–23. doi:10.1002/ptr.2072. PMID 17199238.

[7] "University of Maryland Medical Center - Aromatherapy". *University of Maryland Medical Center*. University of Maryland Medical Center. Retrieved 13 August 2014.

[8] Dioscorides, Pedanius; Goodyer, John (trans.) (1959). Gunther, R.T., ed. *The Greek Herbal of Dioscorides*. New York. Hafner Publishing. OCLC 3570794.

[9] Forbes, R.J. (1970). *A short history of the art of distillation*. Leiden: E.J. Brill. OCLC 2559231.

[10] Ericksen, Marlene (2000). *Healing With Aromatherapy*. New York: McGraw-Hill. p. 9. ISBN 0-658-00382-8.

[11] Gattefossé, R.-M.; Tisserand, R. (1993). *Gattefossé's aromatherapy*. Saffron Walden: C.W. Daniel. ISBN 0-85207-236-8.

[12] "Aromatherapy". University of Maryland Medical Center. Retrieved 24 October 2010.

[13] Valnet, J.; Tisserand, R. (1990). *The practice of aromatherapy: A classic compendium of plant medicines & their healing properties*. Rochester, VT: Healing Arts Press. ISBN 0-89281-398-9.

[14] "Organic Bath Oil". Plaisirs. Retrieved 11 October 2011.

[15] Kingston, Jennifer A. (28 July 2010). "Nostrums: Aromatherapy Rarely Stands Up to Testing". *The New York Times*. Retrieved 29 December 2010.

[16] Nagourney, Eric (11 March 2008). "Skin Deep: In Competition for your Nose". *The New York Times*. Retrieved 29 December 2010.

[17] Mathrani, Vandana (17 January 2008). "The Power of Smell".

[18] Prabuseenivasan, Seenivasan; Jayakumar, Manickkam; Ignacimuthu, Savarimuthu (2006). "In vitro antibacterial activity of some plant essential oils". *BMC Complementary and Alternative Medicine* **6**: 39. doi:10.1186/1472-6882-6-39. PMC 1693916. PMID 17134518.

[19] Barrett, Stephen. "Aromatherapy: Making Dollars out of Scents". *Science & Pseudoscience Review in Mental Health*. Scientific Review of Mental Health Practice. Retrieved 21 February 2013.

[20] Komiya, Migiwa; Takeuchi, Takashi; Harada, Etsumori (2006). "Lemon oil vapor causes an anti-stress effect via modulating the 5-HT and DA activities in mice". *Behavioural Brain Research* **172** (2): 240–9. doi:10.1016/j.bbr.2006.05.006. PMID 16780969.

[21] Kiecolt-Glaser, Janice K.; Graham, Jennifer E.; Malarkey, William B.; Porter, Kyle; Lemeshow, Stanley; Glaser, Ronald (2008). "Olfactory influences on mood and autonomic, endocrine, and immune function". *Psychoneuroendocrinology* **33** (3): 328–39. doi:10.1016/j.psyneuen.2007.11.015. PMC 2278291. PMID 18178322. Lay summary – *Ohio State University Research* (3 March 2008).

[22] Schelz, Zsuzsanna; Molnar, Joseph; Hohmann, Judit (2006). "Antimicrobial and antiplasmid activities of essential oils". *Fitoterapia* **77** (4): 279–85. doi:10.1016/j.fitote.2006.03.013. PMID 16690225.

[23] Melissa Hantman (11 November 2003). "Spicing Up Your Memory". Psychology Today.

[24] "Natural Aphid Control Accomplished Easy and Effectively with Essential Oils!". *Experience Essential Oils*. 2010. Retrieved 14 August 2014.

[25] "Aromatherapy". American Cancer Society. November 2008. Retrieved September 2013.

[26] Kalemba, D.; Kunicka, A. (2003). "Antibacterial and Antifungal Properties of Essential Oils". *Current Medicinal Chemistry* **10** (10): 813–29. doi:10.2174/0929867033457719. PMID 12678685.

[27] Reichling, Jürgen; Schnitzler, Paul; Suschke, Ulrike; Saller, Reinhard (2009). "Essential Oils of Aromatic Plants with Antibacterial, Antifungal, Antiviral, and Cytotoxic Properties – an Overview". *Forschende Komplementärmedizin* **16** (2): 79–80. doi:10.1159/000207196. PMID 19420953.

[28] Soden, Katie; Vincent, Karen; Craske, Stephen; Lucas, Caroline; Ashley, Sue (2004). "A randomized controlled trial of aromatherapy massage in a hospice setting". *Palliative Medicine* **18** (2): 87–92. doi:10.1191/0269216304pm874oa. PMID 15046404.

[29] Ballard, Clive G.; O'Brien, John T.; Reichelt, Katharina; Perry, Elaine K. (2002). "Aromatherapy as a Safe and Effective Treatment for the Management of Agitation in Severe Dementia". *The Journal of Clinical Psychiatry* **63** (7): 553–8. doi:10.4088/JCP.v63n0703. PMID 12143909.

[30] Holmes, Clive; Hopkins, Vivienne; Hensford, Christine; MacLaughlin, Vanessa; Wilkinson, David; Rosenvinge, Henry (2002). "Lavender oil as a treatment for agitated behaviour in severe dementia: A placebo controlled study". *International Journal of Geriatric Psychiatry* **17** (4): 305–8. doi:10.1002/gps.593. PMID 11994882.

[31] Stoeken, Judith E.; Paraskevas, Spiros; Van Der Weijden, Godefridus A. (2007). "The Long-Term Effect of a Mouthrinse Containing Essential Oils on Dental Plaque and Gingivitis: A Systematic Review". *Journal of Periodontology* **78** (7): 1218–28. doi:10.1902/jop.2007.060269. PMID 17608576.

[32] Posadzki P, Alotaibi A, Ernst E (January 2012). "Adverse effects of aromatherapy: a systematic review of case reports and case series". *Int J Risk Saf Med* (Systematic review) **24** (3): 147–61. doi:10.3233/JRS-2012-0568. PMID 22936057.

[33] Grassman, J; Elstner, E F (1973). "Essential Oils". In Caballero, Benjamin; Trugo, Luiz C; Finglas, Paul M. *Encyclopedia of Food Sciences and Nutrition* (2nd ed.). Academic Press. ISBN 0-12-227055-X.

[34] Cather, JC; MacKnet, MR; Menter, MA (2000). "Hyperpigmented macules and streaks". *Proceedings* (Baylor University Medical Center) **13** (4): 405–6. PMC 1312240. PMID 16389350.

[35] Edwards, J.; Bienvenu, F.E. (1999). "Investigations into the use of flame and the herbicide, paraquat, to control peppermint rust in north-east Victoria, Australia". *Australasian Plant Pathology* **28** (3): 212. doi:10.1071/AP99036.

[36] Adamovic, D.S.; et al. "Variability of herbicide efficiency and their effect upon yield and quality of peppermint (Mentha X Piperital L.)". Retrieved 6 June 2009.

[37] The Lavender Cat – Cats and Essential Oil Safety

[38] Bischoff, K.; Guale, F. (1998). "Australian Tea Tree (Melaleuca Alternifolia) Oil Poisoning in Three Purebred Cats". *Journal of Veterinary Diagnostic Investigation* **10**

(2): 208–10. doi:10.1177/104063879801000223. PMID 9576358.

[39] Henley, Derek V.; Lipson, Natasha; Korach, Kenneth S.; Bloch, Clifford A. (2007). "Prepubertal Gynecomastia Linked to Lavender and Tea Tree Oils". *New England Journal of Medicine* **356** (5): 479–85. doi:10.1056/NEJMoa064725. PMID 17267908.

[40] "Oils make male breasts develop". *BBC News* (London). 1 February 2007. Archived from the original on 29 August 2007. Retrieved 2007-09-09.

[41] 'NEITHER LAVENDER OIL NOR TEA TREE OIL CAN BE LINKED TO BREAST GROWTH IN YOUNG BOYS'

[42] 'ATTIA refutes gynecomastia link', Article Date: 21 February 2007

[43] Eucalyptus oil (PIM 031)

[44] Millet, Y.; Jouglard, J.; Steinmetz, M. D. Tognetti, P.; Joanny, P.; Arditti, J. (1981). "Toxicity of Some Essential Plant Oils. Clinical and Experimental Study". *Clinical Toxicology* **18** (12): 1485–98. doi:10.3109/15563658108990357. PMID 7333081.

2.3.11 External links

- Aromatherapy and Essential Oils – health professional and patient PDQ (Physician Data Query) summaries from the National Cancer Institute.

2.4 Artemisia pallens

Artemisia pallens, Dhavanam (Tamil: மரிக்கொழுந்து, தவணம், Marathi: दवणा), is an aromatic herb, In genus of small herbs or shrubs, xerophytic In nature. The flowers are racemose panicles, bear numerous small yellow flower heads or capitula, but the silvery white silky covering of down gives the foliage a grey or white appearance.

Davanam has alternate pinnasect leaves (leaf which is divided into opposite pairs of lobes cut almost to the midrib In narrow divisions) or palmatisect leaves (the green tissue is divided into several segments not fully separated At the base).

2.4.1 Cultivation

It is commercially cultivated for its fragrant leaves and flowers. It has two distinct morphological types, one in which the plants are short in stature and flowering sets in early, and the other in which plants are tall and flowering sets in later. It grows from seeds and cuttings and reaches maturity in four months. The plant is woody in the lower part of the stem, but with yearly branches. Seen mostly grown in Andhra Pradesh, Karnataka, Maharashtra and Tamil Nadu states in India.

Artemisia pallens is a preferred food for the larvae of a number of butterfly species.

2.4.2 Chemistry

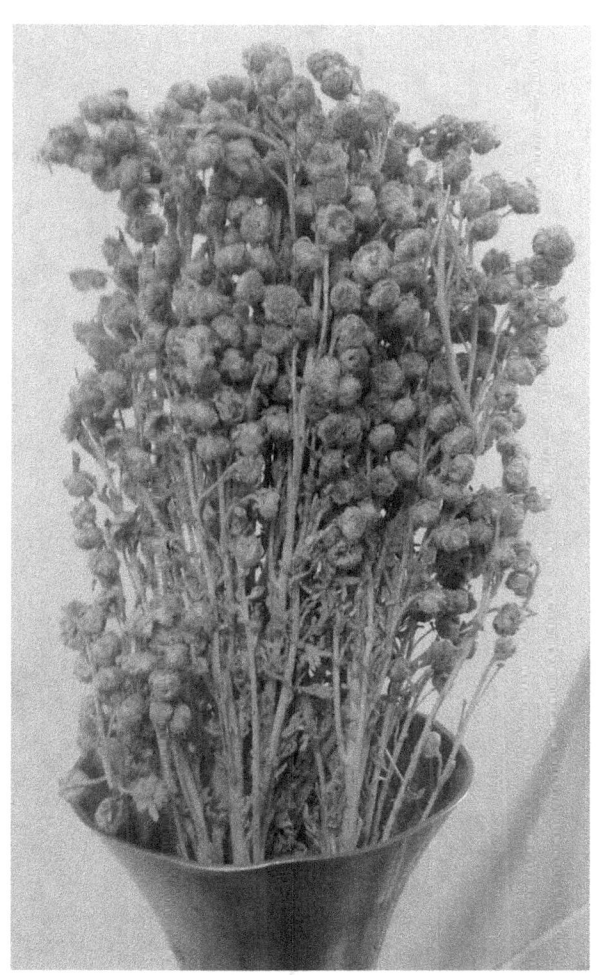

Dired davana plant used as aromatic bouquet.

Davanone, davan ether, davana furan and linalool are the major constituents of davana oil. Methyl cinnamate, ethyl cinnamate, bicyclogermacrene, 2-hydroxyisodavanone, farnesol, geranyl acetate, sesquiterpene lactones, and germacranolides are also found.[1] The amount of davanone and linalool decreased while those of (Z)– and (E)–methyl cinnamate, (E)–ethyl cinnamate, bicyclogermacrene, davana ether, 2-hydroxyisodavanone, and farnesol increased from flower heads emergence stage to the initiation of seed set stage. Five compounds, (Z)– and (E)–methyl cinnamates, (Z)– and (E)–ethyl cinnamates, and geranyl acetate, were identified for the first time in davana oil.[2]

2.4.3   Uses

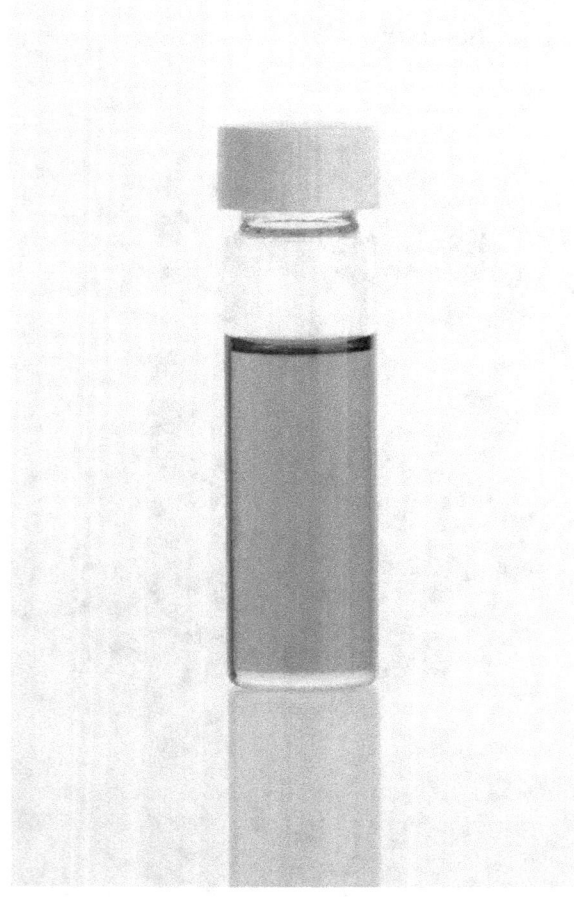

Davana essential oil

The leaves and flowers yield an essential oil known as oil of Davana. Several species yield essential oil and some are used as fodder, some of them are a source of the anthelmintic chemical santonin. Davana blossoms are offered to Shiva, the God of Transformation, by the faithful, and decorate his altar throughout the day. Oral administration of high doses aqueous/methanolic extract from the aerial parts of the plants was observed to reduce blood glucose levels in glucose–fed hyperglycemic and alloxan-treated rabbits and rats.[3]

Uses of Davana oil

- Davana oil is used in making perfumes of sweet and fruity fragrances.

- When applied on the skin, Davana is said to smell differently on different persons. This peculiar property is highly valued in high class perfumery to create fragrances with truly individual notes.

- Davana leaves and stalks are used in making bouquets, garlands, fresh or dry flower arrangements.

2.4.4   Popular culture

- It has even inspired film lyricists ("Madurai Marikozhundu Vasam" is one of the more popular numbers) to come up with romantic numbers.[4]

2.4.5   References

[1] Pujar, PP; Sawaikar, DD; Rojatkar, SR; Nagasampagi, BA (2000). "A new germacranolide from Artemisia pallens". *Fitoterapia* **71** (5): 590–2. doi:10.1016/S0367-326X(00)00168-4. PMID 11449517.

[2] http://www.gardenpoints.org/artpal.html

[3] Subramoniam, A; Pushpangadan, P; Rajasekharan, S; Evans, DA; Latha, PG; Valsaraj, R (1996). "Effects of Artemisia pallens Wall. On blood glucose levels in normal and alloxan-induced diabetic rats". *Journal of Ethnopharmacology* **50** (1): 13–7. doi:10.1016/0378-8741(95)01329-6. PMID 8778502.

[4] "Fragrance that's familiar". *The Hindu* (Chennai, India). 11 June 2005.

2.5   Backhousia citriodora

Backhousia citriodora (common names **lemon myrtle, lemon scented myrtle, lemon scented ironwood**) is a flowering plant in the family Myrtaceae, genus *Backhousia*. It is endemic to subtropical rainforests of central and southeastern Queensland, Australia, with a natural distribution from Mackay to Brisbane.[1] Other common names are sweet verbena tree, sweet verbena myrtle, lemon scented verbena, and lemon scented backhousia.

2.5.1   Growth

It can reach 20 m (66 ft) in height, but is often smaller. The leaves are evergreen, opposite, lanceolate, 5–12 cm (2.0–4.7 in) long and 1.5–2.5 cm (0.59–0.98 in) broad, glossy green, with an entire margin. The flowers are creamy-white, 5–7 mm diameter, produced in clusters at the ends of the branches from summer through to autumn, after petal fall the calyx is persistent.

2.5.2 Etymology

Lemon myrtle was given the botanical name *Backhousia citriodora* in 1853 after the English botanist, James Backhouse.

The common name reflects the strong lemon smell of the crushed leaves. "Lemon scented myrtle" was the primary common name until the shortened trade name, "lemon myrtle", was created by the native foods industry to market the leaf for culinary use. Lemon myrtle is now the more common name for the plant and its products.

Lemon myrtle is sometimes confused with "lemon ironbark", which is *Eucalyptus staigeriana*.

2.5.3 Essential oils

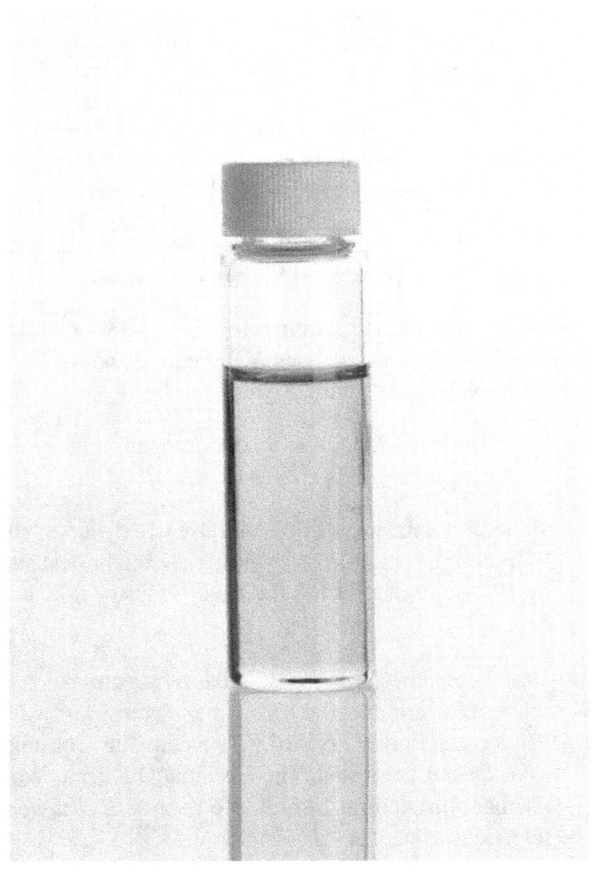

Lemon Myrtle (Backhousia citriodora) *essential oil in a clear glass vial*

B.citriodora has two essential oil chemotypes:

- The citral chemotype is more prevalent and is cultivated in Australia for flavouring and essential oil. Citral as an isolate in steam distilled lemon myrtle oil is

typically 90–98%, and oil yield 1–3% from fresh leaf. It is the highest natural source of citral.

- The citronellal chemotype is uncommon and can be used as an insect repellent.[2][3]

2.5.4 Uses

Indigenous Australians have long used lemon myrtle, both in cuisine and as a healing plant. The oil has the highest citral purity; typically higher than lemongrass. It is also considered to have a "cleaner and sweeter" aroma than comparable sources of citral–lemongrass and *Litsea cubeba*.[4]

Culinary

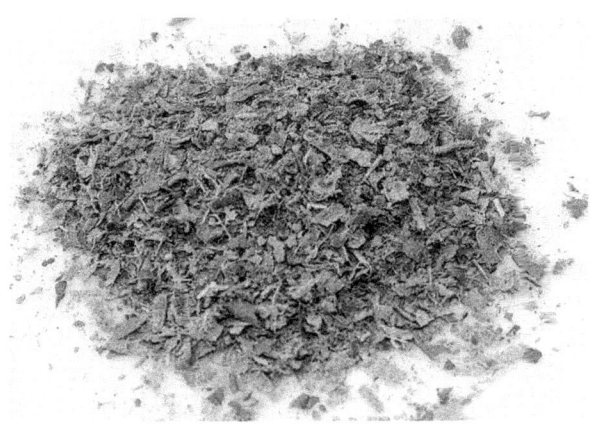

Dried and crushed Lemon myrtle leaves

Lemon myrtle is one of the well known bushfood flavours and is sometimes referred to as the "Queen of the lemon herbs".[5] The leaf is often used as dried flakes, or in the form of an encapsulated flavour essence for enhanced shelf-life. It has a range of uses, such as lemon myrtle flakes in shortbread; flavouring in pasta; whole leaf with baked fish; infused in macadamia or vegetable oils; and made into tea, including tea blends. It can also be used as a lemon flavour replacement in milk-based foods, such as cheesecake, lemon flavoured ice-cream and sorbet without the curdling problem associated with lemon fruit acidity.

The dried leaf has free radical scavenging ability.[6]

Antimicrobial

Lemon myrtle essential oil possesses antimicrobial properties; however the undiluted essential oil is toxic to human cells *in vitro*.[7] When diluted to approximately 1%, absorption through the skin and subsequent damage is thought to be minimal.[8] Lemon myrtle oil has a high Rideal–Walker coefficient, a measure of antimicrobial potency.[9] Use of lemon myrtle oil as a treatment for skin lesions caused by molluscum contagiosum virus (MCV), a disease affecting children and immuno-compromised patients, has been investigated. Nine of sixteen patients who were treated with 10% strength lemon myrtle oil showed a significant improvement, compared to none in the control group.[10] A study in 2003 which investigated the effectiveness of different preparations of lemon myrtle against bacteria and fungi concluded that the plant had potential as an antiseptic or as a surface disinfectant, or as an antimicrobial food additive.[11] The oil is a popular ingredient in health care and cleaning products, especially soaps, lotions, skin-whitening preparations and shampoos.[12]

2.5.5 Cultivation

Lemon myrtle is a cultivated ornamental plant. It can be grown from tropical to warm temperate climates, and may handle cooler districts provided it can be protected from frost when young.[1] In cultivation it rarely exceeds about 5 metres (16 ft) and usually has a dense canopy. The principal attraction to gardeners is the lemon smell which perfumes both the leaves and flowers of the tree. Lemon myrtle is a hardy plant which tolerates all but the poorest drained soils.[1] It can be slow growing but responds well to slow release fertilisers.

Seedling lemon myrtle go through a shrubby, slow juvenile growth stage, before developing a dominant trunk. Lemon myrtle can also be propagated from cutting, but is slow to strike.[1] A study into the plant growing adventitious roots found that "actively growing axillary buds, wide stems and mature leaves" are good indicators that a cutting will take root successfully and survive.[13] A further study on temperature recommended glasshouses for growing cuttings throughout the year.[14] Growing cuttings from mature trees bypasses the shrubby juvenile stage. Cutting propagation is also used to provide a consistent product in commercial production.

In plantation cultivation the tree is typically maintained as a shrub by regular harvesting from the top and sides. Mechanical harvesting is used in commercial plantations. It is important to retain some lower branches when pruning for plant health. The harvested leaves are dried for leaf spice, or distilled for the essential oil.

The majority of commercial lemon myrtle is grown in Queensland and the north coast of New South Wales, Australia.

A 2009 study has suggested that drying lemon myrtle leaves at higher temperatures improves the citral content of the dried leaves, but discolours the leaves more.[15]

2.5.6 Myrtle Rust

A significant fungal pathogen, myrtle rust (*Uredo rangelii*) was detected in lemon myrtle plantations in January 2011.[16][17] Myrtle rust severely damages new growth and threatens lemon myrtle production. Controls are being developed.

2.5.7 Lemon myrtle history

- Pre-1788 – Aboriginal people use *B.citriodora* for medicine and flavouring.

- 1853 – Scientifically named *Backhousia citriodora* by botanist, Ferdinand von Mueller, with the genus named after friend, James Backhouse, quaker missionary and botanist.

- 1888 – Bertram isolates citral from *B.citriodora* oil,[18] and Messrs. Schimmel and Co., Dresden, write about the essential oil as having "...probably a future."

- 1900s–1920s – *B.citriodora* distilled on a small-scale commercial basis around Eumundi, Queensland.

- 1920s – Discovery of antimicrobial qualities of steam-distilled *B.citriodora* oil, by A.R. Penfold and R.Grant, Technological Museum, Sydney.

- 1940s – Tarax Co. use *B.citriodora* oil as a lemon flavouring during World War II.

- 1950s – Some production of oil carried out in the Maryborough and Miriam Vale areas from bush stands by JR Archibold,[19] but the small industry falls into decline.

- 1989 – *B.citriodora* investigated as a potential leaf spice and commercial crop by Peter Hardwick, Wilderness Foods Pty Ltd. The company commissions Dr Ian Southwell, The Essential Oils Unit, Wollongbar Agricultural Institute, to analyse *B.citriodora* selections using gas chromatography.[20]

- 1990 – Restaurants and food manufacturers supplied with dried *B.citriodora* leaf by Vic Cherikoff, Bush Tucker Supply Pty Ltd, produced by Russel and Sharon Costin, Limpinwood Gardens.

- 1991 – *B.citriodora* plantation established by Dennis Archer and Rosemary Cullen-Archer, Toona Essential Oils Pty Ltd, ; and subsequent commercial supply of plantation produced *B.citriodora* oil in 1993.

- 1997 – Large-scale plantations of *B.citriodora* established in north Queensland, by Australian Native Lemon Myrtle Ltd.

- Late 1990s – *B.citriodora* begins to be supplied internationally for a range of flavouring, cosmetic and anti-microbial products. Agronomic production of *B.citriodora* starts to exceed demand.

- 2001 – Standards for Oil of *B.citriodora* established by The Essential Oils Unit, Wollongbar, and Standards Australia.[21]

- 2004 – Monograph published on *B.citriodora* by Toona Essential Oils pty Ltd.

- 2010 – Lemon myrtle sells out in London after Jamie Oliver describes it as "pukka" on his TV show.

2.5.8 See also

- Citral

- Lemon verbena

2.5.9 References

[1] Jones, J. L. (1986), *Ornamental Rainforest Plants of Australia*, Reed Books, ISBN 978-0-7301-0113-0

[2] Doran, J. C.; Brophy, J. J.; Lassak, E. V. & House, A. P. N. (2001), "*Backhousia citriodora* F. Muell. – Rediscovery and chemical characterization of the L-citronellal form and aspects of its breeding system", *Flavour and Fragrance Journal* 16 (5): 325–328, doi:10.1002/ffj.1003

[3] http://onlinelibrary.wiley.com/doi/10.1111/j.1440-6055.2009.00736.x/full

[4] The Aromatic Plant Project

[5] The Cook and the Chef, ABC TV.

[6] Zhao, J., Agboola, S., *Functional Properties of Australian Bushfoods – A Report for the Rural Industries Research and Development Corporation*, 2007, RIRDC Publication No 07/030

[7] Hayes, A. J. & Markovic, B. (2002), "Toxicity of Australian essential oil Backhousia citriodora (Lemon myrtle). Part 1. Antimicrobial activity and in vitro cytotoxicity", *Food and Chemical Toxicology* 40 (4): 535–543, doi:10.1016/S0278-6915(01)00103-X, PMID 11893412

[8] Hayes, A. J. & Markovic, B. (2003), "Toxicity of Australian essential oil Backhousia citriodora (lemon myrtle). Part 2. Absorption and histopathology following application to human skin", *Food and Chemical Toxicology* 41 (10): 1409–1416, doi:10.1016/S0278-6915(03)00159-5, PMID 12909275

[9] Lassak, E. V. & McCarthy, T. (1983), *Australian Medicinal Plants*, Australia: Methuen, p. 98, ISBN 0-454-00438-9

[10] Burke, B. E.; Baillie, J. E. & Olson, R. D. (2004), "Essential oil of Australian lemon myrtle (Backhousia citriodora) in the treatment of molluscum contagiosum in children", *Biomed Pharmacother.* 58 (4): 245–247, doi:10.1016/j.biopha.2003.11.006, PMID 15183850

[11] Wilkinson, J. M.; Hipwell, M.; Ryan, T.; Cavanagh, H. M. A. (2003). "Bioactivity of Backhousia citriodora: Antibacterial and Antifungal Activity". *Journal of Agricultural and Food Chemistry* 51 (1): 76–81. doi:10.1021/jf0258003. PMID 12502388.

[12] Lemon Myrtle Uses, Products and Patents

[13] Kibbler, H.; Johnston, M. E.; Williams, R. R. (2004). "Adventitious root formation in cuttings of Backhousia citriodora F. Muell". *Scientia Horticulturae* 102: 133. doi:10.1016/j.scienta.2003.12.012.

[14] Kibbler, H.; Johnston, M. E.; Williams, R. R. (2004). "Adventitious root formation in cuttings of Backhousia citriodora F. Muell". *Scientia Horticulturae* 102 (3): 343. doi:10.1016/j.scienta.2004.02.007.

[15] Buchaillot, A ; Caffin, N.; Bhandari, B. (2009). "Drying of Lemon Myrtle (Backhousia citriodora) Leaves: Retention of Volatiles and Color". *Drying Technology* 27 (3). 445. doi:10.1080/07373930802683740.

[16] Myrtle rust host list, NSW Primary Industries

[17] *Myrtle rust confirmed on lemon myrtle plantation*, ABC Rural

[18] Simonsen, J. L. (1953), *The Terpenes, Vol. I* (Second ed.), Cambridge University Press, pp. 83–100

[19] Rainforest fragrances

[20] Archived analysis results, Wollongbar Agricultural Institute, Department of Primary Industry, NSW

[21] Standards Australia, "Australia Standard, Oil of *Backhousia citriodora*, citral type (lemon myrtle oil)", AS 4941-2001.

2.5.10 Further reading

1. Atkinson W, Brice H. (1955), "Antibacterial substances produced by flowering plants.", *Aust. J. Exp. Biology* 33 (5): 547–54, doi:10.1038/icb.1955.56.

2. APNI Australian Plant Name Index

2.5.11 External links

- Australian Bushfood and Native Medicine Forum

- Broad range of lemon myrtle products and recipes

- Lemon Myrtle from Vic Cherikoff

2.6 Benzoin resin

Not to be confused with benzoin.
Benzoin resin is a balsamic resin obtained from the bark

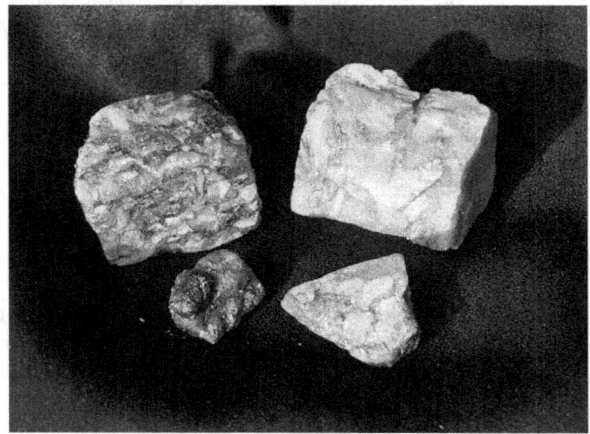

Kemenyan, *benzoin resin as sold in Gombong, Central Java*

of several species of trees in the genus *Styrax*. It is used in perfumes, some kinds of incense, as a flavoring, and medicine (see tincture of benzoin). Commonly called "benzoin", it is called "benzoin resin" here to distinguish it from the chemical compound benzoin. Benzoin resin does *not* contain this crystalline compound.

Benzoin is also called **gum benzoin** or **gum benjamin**, but "gum" is incorrect as benzoin is not a polysaccharide. Its name came via the Italian from the Arabic *lubān jāwī* (لبان جاوي, "frankincense from Java").[1]

Benzoin resin is also called **styrax balsam** or **styrax resin**, but wrongly, since those resins are obtained from a different plant family, Hamamelidaceae.

Benzoin resin is a common ingredient in incense-making and perfumery because of its sweet vanilla-like aroma and fixative properties. Gum benzoin is a major component of the type of church incense used in Russia and some other Orthodox Christian societies, as well as Western Catholic Churches.[2] Most benzoin is used in Arab States of the Persian Gulf and India, where it is burned on charcoal as an incense. It is also used in the production of Bakhoor (Arabic بخور - scented wood chips) as well as various mixed resin incense in the Arab countries and the Horn of Africa. Benzoin resin is also used in blended types of Japanese incense, Indian incense, Chinese incense (known as Anxi xiang; 安息香), and Papier d'Arménie as well as incense sticks.

There are two common kinds of benzoin resin, benzoin Siam and benzoin Sumatra. Benzoin Siam is obtained from *Styrax tonkinensis*, found across Thailand, Laos, Cambodia, and Vietnam. Benzoin Sumatra is obtained from *Styrax benzoin*, which grows predominantly on the island

of Sumatra.[3] Unlike Siamese benzoin, Sumatran benzoin contains cinnamic acid in addition to benzoic acid.[4] In the United States, Sumatra benzoin (Styrax benzoin and Styrax paralleoneurus) is more customarily used in pharmaceutical preparations, Siam benzoin (Styrax tonkinensis et al.) in the flavor and fragrance industries.[5]

In perfumery, benzoin is used as a fixative, slowing the dispersion of essential oils and other fragrance materials into the air.[3] Benzoin resin is used in cosmetics, veterinary medicine, and scented candles.[4] It is used as a flavoring in alcoholic and nonalcoholic beverages, baked goods, chewing gum, frozen dairy, gelatins, puddings, and soft candy.[6]

2.6.1 References

[1] A. Dietrich (1986), "LUBĀN", *The Encyclopaedia of Islam* **5** (2nd ed.), Brill, p. 786a

[2] St. Alban Blend

[3] Karl-Georg Fahlbusch; et al. (2007), "Flavors and Fragrances", *Ullmann's Encyclopedia of Industrial Chemistry* (7th ed.), Wiley, p. 87

[4] Klemens Fielbach; Dieter Grimm (2007), "Resins, Natural", *Ullmann's Encyclopedia of Industrial Chemistry* (7th ed.), Wiley, p. 4

[5] James A. Duke (2008), "Benzoin (Styrax benzoin Dryander.)", *Duke's Handbook of Medicinal Plants of the Bible*, Taylor & Francis, p. 446

[6] George A. Burdock (2010), "Benzoin Resin", *Fenaroli's Handbook of Flavor Ingredients* (6th ed.), Taylor & Francis, pp. 139–140

2.6.2 External links

2.7 Bergamot essential oil

Bergamot essential oil is a cold-pressed essential oil produced by cells inside the rind of a bergamot orange fruit. It is a common top note in perfumes.

Bergamot essential oil is a major component of the original Eau de Cologne composed by Farina at the beginning of 18th-century Germany. The first record of bergamot oil as fragrance ingredient is 1714, to be found in the Farina Archive in Cologne. One hundred bergamot oranges will yield about three ounces (85 grams) of bergamot oil.[1] The scent of bergamot essential oil is similar to a sweet light orange peel oil with a floral note.[2]

"Earl Grey tea" is a type of black tea that contains bergamot essential oil as a flavouring.

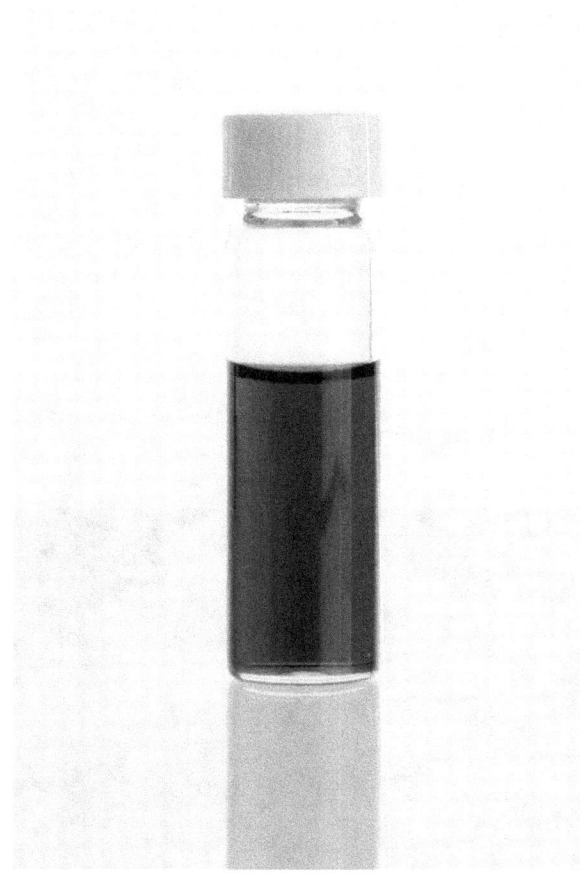

Bergamot essential oil

2.7.1 Production

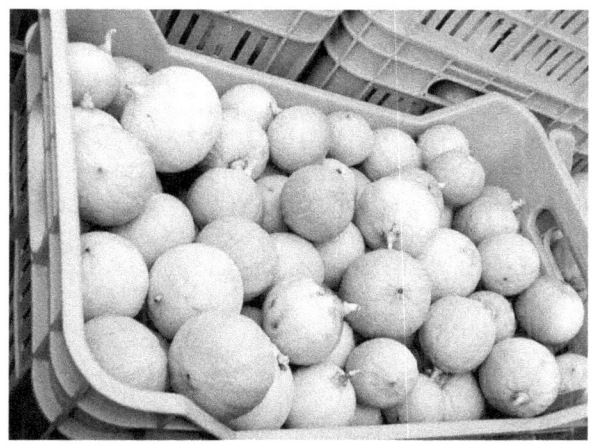

Bergamot fruits harvested for the production of essential oil.

The *sfumatura* or slow-folding process was the traditional technique for manually extracting the bergamot oil.[3]

Today the oil is extracted mechanically with machines

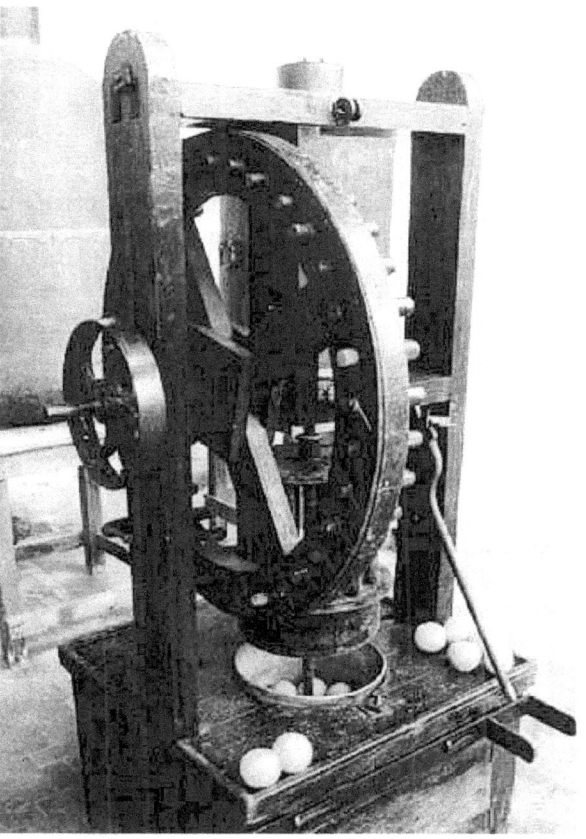

The Macchina calabrese *peeler, invented in 1840 by Nicola Barillà*

called "peelers", these machines "scrape" the outside of the fruit under running water to get an emulsion channeled into centrifuges for separating the essence from the water.

2.7.2 Constituents

A clear liquid (sometimes there is a deposit consisting of waxes) in color from green to greenish yellow, bergamot essential oil consists for the most part (average 95%) of a volatile fraction and for the remaining (5%) of a non-volatile fraction (or residual). Chemically it is a highly complex mixture of many classes of organic substances, particularly for the volatile fraction terpenes, esters, alcohols and aldehydes, and for the non-volatile fraction, oxygenated heterocyclic compounds as coumarins and furanocoumarins.

Volatile fraction

The main compounds in the oil are limonene, linalyl acetate, linalool, γ-terpinene and β-pinene,[4] and in smaller quantities geranial and β-bisabolene.

Linalyl acetate and linalool are qualitatively the most important components of the bergamot oil.

Non-volatile fraction

The main compounds are coumarins (citropten, 5-geranyloxy-7-methoxycoumarin) and furanocoumarins (bergapten, bergamottin).[5][6][7][8]

2.7.3 Adulteration

The bergamot essential oil is particularly subject to adulteration being an essential oil produced in relatively small quantities. Generally adulteration is to "cut" the oil, i.e. adding distilled essences of poor quality and low cost, for example of bitter orange and bergamot mint and/or mixtures of terpenes, natural or synthetic, or "reconstruct" the essence from synthetic chemicals, coloring it with chlorophyll. Worldwide, each year, around three thousand tonnes of declared essence of bergamot are marketed, while the genuine essence of bergamot produced annually amounts to no more than one hundred tons.[9]

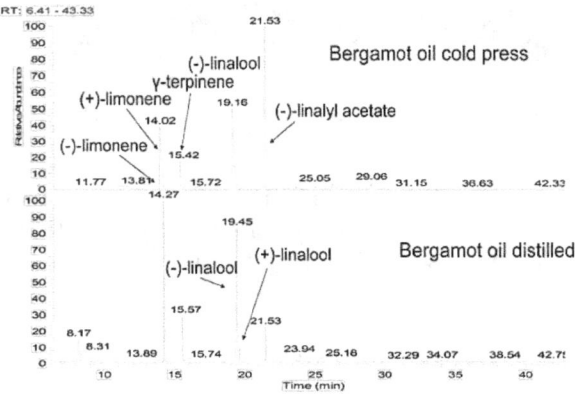

Comparison of bergamot oil obtained from the same raw plant material either by cold pressing or by hydrodistillation (Peratoner) using GC-MS analysis with enantiomeric column

Gas chromatography with columns having a chiral stationary phase allows to analyze mixtures of enantiomers. The analysis of the enantiomeric distribution of various compounds, such as linalyl acetate and linalool, allows the characterization of the bergamot oil according to the manufacturing process and allows for the detection of possible adulteration.[10][11][12][13]

The combined use of isotope ratio mass spectrometry and SNIF-NMR (Site-Specific Natural Isotope Fractionation-Nuclear Magnetic Resonance) allows to discover adulteration otherwise undetectable even allowing for the identification of the geographical origin of the essential oil.[14]

The GC-C-IRMS (Gas Chromatography-Combustion – Isotope Ratio Mass Spectrometer) technique, the most recently used, allows to obtain similar results.[15]

Reference analytical values

Analytical values take as reference for genuinity evalutation of bergamot essential oil by the *Experimental Station for the Industry of the Essential oils and Citrus products*, in Reggio Calabria, Italy.[16]

2.7.4 Toxicology

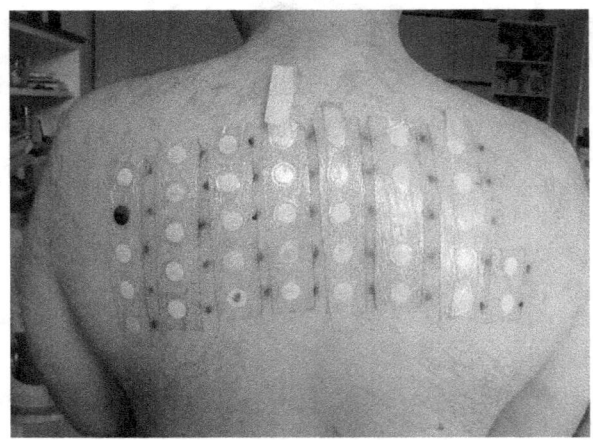

Patch test

In several studies, application of some sources of bergamot oil directly to the skin via patch test was shown to have a concentration-dependent phototoxic effect of increasing redness after exposure to ultraviolet light (due to the chemical bergapten, and possibly also citropten, bergamottin, geranial, and neral).[17][18] This is a property shared by many other citrus fruits. Bergapten has also been implicated as a potassium channel blocker; in one case study, a patient who consumed four liters of Earl Grey tea per day suffered paresthesias, fasciculations and muscle cramps.[19]

2.7.5 Notes

[1] Brannt, William Theodore; Schaedler, Karl. *A Practical Treatise on Animal and Vegetable Fats and Oils*

[2] http://www.fragrantica.com/notes/Bergamot-75.html

[3] Angelo Di Giacomo e Biagio Mincione (1994). *Gli Olii Essenziali Agrumari in Italia* (in Italian). Reggio Calabria: Laruffa Editore.

[4] Sawamura, Masayoshi; Onishi, Yuji; Ikemoto, Junko; Tu, Nguyen Thi Minh; Phi, Nguyen Thi Lan (2006). "Characteristic odour components of bergamot (Citrus bergamia Risso) essential oil". *Flavour and Fragrance Journal* **21** (4): 609–615. doi:10.1002/ffj.1604. ISSN 0882-5734.

[5] Benincasa, M.; Buiarelli, F.; Cartoni, G. P.; Coccioli, F. (1990). "Analysis of lemon and bergamot essential oils by HPLC with microbore columns". *Chromatographia* **30** (5–6): 271–276. doi:10.1007/BF02319706. ISSN 0009-5893.

[6] Mondello, Luigi; Stagno d'Alcontres, Ildefonsa; Del Duce, Rosa; Crispo, Francesco (1993). "On the genuineness of citrus essential oils. Part XL. The composition of the coumarins and psoralens of Calabrian bergamot essential oil (Citrus bergamia Risso)". *Flavour and Fragrance Journal* **8** (1): 17–24. doi:10.1002/ffj.2730080105. ISSN 0882-5734.

[7] Cavazza, A.; Bartle, K. D.; Dugo, P. Mondello, L. (2001). "Analysis of oxygen heterocyclic compounds in citrus essential oils by capillary electrochromatography and comparison with HPLC". *Chromatographia* **53** (1–2): 57–62. doi:10.1007/BF02492428. ISSN 0009-5893.

[8] Dugo, Paola; Piperno, Anna; Romeo, Roberto; Cambria, Maria; Russo, Marina; Carnovale, Caterina; Mondello, Luigi (2009). "Determination of Oxygen Heterocyclic Components in Citrus Products by HPLC with UV Detection". *Journal of Agricultural and Food Chemistry* **57** (15): 6543–6551. doi:10.1021/jf901209r. ISSN 0021-8561.

[9] (Italian) Tonio Licordari *La riflessione Valorizzare ora questa risorsa sulla scia dell'onda... profumata* Gazzetta del Sud Cronaca di Reggio 18-02-2010

[10] Mondello, Luigi; Verzera, Antonella; Previti, Piero; Crispo, Francesco; Dugo, Giovanni (1998). "Multidimensional Capillary GC–GC for the Analysis of Complex Samples. 5. Enantiomeric Distribution of Monoterpene Hydrocarbons, Monoterpene Alcohols, and Linalyl Acetate of Bergamot (Citrus bergamia Risso et Poiteau) Oils". *Journal of Agricultural and Food Chemistry* **46** (10): 4275–4282. doi:10.1021/jf980228u. ISSN 0021-8561.

[11] Eleni, Melliou; Antonios, Michaelakis; George, Koliopoulos; Alexios-Leandros, Skaltsounis; Prokopios, Magiatis (2009). "High Quality Bergamot Oil from Greece. Chemical Analysis Using Chiral Gas Chromatography and Larvicidal Activity against the West Nile Virus Vector". *Molecules* **14** (2): 839–849. doi:10.3390/molecules14020839. ISSN 1420-3049.

[12] Burfield, Tony. "The Adulteration of Essential Oils – and the Consequences to Aromatherapy & Natural Perfumery Practice.". *Presented to the International Federation of Aromatherapists Annual AGM London Oct 11th 2003.* Retrieved 16 June 2013.

[13] Cotroneo, Antonella; Stagno d'Alcontres, Ildefonsa; Trozzi, Alessandra (1992). "On the genuineness of citrus essential oils. Part XXXIV. Detection of added reconstituted bergamot oil in genuine bergamot essential oil by high resolution gas chromatography with chiral capillary columns'. *Flavour and Fragrance Journal* **7** (1): 15–17. doi:10.1002/ffj.2730070104. ISSN 0882-5734.

[14] Hanneguelle, Sophie.; Thibault, Jean Noel.; Naulet, Norbert.; Martin, Gerard J. (1992). "Authentication of essential oils containing linalool and linalyl acetate by isotopic methods". *Journal of Agricultural and Food Chemistry* **40** (1): 81–87. doi:10.1021/jf00013a016. ISSN 0021-8561.

[15] Luisa Schipilliti, G. Dugo, L. Santi, P Dugo and L. Mondello (2011). "Authentication of Bergamot Essential Oil by Gas Chromatography-Combustion-Isotope Ratio Mass Spectrometer (GC-C-IRMS)". *Journal of Essential Oil Research* **23** (2): 60–71. doi:10.1080/10412905.2011.9700447.

[16] (Italian) (English) Francesco Gionfriddo e Domenico Castaldo (2004). "Ridefinizione dei parametri analico-composizionali dell'olio essenziale di bergamotto estratto a freddo / Ridefinition of analitycal compositional parameters for "cold pressed" bergamot essential oil". *Essenze Derivati Agrumari* (74): 151–152.

[17] Girard J, Unkovic J, Delahayes J, Lafille C (1979). "Phototoxicity of Bergamot oil. Comparison between humans and guinea pigs". *Dermatologica* (in French) **158** (4): 229–43. doi:10.1159/000250763. PMID 428611.

[18] Kejlova K, Jirova D, Bendova H, Kandarova H, Weidenhoffer Z, Kolarova H, Liebsch M (2007). "Phototoxicity of bergamot oil assessed by in vitro techniques in combination with human patch tests". *Toxicology in Vitro* **21** (7): 1298–1303. doi:10.1016/j.tiv.2007.05.016. PMID 17569618.

[19] Finsterer, J (2002). "Earl Grey tea intoxication". *Lancet* **359** (9316): 1484. doi:10.1016/S0140-6736(02)08436-2. PMID 11983248.

2.7.6 Bibliography

• Dugo, Giovanni; Bonaccorsi, Ivana (2013). *Citrus bergamia: Bergamot and its Derivatives.* Medicinal and Aromatic Plants – Industrial Profiles (Book 51). CRC Press. ISBN 978-1439862278.

• Costa, Rosaria; Dugo, Paola; Navarra, Michele; Raymo, Vilfredo; Dugo, Giovanni; Mondello, Luigi (2010). "Study on the chemical composition variability of some processed bergamot (Citrus bergamia) essential oils". *Flavour and Fragrance Journal* **25** (1): 4–12. doi:10.1002/ffj.1949. ISSN 0882-5734.

• Carlo Mangola, Enrico Postorino, Francesco Gionfriddo, Maurizio Catalfamo, Renato Manganaro and Giuseppe Calabrò (October 2009). "Evaluation of the Genuineness of Cold-pressed Bergamot Oil". *Perfumer & Flavorist*: 26–31.

- Alp Kunkar and Ennio Kunkar, "Bergamotto e le sue essenze", Edizioni A Z

- A. Kunkar, C. Kunkar: Supercritical CO2 extraction of bergamot oil from peel ; Int. Cong. Medicinal plants and essential oils- Anadolu üniversıtesi-Eskişehir Turkey

2.7.7 External links

- Committee on Herbal Medicinal Products (HMPC) (22 May 2012). "Assessment report on Citrus bergamia Risso et Poiteau, aetheroleum Final" (PDF). European Medicines Agency (EMA). Retrieved 7 April 2014.

- Committee on Herbal Medicinal Products (HMPC) (22 May 2012). "List of references supporting the assessment of Citrus bergamia Risso et Poiteau, aetheroleum Final" (PDF). European Medicines Agency (EMA). Retrieved 7 April 2014.

2.8 Black pepper

"Peppercorn" redirects here.   For other uses, see Peppercorn (disambiguation).

Black pepper (*Piper nigrum*) is a flowering vine in the family Piperaceae, cultivated for its fruit, which is usually dried and used as a spice and seasoning. When dried, the fruit is known as a peppercorn. When fresh and fully mature, it is approximately 5 millimetres (0.20 in) in diameter, dark red, and, like all drupes, contains a single seed. Peppercorns, and the ground pepper derived from them, may be described simply as pepper, or more precisely as **black pepper** (cooked and dried unripe fruit), **green pepper** (dried unripe fruit) and **white pepper** (ripe fruit seeds).

Black pepper is native to south India, and is extensively cultivated there and elsewhere in tropical regions. Currently Vietnam is the world's largest producer and exporter of pepper and producing 34% of the world's *Piper nigrum* crop as of 2008.

Dried ground pepper has been used since antiquity for both its flavour and as a traditional medicine. Black pepper is the world's most traded spice. It is one of the most common spices added to European cuisine and its descendants. The spiciness of black pepper is due to the chemical piperine, not to be confused with the capsaicin that gives fleshy peppers theirs. It is ubiquitous in the modern world as a seasoning and is often paired with salt.

2.8.1 Etymology

The word "pepper" has its roots in the Dravidian word for long pepper, *pippali*.[2][3][4] Ancient Greek and Latin turned *pippali* into the Latin *piper*, which was used by the Romans to refer both to black pepper and long pepper, as the Romans erroneously believed that both of these spices were derived from the same plant.[5] Today's "pepper" derives from the Old English *pipor*. The Latin word is also the source of Romanian *piper*, Italian *pepe*, Dutch *peper*, German *Pfeffer*, French *poivre*, and other similar forms.

In the 16th century, *pepper* started referring to the unrelated New World chili pepper as well. "Pepper" was used in a figurative sense to mean "spirit" or "energy" at least as far back as the 1840s; in the early 20th century, this was shortened to *pep*.[6]

2.8.2 Varieties

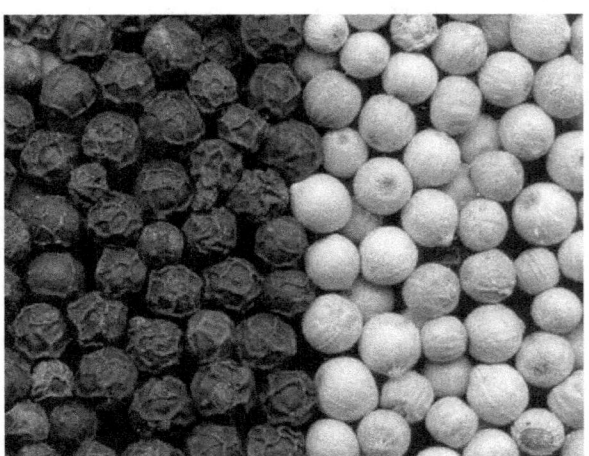

Black and white peppercorns

Black pepper

Black pepper is produced from the still-green, unripe drupes of the pepper plant. The drupes are cooked briefly in hot water, both to clean them and to prepare them for drying. The heat ruptures cell walls in the pepper, speeding the work of browning enzymes during drying. The drupes are dried in the sun or by machine for several days, during which the pepper around the seed shrinks and darkens into a thin, wrinkled black layer. Once dried, the spice is called black peppercorn. On some estates, the berries are separated from the stem by hand and then sun-dried without the boiling process.

Once the peppercorns are dried, pepper spirit and oil can be extracted from the berries by crushing them. Pepper spirit is used in many medicinal and beauty products. Pepper oil is also used as an ayurvedic massage oil and used in certain beauty and herbal treatments.

- Black pepper (*Piper nigrum*) essential oil in a clear glass vial

- Ground black pepper and a plastic pepper shaker

- Roughly cracked black peppercorns, also known as *mignonette* or *poivre mignonette*

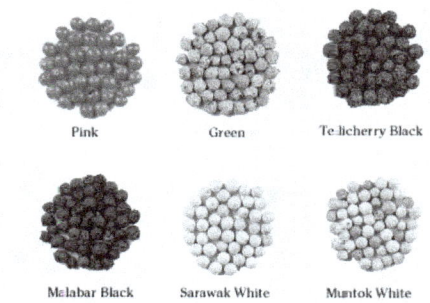

The six variants of pepper

White pepper

"White pepper" redirects here. For the Ween album, see White Pepper.

White pepper consists of the seed of the pepper plant

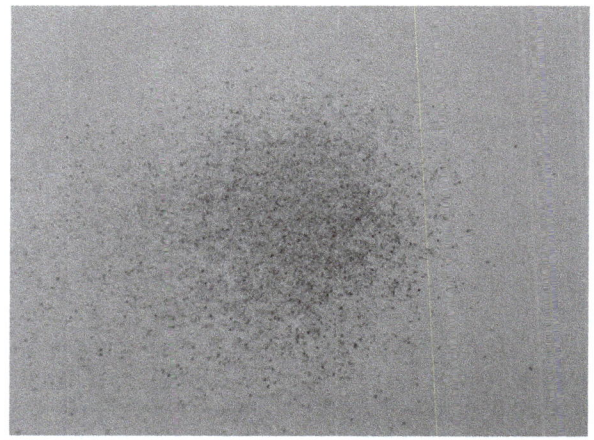

White pepper grains

alone, with the darker-coloured skin of the pepper fruit removed. This is usually accomplished by a process known as retting, where fully ripe red pepper berries are soaked in water for about a week, during which the flesh of the pepper softens and decomposes. Rubbing then removes what

remains of the fruit, and the naked seed is dried. Sometimes alternative processes are used for removing the outer pepper from the seed, including removing the outer layer through mechanical, chemical or biological methods.[7]

Ground white pepper is often used in cream sauces, Chinese and Thai cuisine, and dishes like salad, light-coloured sauces and mashed potatoes, where black pepper would visibly stand out. White pepper has a slightly different flavour from black pepper, due to the lack of certain compounds present in the outer fruit layer of the drupe, but not found in the seed. A slightly sweet version of white pepper from India is sometimes called *safed golmirch* (Hindi), *shada golmorich* (Bengali), or *safed golmirch* (Punjabi).

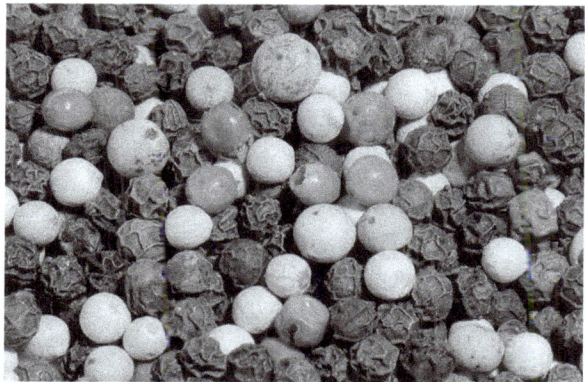

Black, green, pink (Schinus terebinthifolius), and white peppercorns

Green pepper

Green pepper, like black, is made from the unripe drupes. Dried green peppercorns are treated in a way that retains the green colour, such as treatment with sulphur dioxide, canning or freeze-drying. Pickled peppercorns, also green, are unripe drupes preserved in brine or vinegar. Fresh, unpreserved green pepper drupes, largely unknown in the West, are used in some Asian cuisines, particularly Thai cuisine.[8] Their flavour has been described as spicy and fresh, with a bright aroma.[9] They decay quickly if not dried or preserved.

Wild pepper

Wild pepper grows in the Western Ghats region of India. Into the 19th century, the forests contained expansive wild pepper vines, as recorded by the Scottish physician Francis Buchanan (also a botanist and geographer) in his book *A journey from Madras through the countries of Mysore, Canara and Malabar* (Volume III).[10] However, deforestation resulted in wild pepper growing in more limited forest patches from Goa to Kerala, with the wild source gradually decreasing as the quality and yield of the cultivated variety improved. No successful grafting of commercial pepper on wild pepper has been achieved to date.[10]

Orange pepper and red pepper

Orange pepper or red pepper usually consists of ripe red pepper drupes preserved in brine and vinegar. Ripe red peppercorns can also be dried using the same colour-preserving techniques used to produce green pepper.[11]

Pink pepper and other plants used as pepper

Pink pepper from *Piper nigrum* is distinct from the more-common dried "pink peppercorns", which are actually the fruits of a plant from a different family, the Peruvian pepper tree, *Schinus molle*, or its relative the Brazilian pepper tree, *Schinus terebinthifolius*. A pink peppercorn (French: baie rose, "pink berry") is a dried berry of the shrub Schinus molle, commonly known as the Peruvian peppertree. As they are members of the cashew family, they may cause allergic reactions including anaphylaxis for persons with a tree nut allergy.

The bark of *Drimys winteri* ("Canelo" or "Winter's Bark") is used as a substitute for pepper in cold and temperate regions of Chile and Argentina where it is easily available.

In New Zealand the seeds of Kawakawa (*Macropiper excelsum*), a relative of black pepper, are sometimes used as pepper and the leaves of *Pseudowintera colorata* (mountain horopito) are another replacement for pepper.

Several plants in the United States are used also as pepper substitutes, such as *Lepidium campestre*, *Lepidium virginicum*, shepherd's purse, horseradish, and field Pennycress.

Region of origin

Peppercorns are often categorized by their place of origin. Two types come from India's Malabar Coast: *Malabar* and *Tellicherry*. Tellicherry comes from grafted Malabar plants grown on Mount Tellicherry.[12]

Sarawak pepper is native to the Malaysian portion of Borneo. White Muntok pepper comes from Indonesia and Lampung hails its island of Sumatra. Vietnam produces both white and black pepper in the provinces of Bà Rịa–Vũng Tàu, Chu Se District, Bình Phước, and Phú Quốc Island in Kiên Giang Province.[13]

Kampot Pepper is native to Kampot, Cambodia and received Geographical indication (GI) status in 2008. This

pepper is grown in a limited geographical region in four varieties: black, green, red, and white.[14]

2.8.3   Plant

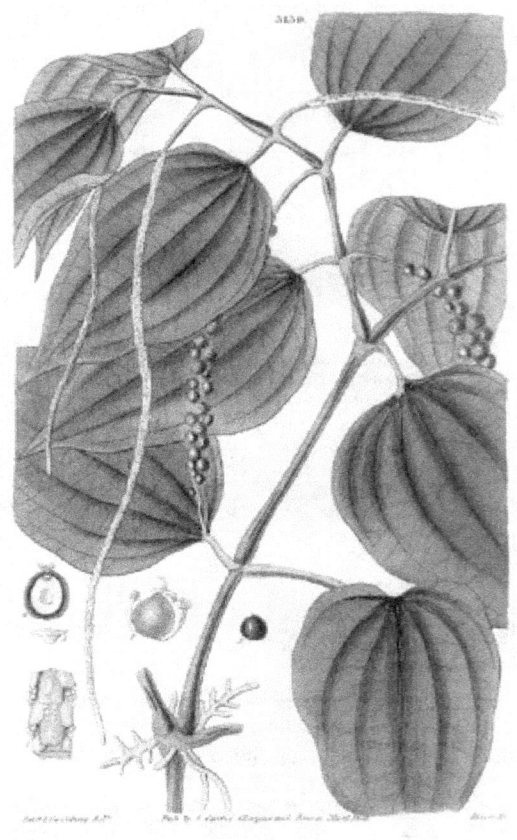

Piper nigrum *from an 1832 print*

The pepper plant is a perennial woody vine growing up to 4 metres (13 ft) in height on supporting trees, poles, or trellises. It is a spreading vine, rooting readily where trailing stems touch the ground. The leaves are alternate, entire, 5 to 10 centimetres (2.0 to 3.9 in) long and 3 to 6 centimetres (1.2 to 2.4 in) across. The flowers are small, produced on pendulous spikes 4 to 8 centimetres (1.6 to 3.1 in) long at the leaf nodes, the spikes lengthening up to 7 to 15 centimetres (2.8 to 5.9 in) as the fruit matures.[15] The fruit of the black pepper is called a drupe and when dried is known as a peppercorn.

Pepper can be grown in soil that is neither too dry nor susceptible to flooding, moist, well-drained and rich in organic matter (the vines do not do too well over an altitude of 900 m (3,000 ft) above sea level). The plants are propagated by cuttings about 40 to 50 centimetres (16 to 20 in) long,

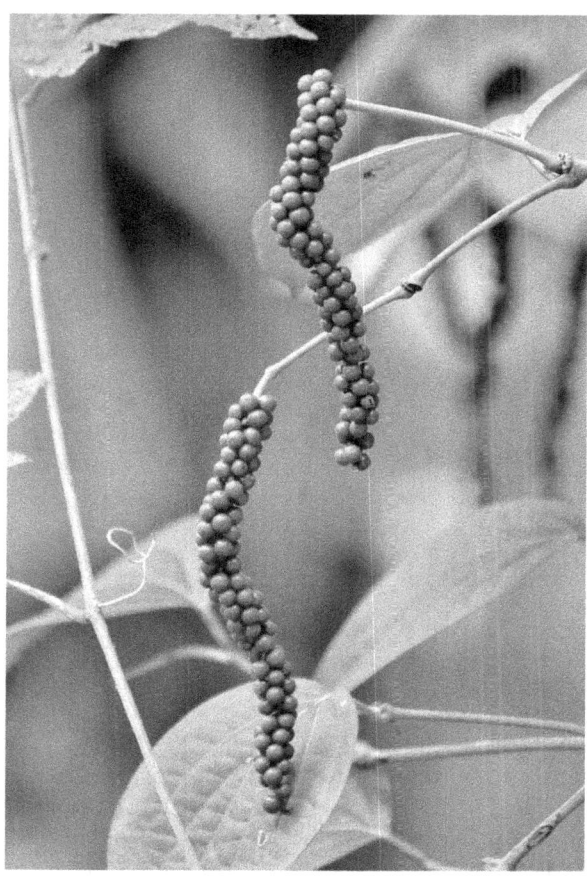

*Unripe drupes of Black Pepper (*Piper nigrum*) at Trivandrum, Kerala, India*

tied up to neighbouring trees or climbing frames at distances of about 2 metres (6 ft 7 in) apart; trees with rough bark are favoured over those with smooth bark, as the pepper plants climb rough bark more readily. Competing plants are cleared away, leaving only sufficient trees to provide shade and permit free ventilation. The roots are covered in leaf mulch and manure, and the shoots are trimmed twice a year. On dry soils the young plants require watering every other day during the dry season for the first three years. The plants bear fruit from the fourth or fifth year, and typically continue to bear fruit for seven years. The cuttings are usually cultivars, selected both for yield and quality of fruit.

A single stem will bear 20 to 30 fruiting spikes. The harvest begins as soon as one or two fruits at the base of the spikes begin to turn red, and before the fruit is fully mature, and still hard; if allowed to ripen completely, the fruit lose pungency, and ultimately fall off and are lost. The spikes are collected and spread out to dry in the sun, then the peppercorns are stripped off the spikes.[15]

Black pepper is either native to Southeast Asia[16] or South Asia.[17] Within the genus *Piper*, it is most closely related to other Asian species such as *Piper caninum*.[17]

- *Piper nigrum* on tree support in Goa, India
- Pepper vine, Tiruvannamalai, Tamil Nadu, India

2.8.4 History

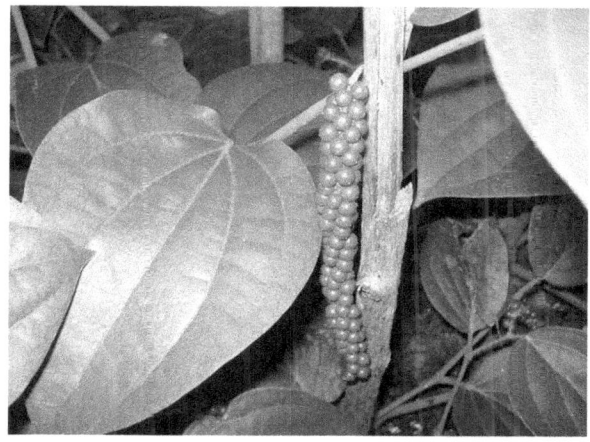

Pepper in Kerala, India

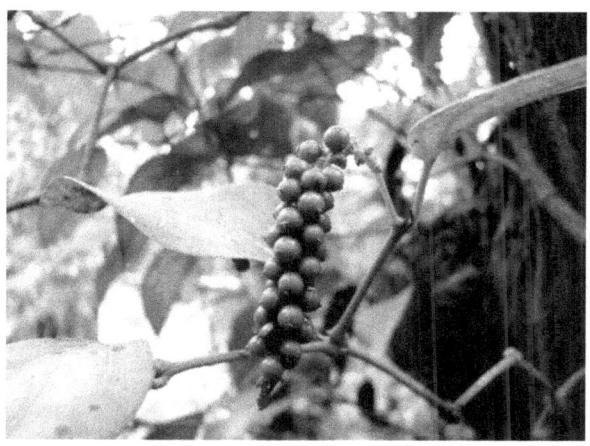

Pepper before ripening

Pepper is native to South Asia and Southeast Asia and has been known to Indian cooking since at least 2000 BCE.[18] J. Innes Miller notes that while pepper was grown in southern Thailand and in Malaysia, its most important source was India, particularly the Malabar Coast, in what is now the state of Kerala.[19] Peppercorns were a much-prized trade good, often referred to as "black gold" and used as a form of commodity money. The legacy of this trade remains in some Western legal systems which recognize the term "peppercorn rent" as a form of a token payment made for something that is in fact being given.

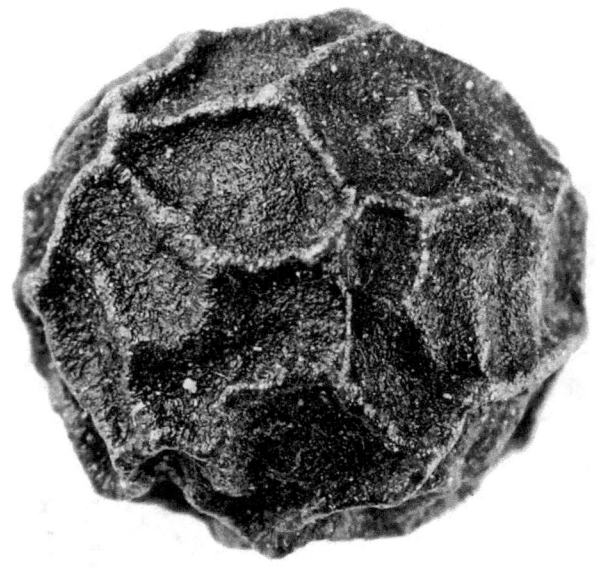

Peppercorn close-up

The ancient history of black pepper is often interlinked with (and confused with) that of long pepper, the dried fruit of closely related *Piper longum*. The Romans knew of both and often referred to either as just "piper". In fact, it was not until the discovery of the New World and of chili peppers that the popularity of long pepper entirely declined. Chili peppers, some of which when dried are similar in shape and taste to long pepper, were easier to grow in a variety of locations more convenient to Europe.

Before the 16th century, pepper was being grown in Java, Sunda, Sumatra, Madagascar, Malaysia, and everywhere in Southeast Asia. These areas traded mainly with China, or used the pepper locally.[20] Ports in the Malabar area also served as a stop-off point for much of the trade in other spices from farther east in the Indian Ocean. Following the British hegemony in India, virtually all of the black pepper found in Europe, the Middle East, and North Africa was traded from Malabar region.

Ancient times

Black peppercorns were found stuffed in the nostrils of Ramesses II, placed there as part of the mummification rituals shortly after his death in 1213 BCE.[21] Little else is known about the use of pepper in ancient Egypt and how it reached the Nile from South Asia.

Pepper (both long and black) was known in Greece at least as early as the 4th century BCE, though it was probably an uncommon and expensive item that only the very rich could afford. Trade routes of the time were by land, or in ships which hugged the coastlines of the Arabian Sea. Long pep-

per, growing in the north-western part of India, was more accessible than the black pepper from further south; this trade advantage, plus long pepper's greater spiciness, probably made black pepper less popular at the time.

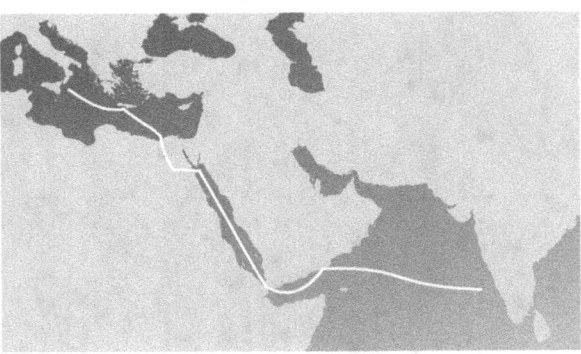

A Roman era trade route from India to Italy

By the time of the early Roman Empire, especially after Rome's conquest of Egypt in 30 BCE, open-ocean crossing of the Arabian Sea direct to southern India's Malabar Coast was near routine. Details of this trading across the Indian Ocean have been passed down in the *Periplus of the Erythraean Sea*. According to the Roman geographer Strabo, the early Empire sent a fleet of around 120 ships on an annual one-year trip to China, Southeast Asia, India and back. The fleet timed its travel across the Arabian Sea to take advantage of the predictable monsoon winds. Returning from India, the ships travelled up the Red Sea, from where the cargo was carried overland or via the Nile-Red Sea canal to the Nile River, barged to Alexandria, and shipped from there to Italy and Rome. The rough geographical outlines of this same trade route would dominate the pepper trade into Europe for a millennium and a half to come.

With ships sailing directly to the Malabar coast, black pepper was now travelling a shorter trade route than long pepper, and the prices reflected it. Pliny the Elder's *Natural History* tells us the prices in Rome around 77 CE: "Long pepper ... is fifteen denarii per pound, while that of white pepper is seven, and of black, four." Pliny also complains "there is no year in which India does not drain the Roman Empire of fifty million sesterces," and further moralizes on pepper:

> It is quite surprising that the use of pepper has come so much into fashion, seeing that in other substances which we use, it is sometimes their sweetness, and sometimes their appearance that has attracted our notice; whereas, pepper has nothing in it that can plead as a recommendation to either fruit or berry, its only desirable quality being a certain pungency; and yet it is for this that we import it all the way from India! Who was the

first to make trial of it as an article of food? and who, I wonder, was the man that was not content to prepare himself by hunger only for the satisfying of a greedy appetite? (*N.H.* 12.14)[22]

Black pepper was a well-known and widespread, if expensive, seasoning in the Roman Empire Apicius' De re coquinaria, a 3rd-century cookbook probably based at least partly on one from the 1st century CE, includes pepper in a majority of its recipes. Edward Gibbon wrote, in *The History of the Decline and Fall of the Roman Empire*, that pepper was "a favorite ingredient of the most expensive Roman cookery".

Postclassical Europe

Pepper was so valuable that it was often used as collateral or even currency. In the Dutch language, "pepper expensive" (*peperduur*) is an expression for something very expensive. The taste for pepper (or the appreciation of its monetary value) was passed on to those who would see Rome fall. Alaric the Visigoth included 3,000 pounds of pepper as part of the ransom he demanded from Rome when he besieged the city in 5th century.[23] After the fall of Rome, others took over the middle legs of the spice trade, first the Persians and then the Arabs; Innes Miller cites the account of Cosmas Indicopleustes, who travelled east to India, as proof that "pepper was still being exported from India in the sixth century".[24] By the end of the Early Middle Ages, the central portions of the spice trade were firmly under Islamic control. Once into the Mediterranean, the trade was largely monopolized by Italian powers, especially Venice and Genoa. The rise of these city-states was funded in large part by the spice trade.

A riddle authored by Saint Aldhelm, a 7th-century Bishop of Sherborne, sheds some light on black pepper's role in England at that time:

I am black on the outside, clad in a wrinkled cover,
Yet within I bear a burning marrow.
I season delicacies, the banquets of kings, and the luxuries of the table,
Both the sauces and the tenderized meats of the kitchen.
But you will find in me no quality of any worth,
Unless your bowels have been rattled by my gleaming marrow.[1]

1. ^ Translation from Turner, p 94. The riddle's answer is of course *pepper*.

It is commonly believed that during the Middle Ages, pepper was used to conceal the taste of partially rotten meat.

There is no evidence to support this claim, and historians view it as highly unlikely: in the Middle Ages, pepper was a luxury item, affordable only to the wealthy, who certainly had unspoiled meat available as well.[25] In addition, people of the time certainly knew that eating spoiled food would make them sick. Similarly, the belief that pepper was widely used as a preservative is questionable: it is true that piperine, the compound that gives pepper its spiciness, has some antimicrobial properties, but at the concentrations present when pepper is used as a spice, the effect is small.[26] Salt is a much more effective preservative, and salt-cured meats were common fare, especially in winter. However, pepper and other spices certainly played a role in improving the taste of long-preserved meats.

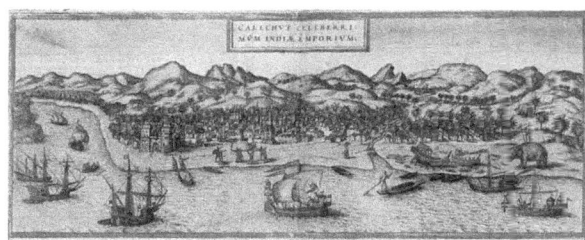

A depiction of Calicut, India published in 1572 during Portugal's control of the pepper trade

Its exorbitant price during the Middle Ages—and the monopoly on the trade held by Italy—was one of the inducements which led the Portuguese to seek a sea route to India. In 1498, Vasco da Gama became the first person to reach India by sailing around Africa (see Age of Discovery); asked by Arabs in Calicut (who spoke Spanish and Italian) why they had come, his representative replied, "we seek Christians and spices". Though this first trip to India by way of the southern tip of Africa was only a modest success, the Portuguese quickly returned in greater numbers and eventually gained much greater control of trade on the Arabian sea. It was given additional legitimacy (at least from a European imperialistic perspective) by the 1494 Treaty of Tordesillas, which granted Portugal exclusive rights to the half of the world where black pepper originated.

The Portuguese proved unable to maintain their stranglehold on the spice trade for long. The old Arab and Venetian trade networks successfully 'smuggled' enormous quantities of spices through the patchy Portuguese blockade, and pepper once again flowed through Alexandria and Italy, as well as around Africa. In the 17th century, the Portuguese lost almost all of their valuable Indian Ocean trade to the Dutch and the English who, taking advantage from the Spanish ruling over Portugal (1580–1640), occupied by force almost all Portuguese dominations in the area. The pepper ports of Malabar began to trade increasingly with the Dutch in the period 1661–1663.

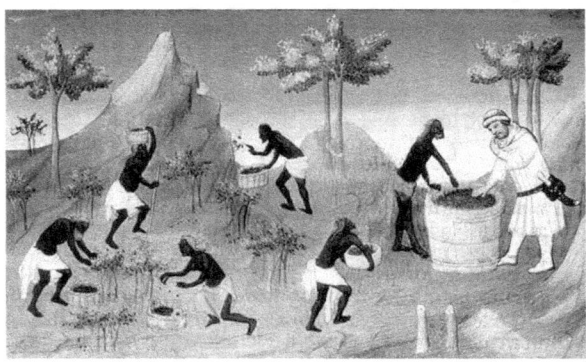

Pepper harvested for the European trader, from a manuscript Livre des merveilles de Marco Polo (*The book of the marvels of Marco Polo*)

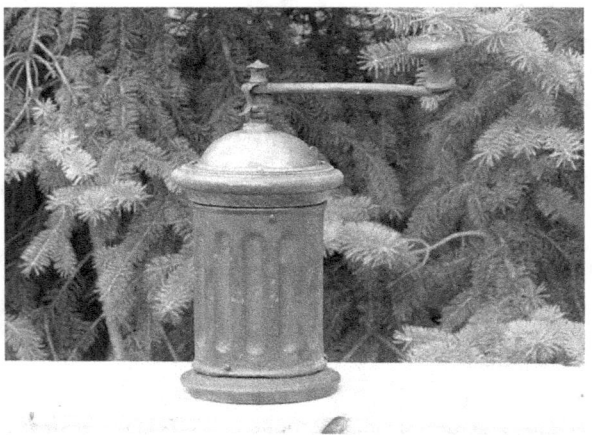

Pepper mill

As pepper supplies into Europe increased, the price of pepper declined (though the total value of the import trade generally did not). Pepper, which in the early Middle Ages had been an item exclusively for the rich, started to become more of an everyday seasoning among those of more average means. Today, pepper accounts for one-fifth of the world's spice trade.[27]

China

It is possible that black pepper was known in China in the 2nd century BCE, if poetic reports regarding an explorer named Tang Meng (??) are correct. Sent by Emperor Wu to what is now south-west China, Tang Meng is said to have come across something called *jujiang* or "sauce-betel". He was told it came from the markets of Shu, an area in what is now the Sichuan province. The traditional view among historians is that "sauce-betel" is a sauce made from betel leaves, but arguments have been made that it actually refers to pepper, either long or black.[28]

In the 3rd century CE, black pepper made its first definite appearance in Chinese texts, as *hujiao* or "foreign pepper". It does not appear to have been widely known at the time, failing to appear in a 4th-century work describing a wide variety of spices from beyond China's southern border, including long pepper.[29] By the 12th century, however, black pepper had become a popular ingredient in the cuisine of the wealthy and powerful, sometimes taking the place of China's native Sichuan pepper (the tongue-numbing dried fruit of an unrelated plant).

Marco Polo testifies to pepper's popularity in 13th-century China when he relates what he is told of its consumption in the city of Kinsay (Hangzhou): "... Messer Marco heard it stated by one of the Great Kaan's officers of customs that the quantity of pepper introduced daily for consumption into the city of Kinsay amounted to 43 loads, each load being equal to 223 lbs."[30] Marco Polo is not considered a very reliable source regarding China, and this second-hand data may be even more suspect, but if this estimated 10,000 pounds (4,500 kg) a day for one city is anywhere near the truth, China's pepper imports may have dwarfed Europe's.

During the course of the treasure voyages in the early 15th century, Admiral Zheng He and his expeditionary fleets returned with such a large amount of black pepper that the once-costly luxury became a common commodity.[31]

2.8.5   Phytochemicals, folk medicine and research

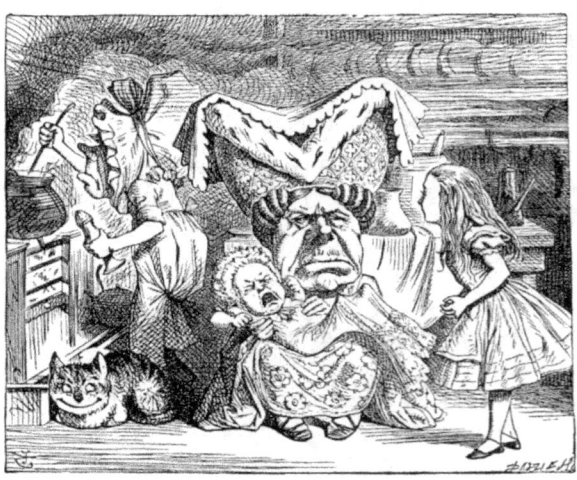

'There's certainly too much pepper in that soup!' Alice said to herself, as well as she could for sneezing. — Alice in Wonderland (*1865). Chapter VI: Pig and Pepper. Note the cook's pepper mill.*

Like many eastern spices, pepper was historically both a seasoning and a folk medicine. Long pepper, being stronger, was often the preferred medication, but both were used. Black pepper (or perhaps long pepper) was believed to cure several illnesses, such as constipation, insomnia, oral abscesses, sunburn and toothaches, among others.[32] Various sources from the 5th century onward recommended pepper to treat eye problems, often by applying salves or poultices made with pepper directly to the eye. There is no current medical evidence that any of these treatments has any benefit.[33] Nevertheless, black pepper, either powdered or its decoction, is widely used in traditional Indian medicine and as a home remedy for relief from sore throat, throat congestion, cough, etc.

Pepper is known to cause sneezing. Some sources say that piperine, a substance present in black pepper, irritates the nostrils, causing the sneezing.[34] Few, if any, controlled studies have been carried out to answer the question.

Piperine is under study for its potential to increase absorption of selenium, vitamin B, beta-carotene and curcumin, as well as other compounds.[35] As a folk medicine, pepper appears in the Buddhist Samaññaphala Sutta, chapter five, as one of the few medicines allowed to be carried by a monk.[36] Pepper contains phytochemicals,[37] including amides, piperidines, pyrrolidines and trace amounts of safrole which may be carcinogenic in laboratory rodents.[38]

Piperine is under study for a variety of possible physiological effects,[39] although this work is preliminary and mechanisms of activity for piperine in the human body remain unknown.

Nutrition

One tablespoon (6 grams) of ground black pepper contains moderate amounts of vitamin K (13% of the daily value or DV), iron (10% DV) and manganese (18% DV), with trace amounts of other essential nutrients, protein and dietary fibre.[40]

2.8.6 Flavor

Pepper gets its spicy heat mostly from piperine derived both from the outer fruit and the seed. Black pepper contains between 4.6% and 9.7% piperine by mass, and white pepper slightly more than that.[41] Refined piperine, by weight, is about one percent as hot as the capsaicin found in chili peppers.[42] The outer fruit layer, left on black pepper, also contains important odour-contributing terpenes including pinene, sabinene, limonene, caryophyllene, and linalool, which give citrusy, woody, and floral notes. These scents are mostly missing in white pepper, which is stripped of the fruit layer. White pepper can gain some different odours (including musty notes) from its longer fermentation stage.[43] The aroma of pepper is attributed to

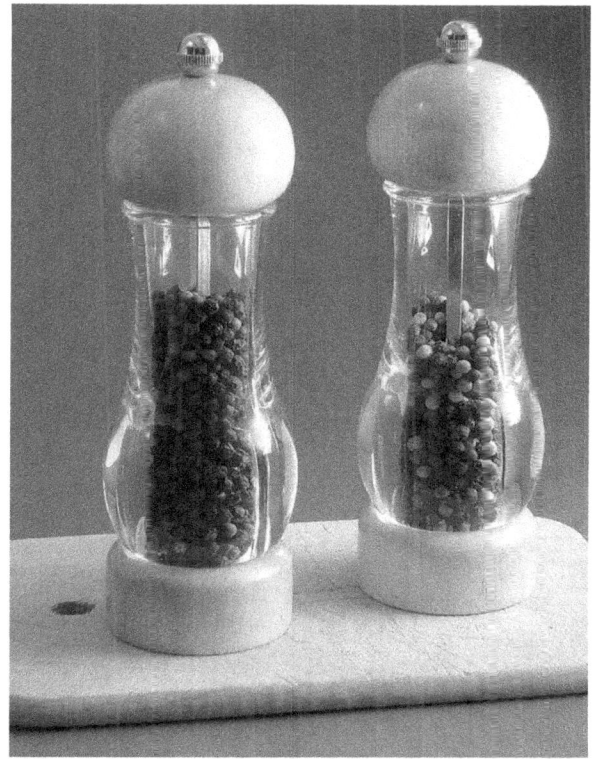

Handheld pepper mills

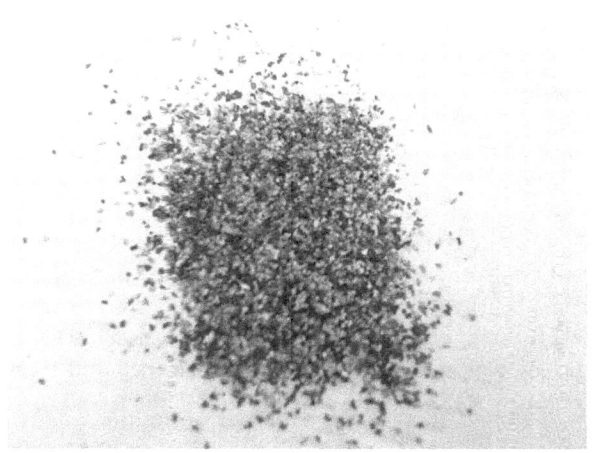

Black pepper grains

rotundone (3,4,5,6,7,8-Hexahydro-3α,8α-dimethyl-5α-(1-methylethenyl)azulene−1(2H)-one), a sesquiterpene originally discovered in the tubers of cyperus rotundus, which can be detected in concentrations of 0.4 nanograms/L in water and in wine: rotundone is also present in marjoram, oregano, rosemary, basil, thyme, and geranium, as well as in some Shiraz wines.[44]

Pepper loses flavour and aroma through evaporation, so airtight storage helps preserve its spiciness longer. Pepper can

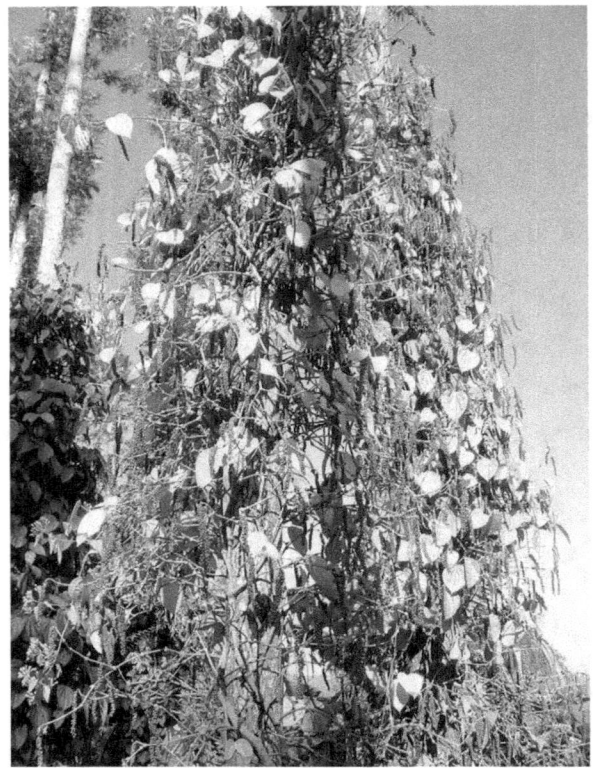

Pepper in Kolli Hills in India

also lose flavour when exposed to light, which can transform piperine into nearly tasteless isochavicine.[43] Once ground, pepper's aromatics can evaporate quickly; most culinary sources recommend grinding whole peppercorns immediately before use for this reason. Handheld pepper mills or grinders, which mechanically grind or crush whole peppercorns, are used for this, sometimes instead of pepper shakers that dispense pre-ground pepper. Spice mills such as pepper mills were found in European kitchens as early as the 14th century, but the mortar and pestle used earlier for crushing pepper have remained a popular method for centuries as well.[45]

2.8.7   World trade

Peppercorns (dried black pepper) are, by monetary value, the most widely traded spice in the world, accounting for 20 percent of all spice imports in 2002. The price of pepper can be volatile, and this figure fluctuates a great deal year to year; for example, pepper made up 39 percent of all spice imports in 1998.[46] By weight, slightly more chili peppers are traded worldwide than peppercorns.

The International Pepper Exchange is located in Kochi, India. Participation in the IPE however is domestic with regulatory restrictions on international membership on local ex-

changes; something common to almost all Asian commodity exchanges.

As of 2008, Vietnam is the world's largest producer and exporter of pepper, producing 34% of the world's *Piper nigrum*. Other major producers include India (19%), Brazil (13%), Indonesia (9%), Malaysia (8%), Sri Lanka (6%), China (6%), and Thailand (4%). Global pepper production peaked in 2003 with over 355,000 t (391,000 short tons), but has fallen to just over 271,000 t (299,000 short tons) by 2008 due to a series of issues including poor crop management, disease and weather. Vietnam dominates the export market, using almost none of its production domestically; however its 2007 crop fell by nearly 10% from the previous year to about 90,000 t (99,000 short tons). Similar crop yields occurred in 2007 across the other pepper producing nations as well.[47] Nowadays, in England, industrial buyers mix Peppers of different origin to maintain a balance between price, taste and other factors. Malabar black peppers are used for weight and taste, Sumatra for colour, and Penang for strength.[48]

2.8.8   See also

- Peppercorn sauce
- Salt

2.8.9   Notes and references

[1] "Piper nigrum information from NPGS/GRIN". www.ars-grin.gov. Retrieved 2 March 2008.

[2] Dravidian India - T.R. Sesha Iyengar - Google Books. Books.google.com. Retrieved on 31 October 2012.

[3] Intercourse Between India and the Western World - H. G. Rawlinson - Google Books. Books.google.com. Retrieved on 31 October 2012.

[4] Antiquities of India: An Account of the History and Culture of Ancient Hindustan - Lionel D. Barnett - Google Books. Books.google.com. Retrieved on 31 October 2012.

[5] "Pepper". Tamilnadu.com. 30 October 2012.

[6] Douglas Harper's *Online Etymology Dictionary* entries for *pepper* and *pep*. Retrieved 13 November 2005.

[7] "Cleaner technology for white pepper production". *The Hindu Business line*. 27 March 2008. Retrieved 29 January 2009.

[8] See Thai Ingredients Glossary. Retrieved 6 November 2005.

[9] Ochef, Using fresh green peppercorns. Retrieved 6 November 2005.

[10] Manjunath Hegde, Bomnalli (19 October 2013). "Meet the pepper queen" (Bangalore). Deccan Herald. Retrieved 22 January 2015.

[11] Katzer, Gernot (2006). Pepper. Gernot Katzer's Spice Pages. Retrieved 2 December 2012.

[12] Peppercorns, from Penzeys Spices. Retrieved 17 October 2006.

[13] Pepper varieties information from A Cook's Wares. Retrieved 6 November 2005.

[14] *Cambodia*. Lonely Planet. 1988. p. 225. GGKEY: ALKFLS6LY8Y.

[15] "Black Pepper Cultivation and Harvest". Thompson Martinez. Retrieved 14 May 2014.

[16] "Piper nigrum Linnaeus". *Flora of China*.

[17] Jaramillo, M. Alejandra; Manos (2001). "Phylogeny and Patterns of Floral Diversity in the Genus Piper (Piperaceae)". *American Journal of Botany* **88** (4): 706–16. doi:10.2307/2657072. PMID 11302858.

[18] Davidson & Saberi 178

[19] J. Innes Miller, *The Spice Trade of the Roman Empire* (Oxford: Clarendon Press, 1969), p. 80

[20] Dalby p. 93.

[21] Stephanie Fitzgerald (8 September 2008). *Ramses II, Egyptian Pharaoh, Warrior, and Builder*. Compass Point Books. p. 88. ISBN 0-7565-3836-X. Retrieved 29 January 2008.

[22] From Bostock and Riley's 1855 translation. Text online.

[23] J. Norwich, Byzantium: The Early Centuries, 134

[24] Innes Miller, *The Spice Trade*, p. 83

[25] Dalby p. 156; also Turner pp. 108–109, though Turner does go on to discuss spices (not pepper specifically) being used to disguise the taste of partially spoiled wine or ale.

[26] H. J. D. Dorman and S. G. Deans (2000). "Antimicrobial agents from plants: antibacterial activity of plant volatile oils". *Journal of Applied Microbiology* **88** (2): 308–16. doi:10.1046/j.1365-2672.2000.00969.x. PMID 10736000.. Full text at Blackwell website; purchase required. "Spices, which are used as integral ingredients in cuisine or added as flavouring agents to foods, are present in insufficient quantities for their antimicrobial properties to be significant."

[27] Jaffee, p. 10.

[28] Dalby pp. 74–75. The argument that *jujiang* was long pepper goes back to the 4th century CE botanical writings of Ji Han; Hui-lin Li's 1979 translation of and commentary on Ji Han's work makes the case that it was *piper nigrum*.

[29] Dalby p. 77.

[30] Yule, Henry; Cordier, Henri, Translation from *The Travels of Marco Polo: The Complete Yule-Cordier Edition*. Vol. 2, Dover. ISBN 0-486-27587-6. *p. 204.*

[31] Finlay, Robert (2008). "The Voyages of Zheng He: Ideology, State Power, and Maritime Trade in Ming China". *Journal of the Historical Society* **8** (3): 337. doi:10.1111/j.1540-5923.2008.00250.x.

[32] Turner p. 160.

[33] Turner p. 171.

[34] U.S. Library of Congress Science Reference Services "Everyday Mysteries", Why does pepper make you sneeze?. Retrieved 12 November 2005.

[35] Dudhatra, GB; Mody, SK; Awale, MM; Patel, HB; Modi, CM; Kumar, A; Kamani, DR; Chauhan, BN (2012). "A comprehensive review on pharmacotherapeutics of herbal bioenhancers". *The Scientific World Journal* **2012** (637953): 637953. doi:10.1100/2012/637953. PMC 3458266. PMID 23028251.

[36] Thanissaro Bhikkhu (30 November 1990). *Buddhist Monastic Code II*. Cambridge University Press. ISBN 0-521-36708-5. Retrieved 29 January 2008.

[37] Dawid, Corinna; Henze, Andrea; Frank, Oliver; Glabasnia, Anneke; Rupp, Mathias; Büning, Kirsten; Orlikowski, Diana; Bader, Matthias; Hofmann, Thomas (2012). "Structural and Sensory Characterization of Key Pungent and Tingling Compounds from Black Pepper (*Piper nigrum* L.)". *Journal of Agricultural and Food Chemistry* **60** (11): 2884–2895. doi:10.1021/jf300036a. PMID 22352449.

[38] James A. Duke (16 August 1993). *CRC Handbook of Alternative Cash Crops*. CRC Press. p. 395. ISBN 0-8493-3620-1. Retrieved 29 January 2009.

[39] Srinivasan K (2007). "Black pepper and its pungent principle-piperine: a review of diverse physiological effects". *Crit Rev Food Sci Nutr* **47** (8): 735–48. doi:10.1080/10408390601062054. PMID 17987447.

[40] "Nutrition facts for black pepper, one tablespoon (6 g); USDA Nutrient Database, version SR-21". Conde Nast. 2014. Retrieved 25 October 2014.

[41] Pepper. Tis-gdv.de. Retrieved on 31 October 2012.

[42] Lawless, Harry T.; Heymann, Hildegarde (2010). *Sensory Evaluation of Food: Principles and Practices*. Springer. p. 43. ISBN 1441964886.

[43] McGee p. 428.

[44] Siebert, Tracey E.; Wood, Claudia; Elsey, Gordon M.; Alan (2008). "Determination of Rotundone, the Pepper Aroma Impact Compound, in Grapes and Wine". *J. Agric. Food Chem* **56** (10): 3745–3748. doi:10.1021/jf800184t. PMID 18461962.

[45] Montagne, Prosper (2001). *Larousse Gastronomique*. Hamlyn. p. 726. ISBN 0-600-60235-4. OCLC 47231315 50747863 83960122. "Mill".

[46] Jaffee p. 12, table 2.

[47] "Karvy's special Reports — Seasonal Outlook Report Pepper" (PDF). Karvy Comtrade Limited. 15 May 2008. Retrieved 29 January 2008.

[48] "Black Pepper". Regency as China Business Limited. 1 January 2014. Retrieved 20 May 2014.

2.8.10 Bibliography

- Dalby, Andrew (2002). *Dangerous Tastes*. Berkeley: University of California Press. ISBN 0-520-23674-2.

- Davidson, Alan (2002). *Wilder Shores of Gastronomy: Twenty Years of the Best Food Writing from the Journal Petits Propos Culinaires*. Berkeley: Ten Speed Press. ISBN 978-1-58008-417-8.

- Jaffee, Steven (2004). "Delivering and Taking the Heat: Indian Spices and Evolving Process Standards" (PDF). *An Agriculture and Rural Development Discussion Paper* (Washington: World Bank).

- McGee, Harold (2004). "Black Pepper and Relatives". *On Food and Cooking (Revised Edition)*. Scribner. pp. 427–429. ISBN 0-684-80001-2. OCLC 56590708.

- Turner, Jack (2004). *Spice: The History of a Temptation*. London: Vintage Books. ISBN 0-375-70705-0. OCLC 61213802.

2.8.11 Further reading

- Black Pepper Chemical List (Dr. Duke's Databases)

- "Black Pepper" from Plant Cultures, a collaboration between NYKRIS and Kew Gardens

- Ravindran, P.N. (2000). *Black pepper: piper nigrum*. Amsterdam: Harwood Academic, CRC. ISBN 978-90-5702-453-5

2.8.12 External links

- Media related to Piper nigrum at Wikimedia Commons

- Data related to Piper nigrum at Wikispecies

- Pepper at Wikibook Cookbooks

2.9 Cajeput oil

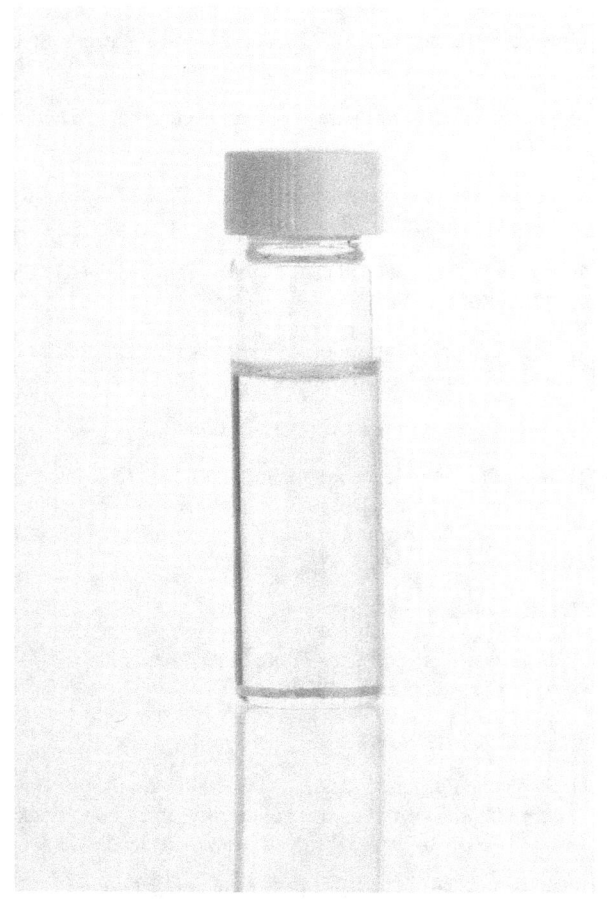

Cajeput essential oil in clear glass vial

Cajeput oil is a volatile oil obtained by distillation from the leaves of the myrtaceous trees *Melaleuca leucadendra*, *Melaleuca cajuputi*, and probably other *Melaleuca* species. The trees yielding the oil are found throughout Maritime Southeast Asia and over the hotter parts of the Australian continent. The majority of the oil is produced on the Indonesian island of Sulawesi. The name "cajeput" is derived from its Indonesian name, "*kayu putih*" or "white wood".

The oil is prepared from leaves collected on a hot dry day, macerated in water, and distilled after fermenting for a night. This oil is extremely pungent, and has the odor of a mixture of turpentine and camphor. It consists mainly of cineol (see terpenes), from which cajuputene, having a hyacinth-like odor, can be obtained by distillation with phosphorus pentoxide. The drug is a typical volatile oil, and is used internally in doses of 2 to 3 minims, for the same purposes as, say, clove oil. It is frequently employed externally as a counterirritant. It is an ingredient in some liniments for sore muscles such as Tiger Balm and Indonesian traditional medicine Minyak Telon.

It is also used as an ingredient in inhalants/decongestants and topical pain/inflammation remedies such as Olbas Oil.

2.9.1 Historical note

In October 1832 while in the port of Manila, the Asiatic or spasmodic cholera suddenly made its appearance on board the USS Peacock (1828). The first case was in a sailor named Peterson, sixty-three years old. The surgeon administered six grains of opium, in three doses; bad symptoms increasing, fifteen drops of cajeput oil were given in brandy and water, and repeated in half an hour. This treatment, however, apparently did not help the patient; Peterson died about eleven hours after being stricken, as did seven others, of "the terrific and appalling effects produced by one of the greatest scourges that ever visited the world."[1]:p. 64

2.9.2 For fish

Cajeput is used for the treatment of bacterial or fungal infections in fish. Common brand names containing Cajeput are Melafix and Bettafix. Melafix is a stronger concentration and Bettafix is a lower concentration that makes it harder to overdose smaller fish, especially bettas. It is most commonly used to promote fin and tissue regrowth, but is also effective in treating other conditions, such as fin rot or velvet. The remedy is used mostly on betta fish.

2.9.3 See also

* Tea tree oil – derived from *Melaleuca alternifolia*

2.9.4 References

[1] Roberts, Edmund (Digitized 12 October 2007) [First published in 1837]. *Embassy to the Eastern courts of Cochin-China, Siam, and Muscat : in the U. S. sloop-of-war Peacock... during the years 1832-3-4.* Harper & brothers. OCLC 12212199. Check date values in: |date= (help)

* This article incorporates text from a publication now in the public domain: Chisholm, Hugh, ed. (1911). *Encyclopædia Britannica* (11th ed.). Cambridge University Press.

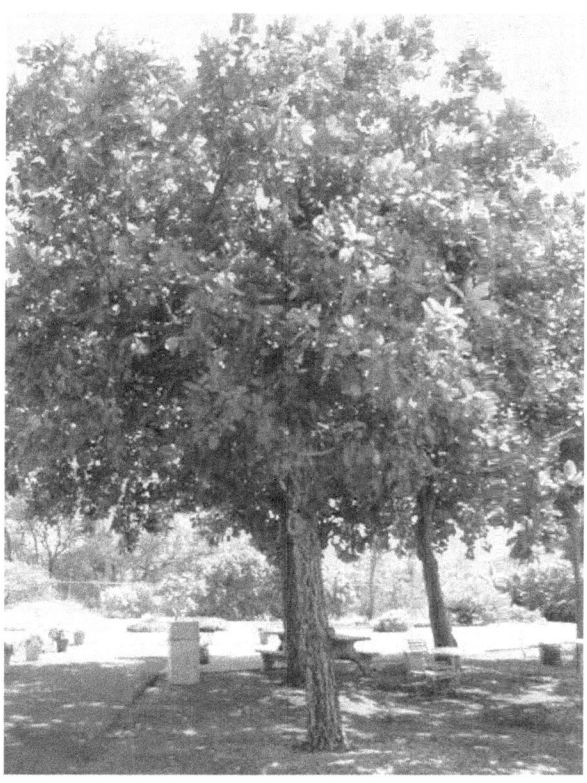

Tree

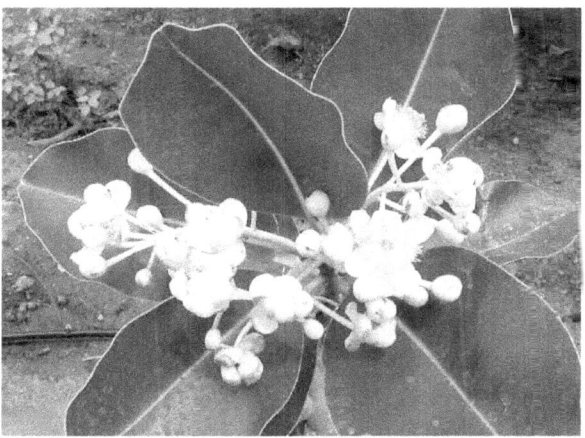

Inflorescence

ing to Guttiferae family. The oil has medicinal value and use as a fuel.

2.10 Calophyllum inophyllum seed oil

Calophyllum inophyllum **seed oil** is the oil extracted from the seed of *Calophyllum inophyllum*, a tropical tree belong-

2.10.1 Fruits

Fruiting takes place twice in a year in May and November. The fruit (the ball nut) is a round, green drupe reaching 2 to 4 cm in diameter and having a single large seed. When ripe, the fruit is wrinkled and its color varies from yellow

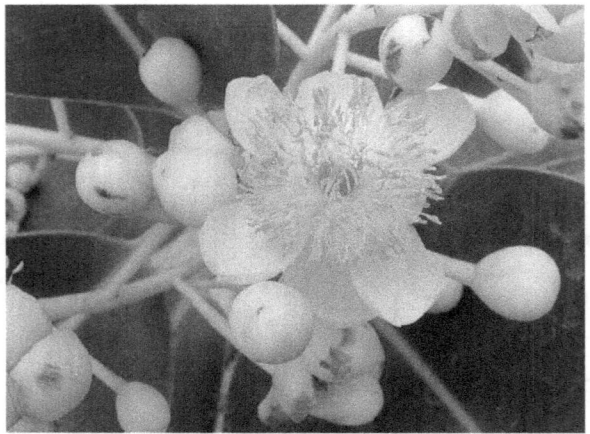

Flower

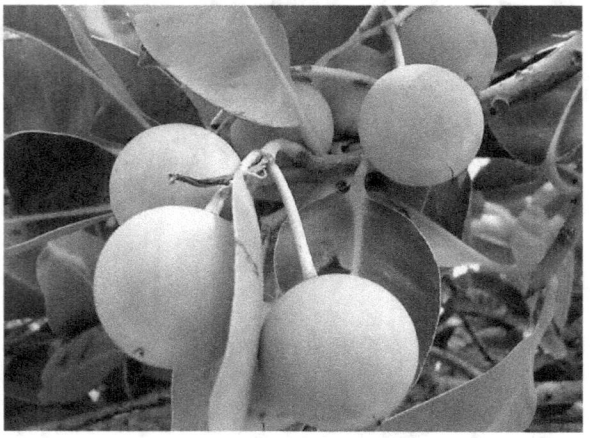

Fruits

to brownish-red. The weight of the small fruit is 9 to 16.0 g when they are fresh. After drying, the weight is reduced to about 4 g. Ripe and fallen fruits are collected from the bottom of the tree, by beating the limbs with a long hand stick, or hand-picked by climbing the tree.

2.10.2   Kernel

The kernel part in the whole dry fruit comprises 43–52% of its weight. The kernel is 1.5 cm diameter, enclosed in a soft seed coat and a hard seed coat. The kernel contains 55–73% of oil and 25% moisture when fresh.[1]

2.10.3   Seed processing and extraction of oil

The seeds are decorticated by wooden mallets or by decorticators or by pressing under planks. Usually, the kernels are pressed in wooden and stone *ghani*.[1]

2.10.4   Properties and fatty acids of oil

The oil is bluish-yellow to dark green viscous, known as domba oil, or pinnai oil, or dilo oil. It has a disagreeable taste or odour, as it contains some resinous material that can easily be removed by refining. The concentration of resinous substances in the oil varies from 10 to 30%.[2] The main compounds of the seed oil are oleic, linoleic, stearic, and palmitic acid.

Physical characteristics[1]

Fatty acids present in oil

2.10.5   Uses

The seeds yield a thick, dark green tamanu oil for medicinal use or hair grease. The first neoflavone isolated in 1951 from natural sources was calophyllolide from *C. inophyllum* seeds.[3]

The fatty acid methyl esters derived from *C. inophyllum* seed oil meets the major biodiesel requirements in the United States (ASTM D 6751), and European Union (EN 14214). The average oil yield is 11.7 kg-oil/tree or 4680 kg-oil/hectare. In the northwest coastal areas of Luzon island in Philippines, the oil was used for night lamps.[4] This widespread use started to decline when kerosene became available, and later on electricity. It was also used as fuel to generate electricity to provide power for radios during World War II.

In Southern India, the oil of the seeds of the plant is used specifically for treating skin diseases. It is also applied topically in cases of rheumatism. The oil may have been useful in waterproofing cloth and is used as a varnish. An extract from the fruit was once used to make a brown dye to colour cloth. The oil can also be used to make soap.[5]

In the most of the South Sea islands, tamanu or sultan champa oil is used as an analgesic medicine(natives use it in frictions for sciatica and rhematism) and to cure ulcers and bad wounds[6] A farmer in Nagappattinam district of Tamil Nadu has successfully used the oil as biodiesel to run his 5-hp pumpset.[7]

External links

- Prospects and potential of fatty acid methyl esters of some non-traditional seed oils for use as biodiesel in India

- http://www.dweckdata.com/Published_papers/ Tamanu.pdf

2.10.6 References

[1] SEAHand Book-2009 by The Solvent Extractors' Association of India

[2] http://www.worldagroforestry.org/sea/Products/ AFDbases/af/asp/SpeciesInfo.asp?SpID=2

[3] Neoflavones. 1. Natural Distribution and Spectral and Biological Properties. M. M. Garazd, Ya. L. Garazd and V. P. Khilya, Chemistry of Natural Compounds, Volume 39, Number 1 / janvier 2003.

[4] http://gardentia.net/2012/12/06/undi-4/

[5] http://www.svlele.com/undie.htm

[6] http://www.dweckdata.com/Published_papers/Tamanu. pdf

[7] http://www.thehindu.com/sci-tech/science/ using-bio-fuel-to-run-an-irrigation-pump-for-five-acres/ article5835856.ece

2.11 Cananga odorata

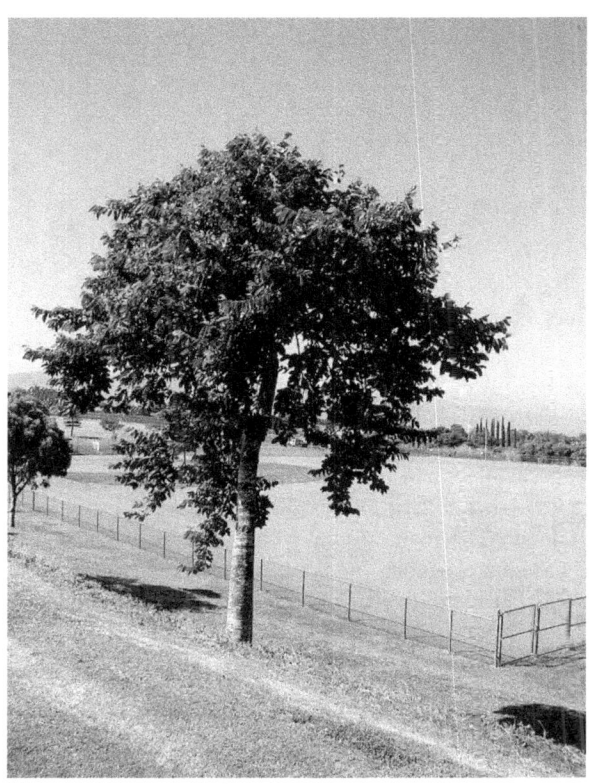

A Cananga odorata *in Maui*

Cananga odorata, known as the **cananga tree** (Indonesian: *kenanga*, Balinese: *sandat*), is a tropical tree that originates in the Philippines.[1] It is valued for the perfume extracted from its flowers, called **ylang-ylang** /'iːlæŋ 'iːlæŋ/ *EE-lang-EE-lang*[2] (a name also sometimes used for the tree itself), which is an essential oil used in aromatherapy. The tree is also called the fragrant cananga, Macassar-oil plant, or perfume tree.[3]

The ylang-ylang vine (*Artabotrys odoratissimus*)[4] and climbing ylang-ylang (*Artabotrys hexapetalus*)[5] are woody, evergreen climbing plants in the same family. *Artabotrys odoratissimus* is also a source of perfume.[4]

2.11.1 Etymology

The name *ylang-ylang* is derived from Tagalog, either from the word *ilang*, meaning "wilderness", alluding to its natural habitat, or the word *ilang-ilan*, meaning "rare", suggestive of its exceptionally delicate scent. A common mistranslation is "flower of flowers".[4]

2.11.2 Description

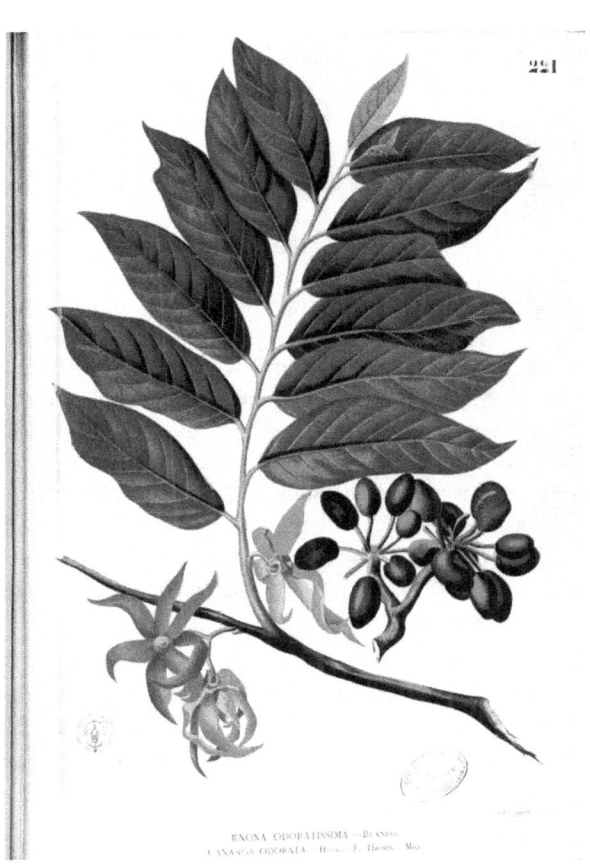

Cananga odorata *illustrated in Francisco Manuel Blanco s Flora de Filipinas*

Cananga odorata is a fast-growing tree of the custard apple family Annonaceae. Its growth exceeds 5 m (15 ft) per year and attains an average height of 12 m (40 ft) in an ideal climate. The evergreen leaves are smooth and glossy, oval, pointed and with wavy margins, and 13–20 cm (5–8 in) long. The flower is drooping, long-stalked, with six narrow, greenish-yellow (rarely pink) petals, rather like a sea star in appearance, and yields a highly fragrant essential oil.

Cananga odorata var. *fruticosa*, dwarf *ylang-ylang*, grows as small tree or compact shrub with highly scented flowers.

2.11.3   Distribution and habitat

The plant is native to the Philippines and Indonesia and is commonly grown in Polynesia, Melanesia, Micronesia and Comoros Islands. It grows in full or partial sun, and prefers the acidic soils of its native rainforest habitat. Ylang-ylang has been cultivated in temperate climates under conservatory conditions.

2.11.4   Ecology

Its clusters of black fruit are an important food item for birds, such as the collared imperial-pigeon, purple-tailed imperial-pigeon, Zoe's imperial-pigeon, superb fruit-dove, pink-spotted fruit-dove, coroneted fruit-dove, orange-bellied fruit-dove, and wompoo fruit-dove.[6] Sulawesi red-knobbed hornbill serves as an effective seed disperser for *C. odorata*.[7]

2.11.5   Uses

The essential oil is used in aromatherapy. It is believed to relieve high blood pressure, normalize sebum secretion for skin problems, and is considered to be an aphrodisiac. According to Margaret Mead, it was used as such by South Pacific natives such as the Samoan Islanders where she did much of her research. The oil from ylang-ylang is widely used in perfumery for oriental or floral themed perfumes (such as Chanel No. 5). Ylang-ylang blends well with most floral, fruit and wood scents.

In Indonesia, ylang-ylang flowers are spread on the bed of newlywed couples. In the Philippines, its flowers, together with the flowers of the sampaguita, are strung into a necklace (*lei*) and worn by women and used to adorn religious images.

Ylang-ylang's essential oil makes up 29% of the Comoros' annual export (1998).

Ylang-ylang is a common flavoring in Madagascar for ice cream.

2.11.6   Ylang-ylang essential oil

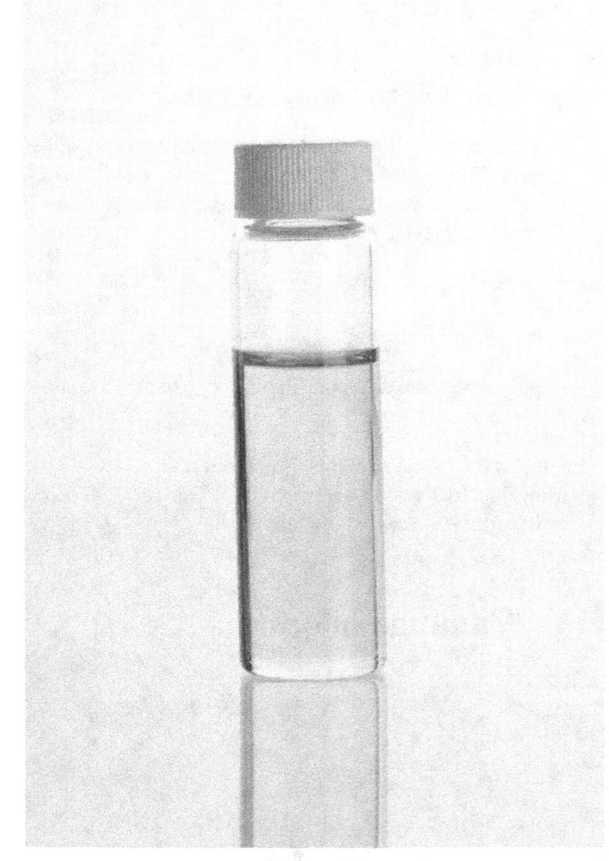

Ylang-ylang (Cananga odorata) *essential oil*

Characteristics

The fragrance of ylang-ylang is rich and deep with notes of rubber and custard, and bright with hints of jasmine and neroli. The essential oil of the flower is obtained through steam distillation of the flowers and separated into different grades (extra, 1, 2, or 3) according to when the distillates are obtained. The main aromatic components of ylang-ylang oil are benzyl acetate, linalool, p-cresyl methyl ether, and methyl benzoate, responsible for its characteristic odor.[8]

Chemical constituents

Typical chemical compositions of the various grades of ylang-ylang essential oil are reported as:[9]

- Linalool

- Germacrene

- Geranyl acetate

- Caryophyllene

- p-cresyl methyl ether

- Methyl benzoate

- Sesquiterpenes

2.11.7 See also

- Dwarf ylang-ylang

- Kananga Water

- Macassar oil

2.11.8 References

[1] "Ylang- Ylang "Flower of Flowers"'. School of Holistic Aromatheraphy. Retrieved 6 October 2013.

[2] OED

[3] "University of Melbourne: multilingual plant names database". Plantnames.unimelb.edu.au. 2004-08-05. Retrieved 2012-12-30.

[4] "Britannica.com". Britannica.com. Retrieved 2012-12-30.

[5] "Tropicos". Tropicos. Retrieved 2012-12-30.

[6] Frith, H.J.; Rome, F.H.J.C. & Wolfe, T.O. (1976): Food of fruit-pigeons in New Guinea. *Emu* 76(2): 49-53. HTML abstract

[7] http://www.researchgate.net/profile/Margaret_Kinnaird/publication/230142476_Evidence_for_Effective_Seed_Dispersal_by_the_Sulawesi_RedKnobbed_Hornbill_Aceros_cassidix1/links/553658d70cf2_8056e941e90.pdf

[8] Manner, Harley and Craig Elevitch,*Traditional Tree Initiative: Species Profiles for Pacific Island Agroforestry* (2006), Permanent Agricultural Resources, Honolulu, Hi.

[9] "Ylang-Ylang Essential Oil - Chemical Composition". scienceofacne.com.

2.11.9 Further reading

- Elevitch, Craig (ed.) (2006): *Traditional Trees of Pacific Islands: Their Culture, Environment and Use*. Permanent Agricultural Resources Publishers, Honolulu. ISBN 0-9702544-5-8

- Manner, Harley & Elevitch, Craig (ed.) (2006): *Traditional Tree Initiative: Species Profiles for Pacific Island Agroforestry*. Permanent Agricultural Resources Publishers, Honolulu.

- Davis, Patricia (2000): *"Aromatherapy An A-Z"*. Vermilion:Ebury Publishing, London.

2.11.10 External links

- Data related to Cananga odorata at Wikispecies

2.12 Cannabis flower essential oil

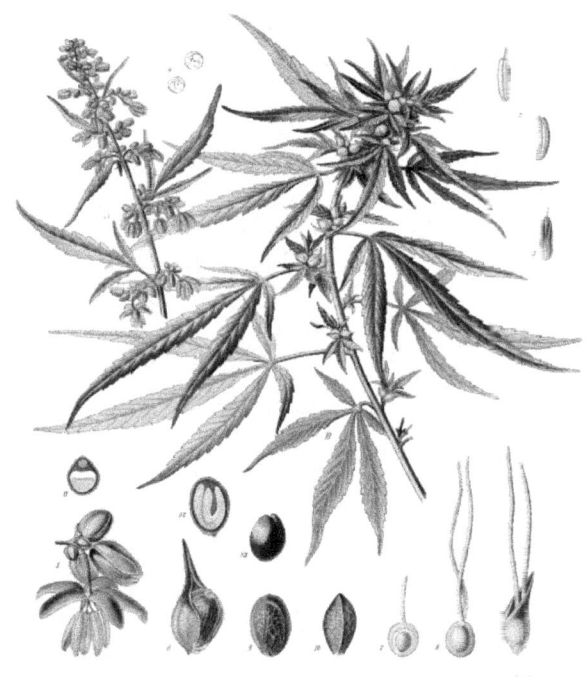

Cannabis plant

Cannabis flower essential oil, also known as **hemp essential oil**, is an essential oil obtained by steam distillation from the flowers and upper leaves of the hemp plant (Cannabis sativa L.) Hemp essential oil is distinct from hemp oil and hash oil: the former is a vegetable oil that is pressed from the seeds of low-THC varieties of hemp, the latter is a THC-rich extract of dried female hemp flowers (marijuana) or resin (hashish).

A pale yellow liquid, cannabis flower essential oil is a volatile oil that is a mixture of monoterpenes, sesquiterpenes, and other terpenoid compounds. The typical scent of hemp results from about 140 different terpenoids. The essential oil is manufactured from both low-THC ("fibre-type") and high-THC ("drug-type") varieties of hemp. Even in "drug-type" hemp, the THC content of the essential oil does not exceed 0.08%.

Hemp essential oil is used as a scent in perfumes, cosmetics, soaps, and candles. It is also used as a flavoring in foods, primarily candy and beverages.

2.12.1 Yield

The yield depends on the hemp type (drug, fiber) and pollination; sex, age, and part of the plant; cultivation (indoor, outdoor etc.); harvest time and conditions; drying; and storage. For example, fresh buds from an Afghani variety yielded 0.29% essential oil. Drying and storage reduced the content from 0.29% to 0.20% after 1 week, and to 0.13% after 3 months. Monoterpenes showed a significantly greater loss than sesquiterpenes, but none of the major components completely disappeared in the drying process.[1]

About 1.3 L of essential oil per ton resulted from freshly harvested outdoor-grown hemp, corresponding to about 10 L/ha. The yield of nonpollinated ("sinsemilla") hemp at 18 L/ha was more than twofold compared with pollinated hemp (8 L/ha).[1]

2.12.2 Constituents

Sixty-eight components were detected by GC and GC/mass spectrometry (MS) in fresh bud oil distilled from high-potency, indoor-grown hemp. The 57 identified constituents were 92% monoterpenes, 7% sesquiterpenes, and approx. 1% other compounds (ketones, esters). The dominating monoterpenes were myrcene (67%) and limonene (16%).[1]

In the essential oil from outdoor-grown hemp, the monoterpene concentration varied between 47.9 and 92.1% of the total terpenoid content. The sesquiterpenes ranged from 5.2 to 48.6%. The most abundant monoterpene was β-myrcene, followed by trans-caryophyllene, α-pinene, trans-ocimene, and α-terpinolene.[1]

Even in "drug-type" hemp, the THC content of the essential oil was not more than 0.08%.[1]

In the essential oil of five different European hemp cultivars, the dominating terpenes were myrcene (21.1–35.0 %), α-pinene (7.2–14.6 %), α-terpinolene (7.0–16.6 %), trans-caryophyllene (12.2.–18.9 %), and α-humulene (6.1–8.7 %). The main differences between the cultivars were found in the contents of α-terpinolene and α-pinene.[1]

Other terpenoids present only in traces are sabinene, α-terpinene, 1,8-cineole (eucalyptol), pulegone, γ-terpinene, terpineol−4-ol, bornyl acetate, α-copaene, alloaromadendrene, viridiflorene, β-bisabolene, γ-cadinene, trans-β-farnesene, trans-nerolidol, and β-bisabolol.[1]

The major alkane present in an essential oil obtained by extraction and steam distillation was the n-C_{29} alkane nonacosane (55.8 and 10.7%, respectively).[1]

2.12.3 See also

- Cannabis

- Cannabis (drug)

- Essential oil

- Hemp oil

- Hash oil

2.12.4 References

[1] Rudolf Brenneisen (2007), "Chemistry and Analysis of Phytocannabinoids and Other Cannabis Constituents", in Mahmoud A. ElSohly, *Marijuana and the Cannabinoids*, Humana Press, pp. 17–49

2.12.5 External links

- Hemp Essential Oil: Sweet Smell of Success

- Essential oil of Cannabis sativa L. strains

2.13 Carrot seed oil

Carrot seed oil is the essential oil extract of the seed from the carrot plant *Daucus carota*. The oil has a woody, earthy sweet smell and is yellow or amber-coloured to pale orange-brown in appearance. The pharmocologically active constituents of carrot seed extract are three flavones: luteolin, luteolin 3'-O-beta-D-glucopyranoside, and luteolin 4'-O-beta-D-glucopyranoside. [1] Rather than the extract the distilled (ethereal) oil is used in perfumery and food aromatization. The main constituent of this oil is carotol. Carrot seed oil can be used as sunscreen, as long as it has a lot of fat and density.

Pressed carrot seed oil is extracted by cold-pressing the seeds of the carrot plant. The properties of pressed carrot seed oil are quite different from those of the essential oil.[2]

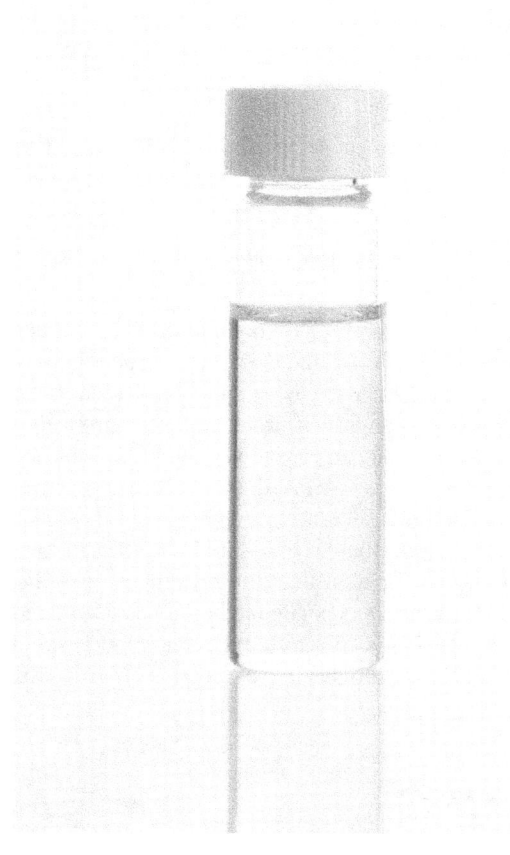

*Carrot seed (*Daucus carota*) essential oil in clear glass vial*

2.13.1 References

[1] Y. Kumarasamy, L. Nahar, M. Byres, A. Delazar, S.D. Sarker (2005). "The assessment of biological activities associated with the major constituents of the methanol extract of 'wild carrot' (Daucus carota L) seeds". *Journal of Herbal Pharmacotherapy* **5** (1): 61–72. doi:10.1080/j157v05n01_07. PMID 16093236.

[2] Lucy Yu Liangli, Kevin Zhou Kequan, Joan Parry (2005). "Antioxidant properties of cold-pressed black caraway, carrot, cranberry, and hemp seed oils". *Food chemistry* **91** (4): 723–729. doi:10.1016/j.foodchem.2004.06.044.

2.14 Cedar oil

Cedar oil, also known as *cedarwood oil*, is an essential oil derived from the foliage, and sometimes the wood and roots, of various types of conifers, most in the pine or cypress botanical families. It has many uses in medicine, art, industry and perfumery, and while the characteristics of oils derived from various species may themselves vary, all have some degree of bactericidal and pesticidal effects.

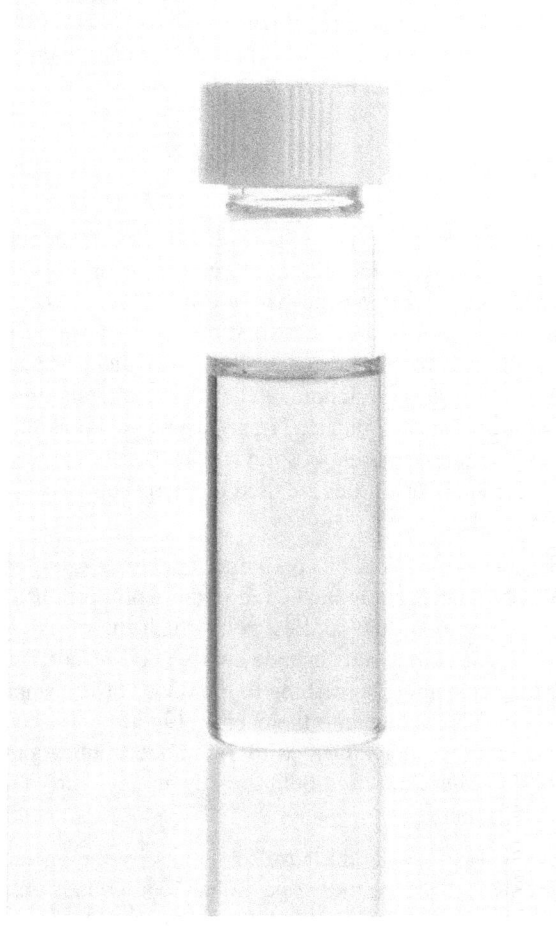

Cedarwood essential oil

2.14.1 Sources and characteristics

Although termed cedar or cedarwood oils, the most important oils of this group are produced from distilling wood of a number of different junipers and cypresses (*Juniperus* and *Cupressus* spp., of the family *Cupressaceae*), rather than true cedars (*Cedrus* spp. of the family *Pinaceae*). A cedar leaf oil is also commercially distilled from the Eastern arborvitae (*Thuja occidentalis*, also of the *Cupressaceae*), and similar oils are distilled, pressed or chemically extracted in small quantities from wood, roots and leaves from plants of the genera *Platycladus*, *Cupressus*, *Taiwania* and *Calocedrus*.[1]

The cedar oil of the ancients, in particular the Sumerians and Egyptians, was derived from the Cedar of Lebanon, a true cedar native to the northern and western mountains of the Middle East. The once-mighty Cedar of Lebanon forests of antiquity have been almost entirely eradicated, and today no commercial oil extraction is based on this species. One of the elements found in many cedarwood trees is cedrol. Depending on the amount of cedrol in a specific species of cedarwood can determine its pesticidal effect on insects. Ancient Egyptians would use the oil from cedarwood trees in the embalming process, which in effect helped to keep the insects from disturbing the body.

2.14.2 Uses

Cedarwood oils each have characteristic woody odours which may change somewhat in the course of drying out. The crude oils are often yellowish or even darker in colour and some, such as Texas cedarwood oil (derived primarily from *Juniperus ashei* and *J. deppeana*), are quite viscous and deposit crystals on standing. They find use (sometimes after *rectification*) in a range of fragrance applications such as soap perfumes, household sprays, floor polishes and insecticides. Small quantities are used in microscope work as a clearing oil.

All the cedarwood oils of commerce contain a group of chemically related compounds, the relative proportions of which depend upon the species from which the oil is obtained. These compounds include cedrol and cedrene, and while they contribute something to the odour of the whole oil they are also valuable to the chemical industry for conversion to other derivatives with fragrance applications. The oils are therefore used both directly and as sources of chemical isolates.

Cedar oil was used as the base for paints by the ancient Sumerians. They would grind cobalt compounds in a mortar and pestle to produce a blue pigment. They could obtain green from copper, yellow from lead antimonate, black from charcoal, and white from gypsum.

Today, cedar oil is often used for its aromatic properties, especially in aromatherapy; it can also be used to renew the smell of natural cedar furniture. Cedar oil is used as an insect repellent, both directly applied to the skin and as an additive to sprays, candles and other products.

In India, oil from the deodar cedar (*Cedrus deodara*, a true cedar) has been shown to possess insecticidal and antifungal properties and to have some potential for control of fungal deterioration of spices during storage. However, its commercial potential for this purpose remains, at present, speculative.

One of three methods of ancient Egyptian embalming practices employs the use of cedar oil. This was a less costly method than the most well known of the ancient Egyptian practices of removing internal organs for separate preservation in canopic jars. The practice

> ...called for the injection of cedar oil into body cavities without evisceration. The body was laid in natrum or natron — a fixed alkali — for

the prescribed period, after which the cedar oil, which had dissolved the soft organs, was released; and the body, its flesh dissolved by the natron, was reduced to preserved skin and bones.[2]

Until the development of synthetic immersion oil in the 1940s, cedar oil was widely used for the oil immersion objective in light microscopy.

Cedar leaf oil from cedrus atlantica does not contain thujone.

Cedarwood oil is a mixture of organic compounds considered generally safe by the FDA as a food additive preservative. The oil is used as an antibacterial and fungicide. Studies have shown that prolonged exposure to high levels of cedarwood oil can cause liver and pulmonary toxicity. The United States EPA does not expect such effects to occur among users of currently registered products because their use and public exposure is at a much lower level and more intermittent than those in the case studies. The EPA believes there is negligible human environmental risk posed by exposure to registered cedarwood pesticide or food preservative products if used in properly prescribed manner.

2.14.3 Notes

[1] Chapter 10: Cedarwood Oils, United Nations Food and Agriculture Organization report

[2] Habenstein, Robert W.; Lamers, William M. (2007). *The History of American Funeral Directing*. Burton & Mayer, Inc.

2.15 Citron

For other uses, see Citron (disambiguation).
Not to be confused with Citroën.
See also: Citrus taxonomy § Citron varieties

The **citron** is a large fragrant citrus fruit with a thick rind, botanically classified as ***Citrus medica*** by both the Swingle and Tanaka botanical name systems. It is one of the four original citrus fruits (the others being pommelo, mandarin and papeda), from which most other citrus types developed through natural hybrid speciation or artificial hybridization.[1]

2.15.1 Etymology

The fruit's English name "citron" derives ultimately from Latin, *citrus*, which is also the origin of the genus name.

Other languages

A source of confusion is that citron or similar words in French, Lithuanian, Hungarian, Finnish, Latvian, the West Slavic languages, and all Germanic languages but English are false friends, as they refer to the lemon. Indeed, into the 16th century, the English name citron included the lemon and perhaps the lime as well.[2]

In most Arabic languages it is called *Turunj*, or similar, but in Syria and many other Muslim countries it is called *Kab-bad*;[3] in Japanese it is called *Bushukan* (maybe referring only to the fingered varieties).[4]

2.15.2 Uses

Culinary

Main article: Succade
While the lemon or orange are peeled to consume their

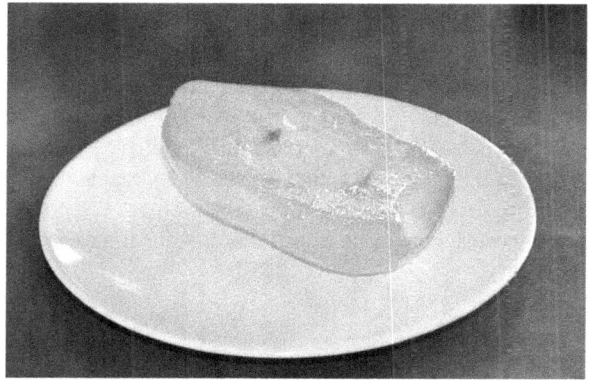

A citron halved and depulped, cooked in sugar

pulpy and juicy segments, the citron's pulp is dry, containing a small quantity of insipid juice, if any. The main content of a citron fruit is the thick white rind, which adheres to the segments and cannot be separated from them easily. The citron gets halved and depulped, then its rind is cooked in sugar, diced, and used as a confection.

Today the citron is used for the fragrance or zest of its flavedo, but the most important part is still the inner rind (known as pith or *albedo*), which is a fairly important article in international trade and is widely employed in the food industry as succade,[5] as it is known when it is candied in sugar.

The dozens of varieties of citron are collectively known as *Lebu* in Bangladesh, where it is the primary citrus fruit.

In Iran, the citron's thick white rind is used to make jam; in Pakistan the fruit is used to make jam but is also pickled; in South Indian cuisine, the citron is widely used in pickles and

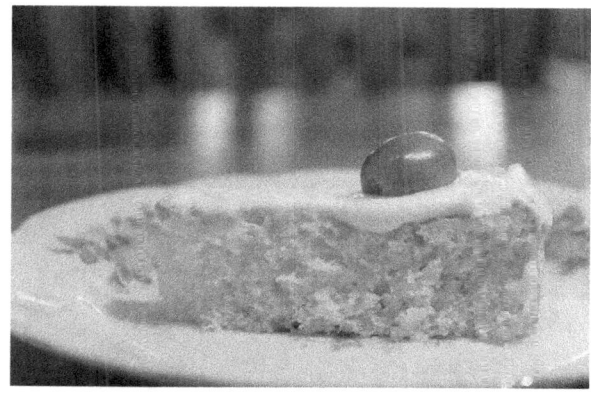

citron torte

preserves. In Korea, citron (called yujacha) is used to make tea, which supposedly helps to suppress coughing, relieve hangovers, and is effective in curing indigestion.[6]

Medicinal

From ancient through medieval times, the citron was used mainly for medical purposes: to combat seasickness, pulmonary troubles, intestinal ailments, scurvy and other disorders. The essential oil of the flavedo (the outermost, pigmented layer of rind) was also regarded as an antibiotic. Citron juice with wine was considered an effective antidote to poison, as Theophrastus reported. In the Ayurvedic system of medicine, the juice is still used for treating conditions like nausea, vomiting, and excessive thirst.

The juice of the citron has a high Vitamin C content and used medicinally as an anthelmintic, appetizer, tonic, in cough, rheumatism, vomiting, flatulence, haemorrhoids, skin diseases and weak eyesight.[7] A recent study has shown that citron has some cardiovascular benefits.[8]

There is an increasing market for the citron for the soluble fiber (pectin) found in its thick albedo.[9] There are also scientific claims that modified citrus pectin can help even against cancer.[10]

Religious

Main article: Etrog

The citron is also used by Jews (the word for it in Hebrew is *etrog*) for a religious ritual during the Feast of Tabernacles; therefore, is considered to be a Jewish symbol which is found on various Hebrew antiques and archaeological findings.[11] Citrons used for ritual purposes cannot be grown by grafting branches.

Main article: Buddha's hand

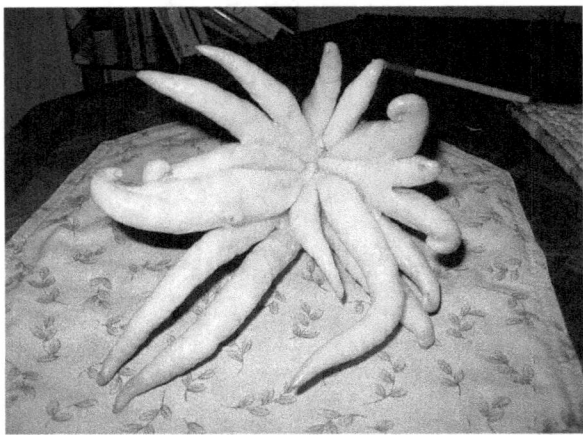

The Fingered Citron

A variety of citron native to China has sections that separate into finger-like parts is used as an offering in Buddhist temples.

Perfumery

For many centuries, citron's fragrant essential oil has been used in perfumery, the same oil that was used medicinally for its antibiotic properties. Its major constituent is limonene.[12]

2.15.3 Description and variation

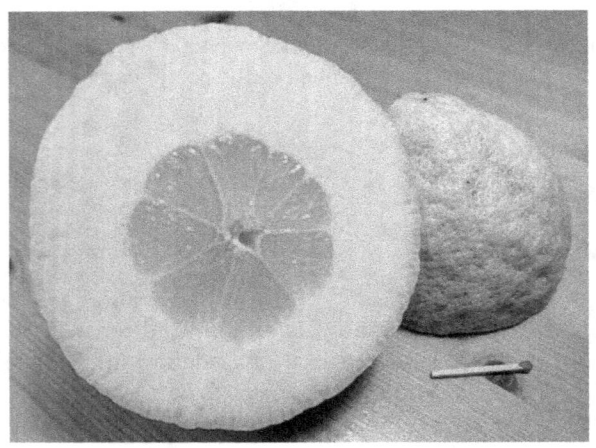

A citron or citron-like hybrid of Italian origin (note the thick rind).

Fruit

The citron fruit is usually ovate or oblong, narrowing towards the stylar end. However, the citron's fruit shape is highly variable, due to the large quantity of albedo, which forms independently according to the fruits' position on the tree, twig orientation, and many other factors. The rind is leathery, furrowed, and adherent. The inner portion is thick, white and hard; the outer is uniformly thin and very fragrant. The pulp is usually acidic, but also can be sweet, and even pulpless varieties are found.

Most citron varieties contain a large number of monoembryonic seeds. They are white, with dark innercoats and red-purplish chalazal spots for the acidic varieties, and colorless for the sweet ones. Some citron varieties are also distinct, having persistent styles, that do not fall off after fecundation. Those are usually promoted for *etrog* use.

Some citrons have medium-sized oil bubbles at the outer surface, medially distant to each other. Some varieties are ribbed and faintly warted on the outer surface. There is also a fingered citron variety called Buddha's hand.

The color varies from green, when unripe, to a yellow-orange when overripe. The citron does not fall off the tree and can reach 8–10 pounds (4–5 kg) if not picked before fully mature.[13] However, they should be picked before the winter, as the branches might bend or break to the ground, and may cause numerous fungal diseases for the tree.

Plant

Citrus medica is a slow-growing shrub or small tree that reaches a height of about 8 to 15 ft (2 to 5 m). It has irregular straggling branches and stiff twigs and long spines at the leaf axils. The evergreen leaves are green and lemon-scented with slightly serrate edges, ovate-lanceolate or ovate elliptic 2.5 to 7.0 inches long. Petioles are usually wingless or with minor wings. The flowers are generally unisexual providing self-pollination, but some male individuals could be found due to pistil abortion. The clustered flowers of the acidic varieties are purplish tinted from outside, but the sweet ones are white-yellowish.

The citron tree is very vigorous with almost no dormancy, blooming several times a year, and is therefore fragile and extremely sensitive to frost.[14]

Varieties and hybrids

The acidic varieties include the Florentine and Diamante citron from Italy, the Greek citron and the Balady citron from Israel. The sweet varieties include the Corsican and

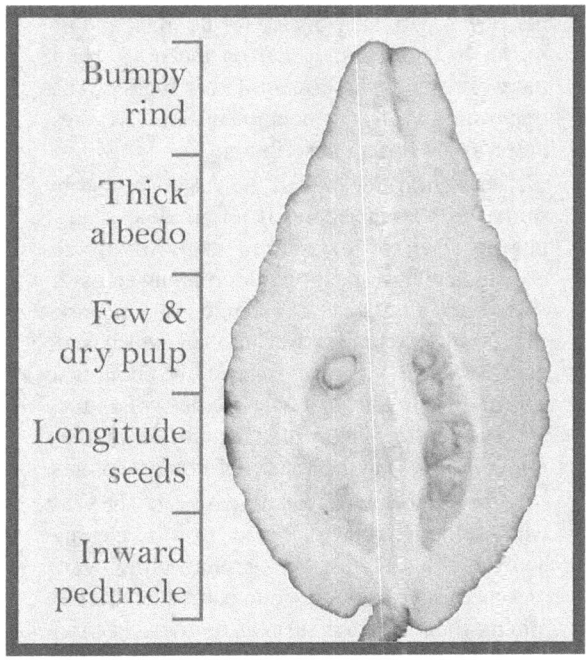

A pure citron, of any kind, has a large portion of albedo, which is important for the production of Succade.

Moroccan citrons. Between the pulpless are also some fingered varieties and the Yemenite citron.

There are also a number of citron hybrids; for example, ponderosa lemon, the lumia and rhobs el Arsa are known citron hybrids, some are claiming that even the Florentine citron is not pure citron, but a citron hybrid.

2.15.4 Origin and distribution

Despite the variation among the cultivars, authorities agree the citron is an old and original species. There is molecular evidence that all other cultivated citrus species arose by hybridization among four ancestral types, which are the citron, pomelo, mandarin and some papedas. The citron is believed to be the purest of them all, since it is usually fertilized by self-pollination, and is therefore generally considered to be a male parent of any citrus hybrid rather than a female one.[15][16][17][18][19][20]

Today, authorities agree that all citrus species are native to Southeast Asia where they are found wild and in an uncultivated form. The story of how they spread to the Mediterranean has been reported by Francesco Calabrese,[21] Henri Chapot,[22] Samuel Tolkowsky,[23] Elizabetta Nicolisi,[24] and others.[25][26][27][28]

The citron could also be native to India where it borders on Burma, in valleys at the foot of the Himalayas, and in the Indian Western Ghats.[29][30] It is thought that by the time of

Theophrastus, the citron was mostly cultivated in the Persian Gulf on its way to the Mediterranean basin, where it was cultivated during the later centuries in different areas as described by Erich Isaac.[31] Many mention the role of Alexander the Great and his armies as they attacked Persia and what is today Pakistan, as being responsible for the spread of the citron westward, reaching the European countries such as Macedonia and Italy.[32][33][34][35][36][37][38][39]

2.15.5 Antiquity

See also: Etrog § Historic cultivation areas

Leviticus mentions the "fruit of the tree hadar" as being required for ritual use during the Feast of Tabernacles (Lev. 23:40). According to Rabbinical tradition, the "fruit of the tree hadar" refers to the citron, which the Israelites brought to Israel from their exile in Egypt, where the Egyptologist and archaeologist Victor Loret claimed to have identified it depicted on the walls of the botanical garden at the Karnak Temple, which dates back to the time of Thutmosis III, approximately 3,000 years ago.[40]

The citron has been cultivated since ancient times, predating the cultivation of other citrus species.[41]

Theophrastus

The following description on citron was given by Theophrastus[42]

> In the east and south there are special plants... i.e. in Media and Persia there are many types of fruit, between them there is a fruit called Median or Persian Apple. The tree has a leaf similar to and almost identical with that of the *andrachn* (*Arbutus andrachne* L.), but has thorns like those of the *apios* (the wild pear, **Pyrus amygdaliformis** Vill.) or the firethorn, *Cotoneaster pyracantha* Spach.), except that they are white, smooth, sharp and strong.
>
> The fruit is not eaten, but is very fragrant, as is also the leaf of the tree; and the fruit is put among clothes, it keeps them from being moth-eaten. It is also useful when one has drunk deadly poison, for when it is administered in wine; it upsets the stomach and brings up the poison. It is also useful to improve the breath, for if one boils the inner part of the fruit in a dish or squeezes it into the mouth in some other medium, it makes the breath more pleasant.
>
> The seed is removed from the fruit and sown in the spring in carefully tilled beds, and it is wa-

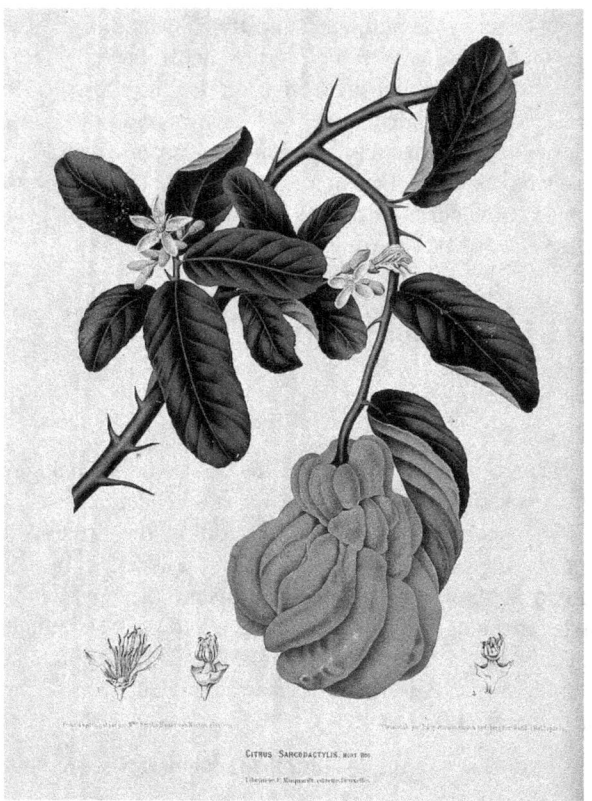

Illustration of fingered citron with the leaves and thorns that are common to all varieties of citron.

tered every fourth or fifth day. As soon the plant is strong it is transplanted, also in the spring, to a soft, well watered site, where the soil is not very fine, for it prefers such places.

And it bears its fruit at all seasons, for when some have gathered, the flower of the others is on the tree and is ripening others. Of the flowers I have said[43] those that have a sort of distaff [meaning the pistil] projecting from the middle are fertile, while those that do not have this are sterile. It is also sown, like date palms, in pots punctured with holes.

This tree, as has been remarked, grows in *Media* and *Persia*.

Pliny the Elder

About 400 years later it was also described by Pliny the Elder, who called it *nata Assyria malus*. The following is from his book Natural History:

There is another tree also with the same name of "citrus," and bears a fruit that is held by some

persons in particular dislike for its smell and remarkable bitterness; while, on the other hand, there are some who esteem it very highly. This tree is used as an ornament to houses; it requires, however, no further description.[44]

The citron tree, called the Assyrian, and by some the Median apple, is an antidote against poisons. The leaf is similar to that of the arbute, except that it has small prickles running across it. As to the fruit, it is never eaten, but it is remarkable for its extremely powerful smell, which is the case, also, with the leaves; indeed, the odour is so strong, that it will penetrate clothes, when they are once impregnated with it, and hence it is very useful in repelling the attacks of noxious insects.

The tree bears fruit at all seasons of the year; while some is falling off, other fruit is ripening, and other, again, just bursting into birth. Various nations have attempted to naturalize this tree among them, for the sake of its medical properties, by planting it in pots of clay, with holes drilled in them, for the purpose of introducing the air to the roots; and I would here remark, once for all, that it is as well to remember that the best plan is to pack all slips of trees that have to be carried to any distance, as close together as they can possibly be placed.

It has been found, however, that this tree will grow nowhere except in Media or Persia. It is this fruit, the pips of which, as we have already mentioned, the Parthian grandees employ in seasoning their ragouts, as being peculiarly conducive to the sweetening of the breath. We find no other tree very highly commended that is produced in Media.[45]

Citrons, either the pulp of them or the pips, are taken in wine as an antidote to poisons. A decoction of citrons, or the juice extracted from them, is used as a gargle to impart sweetness to the breath. The pips of this fruit are recommended for pregnant women to chew when affected with qualmishness. Citrons are good, also, for a weak stomach, but it is not easy to eat them except with vinegar.[46]

2.15.6   See also

- Archaeological finds of citrons in Israel
- Gallery of Etrog citrons
- Gallery of Fingered citrons

2.15.7 Gallery

- In a German market, for culinary use
- In fruit market of Italy
- Naxos citrons and leaf
- Citron or hybrid in Sicily
- A wild citron in India
- Citron flowers
- Unknown citron type in pot
- A Corsican citron

2.15.8 Notes

[1] Klein, J. (2014). "Citron Cultivation, Production and Uses in the Mediterranean Region". In Z. Yaniv; N. Dudai. *Medicinal and Aromatic Plants of the Middle-East* **2**. Springer Netherlands. pp. 199–214. doi:10.1007/978-94-017-9276-9_10.

[2] "Home : Oxford English Dictionary". *oed.com*.

[3] "Citrus medica" (PDF). *plantlives.com*.

[4] "Buddha". *ucr.edu*.

[5] The Purdue University

- The Citron in Crete
- Vine Tree Orchards

[6] "Traditional Drinks – Official Korea Tourism Organization". *visitkorea.or.kr*.

[7] "Matulunga (Citrus medica)". *frlht.org*

[8] "Citrus medica "Otroj": Attenuates Oxidative Stress and Cardiac Dysrhythmia in Isoproterenol-Induced Cardiomyopathy in Rats". *nih.gov*.

[9] Preparation and Characterization of Pectin...

- Pectin extraction from Citron peel (Citrus medica Linn.) and its use in food system
- Pectin extraction...
- Scholarly Document
- Free Patents Online
- Peak of Health
- See also FiberStar and NYU Langone Medical Center

[10] "Researchers demonstrate how modified citrus pectin works against cancer". *News-Medical.net*. 4 June 2013.

[11] See Etrog

[12] Inouye, S.; Takizawa, T.; Yamaguchi, H. (2001). "Antibacterial activity of essential oils and their major constituents against respiratory tract pathogens by gaseous contact". *Journal of Antimicrobial Chemotherapy* **47** (5): 565–573. doi:10.1093/jac/47.5.565. PMID 11328766.

[13] *Un curieux Cedrat marocain*, Chapot 1950.

- The Search for the Authentic Citron: Historic and Genetic Analysis; HortScienc 40(7):1963–1968. 2005

[14] "Website Disabled". *ucr.edu*.

[15] "Citrus phylogeny and genetic origin of important species as investigated by molecular markers". *springerlink.com*.

[16] Assessing genetic diversity and population structure in a citrus germplasm collection utilizing simple sequence repeat markers (SSRs) by: Noelle A. Barkley, Mikeal L. Roose, Robert R. Krueger and Claire T. Federici

[17] Phylogenetic relationships in the "true citrus fruit trees" revealed by PCR-RFLP analysis of cpDNA. 2004

[18] The Search for the Authentic Citron: Historic and Genetic Analysis; HortScienc 40(7):1963–1968. 2005

[19] Chromosome Numbers in the Subfamily Aurantioideae with Special Reference to the Genus Citrus; C. A. Krug. Botanical Gazette, Vol. 104, No. 4 (Jun., 1943), pp. 602–611

[20] The relationships among lemons, limes and citron: a chromosomal comparison. by R. Carvalhoa, W.S. Soares Filhob, A.C. Brasileiro-Vidala, M. Guerraa.

[21] Calabrese, *La favolosa storia degli agrumi*. L'EPOS, 1998, Palerno Italy. English translation in Citrus: the genus citrus

[22] Capot, "The citrus plant", p.6-13. in: *Citrus*. Ciba-Geigy Agrochemicals Tech. Monogr.4. Ciba-Geigy Ltd., 1975, Basle, Switzerland.

[23] Tolkowsky, *Hesperides. A history of the culture and use of citrus fruits*, p.371. John Bale, Sons and Curnow, 1938, London, England.

[24] "Citrus Genetics, Breeding and Biotechnology". *google.com*.

[25] "Website Disabled". *ucr.edu*.

[26] "Citron". *purdue.edu*.

[27] Food in China: a cultural and historical inquiry By Frederick J. Simoons, Google Books

[28] The Search for the Authentic Citron: Historic and Genetic Analysis; HortScienc 40(7):1963–1968. 2005

[29] "The Garden – Sir Joseph Hooker. *Flora of British India*, i. 514". *google.com*.

[30] COUNTRY REPORT TO THE FAO INTERNATIONAL TECHNICAL CONFERENCE ON PLANT GENETIC RESOURCES (Leipzig, 1996); Prepared by: Nepal Agricultural Research Council; Kathmandu, June 1995; CHAPTER 2.2

[31] Isaac, "The Citron in the Mediterranean: a study in religious influences", *Economic Geography*, Vol. 35 No. 1. (Jan. 1959) pp. 71–78

[32] "Citron". *purdue.edu*.

[33] "ethrog". *ucr.edu*.

[34] "Foods & Nutrition Encyclopedia, 2nd Edition". *google.com*.

[35] "Citrus". *google.com*.

[36] Biology of Citrus

[37] "Citrus Fruits and Their Culture". *google.com*.

[38] "Food in China". *google.com*.

[39] "The Cultivated Oranges and Lemons, Etc. of India and Ceylon". *google.com*.

[40] "Journal of the Royal Horticultural Society". *google.com*.

[41] "THE INTRODUCTION OF CULTIVATED CITRUS TO EUROPE VIA NORTHERN AFRICA AND THE IBERIAN PENINSULA". *ebscohost.com*.

[42] *Historia plantarum* 4.4.2-3 (*exc.* Athenaeus *Deipnosophistae* 3.83.d-f); cf. Vergil *Georgics* 2.126-135; Pliny *Naturalis historia* 12.15,16.

[43] *Historia plantarum* 1.13.4.

[44] http://www.perseus.tufts.edu/hopper/text?doc=Perseus%3Atext%3A1999.02.0137%3Abook%3D13%3Achapter%3D31

[45] "Pliny the Elder, The Natural History, BOOK XII. THE NATURAL HISTORY OF TREES, CHAP. 7. (3.)—HOW THE CITRON IS PLANTED.". *tufts.edu*.

[46] "Pliny the Elder, The Natural History, BOOK XXIII. THE REMEDIES DERIVED FROM THE CULTIVATED TREES., CHAP. 56.—CITRONS: FIVE OBSERVATIONS UPON THEM.". *tufts.edu*.

2.15.9 References

- Citrus Fruits and Their Culture By H. Harold Hume

- All Kinds of Scented Wood By Richard S. Barnett

- Food in China: A Cultural and Historical Inquiry By Frederick J. Simoons

- Biology of Citrus By Pinhas Spiegel-Roy, Eliezer E. Goldschmidt

- The Encyclopædia Britannica: "a" Dictionary of Arts, Sciences, Literature ... edited by Hugh Chisholm

- Citrus: The Genus Citrus By Giovanni Dugo, Angelo Di Giacomo

- The Encyclopædia Britannica: A Dictionary of Arts, Sciences, Literature and ... By Hugh Chisholm

- Fruit Breeding in India: Papers By G. S. Nijjar

- Proceedings, Google Book Search

- A Dictionary of Greek and Roman Culture

- International Standard Bible Encyclopedia: A-D By Geoffrey William Bromiley

- The Great Citrus Book: A Guide With Recipes By Allen Susser

- Citrus: The Genus Citrus By Giovanni Dugo, Angelo Di Giacomo - "Peel confection and candying"

- Penny Cyclopaedia of the Society for the Diffusion of Useful Knowledge

- Origin of Cultivated Plants By Alphonse de Candolle

- Evyatar Marienberg and David Carpenter, The Stealing of the 'Apple of Eve' from the 13th century Synagogue of Winchester, Henri III Fine Rolls Project, Fine of the Month: December 2011

2.15.10 External links

- USDA Plants Profile – *Citrus medica*

- Purdue University (U.S.A.): article on citron culture and use.

- Citrus Pages

- University of California- "Citrus Diversity"

- Stuart-exchange_org:*Citrus medica* used as a medicinal plant.

- UCLA: "Give Me A Squeeze"

- Alchemy Works: Citron

- Wildflowers of Israel – Citron

- Differences between Lemon and Citron

- Buddha's Hand citron by David Karp (pomologist)

2.16 Citronella oil

For other uses, see Citronella (disambiguation).

Citronella oil is one of the essential oils obtained from the leaves and stems of different species of *Cymbopogon* (lemongrass). The oil is used extensively as a source of perfumery chemicals such as citronellal, citronellol and geraniol. These chemicals find extensive use in soap, candles and incense, perfumery, cosmetic and flavouring industries throughout the world.[1]

Citronella oil is also a plant-based insect repellent, and has been registered for this use in the United States since 1948.[2] The United States Environmental Protection Agency considers oil of citronella as a biopesticide with a non-toxic mode of action.[3] However, since citronella insect repellant effects were not proven within the EU, the use of citronella as an insecticide is prohibited under the Biocidal Product Directive 2006.

Research also shows that citronella oil has strong antifungal properties,[4][5][6] is effective in calming barking dogs,[7] and has even been used as a successful spray-on deterrent against pets destroying household items.

2.16.1 Types

Citronella oil is classified in trade into two chemotypes:[8]

Ceylon type

- CAS: 89998-15-2

- CAS: 8000-29-1

- EINECS: 289-753-6

- FEMA: 2308

- CoE: 39

- Obtained from: *Cymbopogon nardus* Rendle

- Consists of geraniol (18-20%), limonene (9-11%), methyl isoeugenol (7-11%), citronellol (6-8%), and citronellal (5-15%).

Java type

- CAS: 91771-61-8

- CAS: 8000-29-1

- EINECS: 294-954-7

- FEMA: 2308

- CoE: 2046

- Obtained from: *Cymbopogon winterianus* Jowitt

- Consists of citronellal (32-45%), geraniol (11-13%), geranyl acetate (3-8%), limonene (1-4%).

- The higher proportions of geraniol and citronellal in the Java type make it a better source for perfumery derivatives.[1][9] The name *Cymbopogon winterianus* is given to this selected variety to commemorate Mr. Winter—an important oil distiller of Ceylon, who first cultivated and distilled the Maha Pangeri type of citronella in Ceylon.

Both types probably originated from Mana Grass of Sri Lanka, which according to Finnemore (1962) occurs today in two wild forms--*Cymbopogon nardus* var. *linnae (typicus)* and *C. nardus* var. *confertiflorus*. Neither wild form is known to be used for distillation to any appreciable extent.

Citronella oil from Cymbopogon species should not be confused with other similar lemony oils from *Corymbia citriodora* and *Pelargonium citrosum*.

2.16.2 Health questions

Direct application of citronella oil has been found to raise the heart rate of some people.[10] Health Canada banned the oil's use as an insect repellent in 2012 but later lifted the ban in February 2015.[11][12]

2.16.3 World production

At present, the world production of citronella oil is approximately 4,000 tonnes. The main producers are China and Indonesia - producing 40 percent of the world's supply. The oil is also produced in Taiwan, Guatemala, Honduras, Brazil, Sri Lanka, India, Argentina, Ecuador, Jamaica, Madagascar, Mexico, and South Africa.

The market for natural citronella oil has been eroded by chemicals synthesised from turpentine derived from conifers. However, natural citronella oil and its derivatives are preferred by the perfume industry.[13]

2.16.4 Use as a repellent

Citronella oil is popular as a 'natural' insect repellent. Its mosquito repellent qualities have been verified by

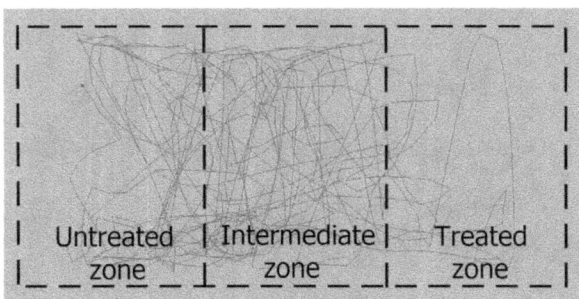

Video tracking of a stable fly, demonstrating repellency of citronella oil [14]

research,[15] including effectiveness in repelling *Aedes aegypti* (dengue fever mosquito).[16] To be continually effective most citronella repellent formulas need to be reapplied to the skin every 30–60 minutes.[17]

Research also indicates that citronella oil is an effective repellent for body louse, head louse and stable flies.[14][18][19] A study conducted by ARPA in 1963 determined that hydroxycitronellal was an effective repellent against both aquatic and terrestrial leeches.[20]

The US Environmental Protection Agency states that citronella oil has little or no toxicity when used as a topical insect repellent, with no reports of adverse effects of concern over a 60-year period.[21] Because some products are applied to human skin, EPA requires proper precautionary labeling to help assure safe use. If used according to label instructions in the US, citronella is not expected to pose health risks to people, including children and other sensitive populations.[2] The US Food & Drug Administration considers citronella oil as generally recognized as safe (GRAS).

Canadian regulatory concerns with citronella as an insect repellent are primarily based on data-gaps in toxicology, not on incidents.[22][23]

In Europe, Ceylon type citronella oil is placed on the category 3 list, with some safety concern regarding methyl eugenol.[8] In the UK, E.U. legislation governing insect repellents came into force in September 2006, which banned citronella as an active ingredient in any insect repellent products.[24] This applied to both insect repellent for humans and animals. It can still be sold as a perfume, but must not be sold as an insect repeller.

2.16.5 References

[1] Lawless, J. (1995). *The Illustrated Encyclopedia of Essential Oils.* ISBN 1-85230-661-0.

[2] "U.S. EPA Citronella Factsheet" (PDF). Retrieved June 9, 2014.

[3] EPA citronella reregistration fact sheet

[4] Nakahara, Kazuhiko; Alzoreky, Najeeb S.; Yoshihashi, Tadashi; Nguyen, Huong T. T.; Trakoontivakorn, Gassinee (October 2003). "Chemical Composition and Antifungal Activity of Essential Oil from *Cymbopogon nardus* (Citronella Grass)". *Japan International Research Center for Agricultural Sciences* **37** (4): 249–52. INIST:15524982.

[5] Pattnaik, S; Subramanyam, VR; Kole, C (1996). "Antibacterial and antifungal activity of ten essential oils in vitro". *Microbios* **86** (349): 237–46. PMID 8893526. INIST:3245986.

[6] Prabuseenivasan, Seenivasan; Jayakumar, Manickkam; Ignacimuthu, Savarimuthu (2006). "In vitro antibacterial activity of some plant essential oils". *BMC Complementary and Alternative Medicine* **6**: 39. doi:10.1186/1472-6882-6-39. PMC 1693916. PMID 17134518.

[7] Segelken, Roger (1996). "Study: 'Nuisance-barking' dogs respond best to citronella spray collars". Cornell Chronicle. Retrieved 2009-04-22.

[8] Chang, Yu Shyun, 2007, *8 Map species from Malaysia for ICS,* Forest Research Institute Malaysia, Workshop on NFP, 28–29 May 2007, Nanchang, PR China

[9] Online referenced article, Torres, R.C., Tio, BDJ, *Citronella oil industry: challenges and breakthroughs*

[10] Citronella

[11] http://commonground.ca/2012/10/health-canada-bans-citronella/

[12] Citronella makes comeback in Canada

[13] FOODNET, The Association for Strengthening Agricultural research in Eastern and Central Africa

[14] Baldacchino, Frédéric; Tramut, Coline; Salem, Ali; Liénard, Emmanuel; Delétré, Emilie; Franc, Michel; Martin, Thibaud; Duvallet, Gérard; Jay-Robert, Pierre (2013). "The repellency of lemongrass oil against stable flies, tested using video tracking". *Parasite* **20**: 21. doi:10.1051/parasite/2013021. PMC 3718533. PMID 23759542.

[15] Kim, Jeong-Kyu; Kang, Chang-Soo; Lee, Jong-Kwon; Kim, Young-Ran; Han, Hye-Yun; Yun, Hwa Kyung (2005). "Evaluation of Repellency Effect of Two Natural Aroma Mosquito Repellent Compounds, Citronella and Citronellal". *Entomological Research* **35** (2): 117–20. doi:10.1111/j.1748-5967.2005.tb00146.x.

[16] Trongtokit, Yuwadee; Rongsriyam, Yupha; Komalamisra, Narumon; Apiwathnasorn, Chamnarn (2005). "Comparative repellency of 38 essential oils against mosquito bites". *Phytotherapy Research* **19** (4): 303–9. doi:10.1002/ptr.1637. PMID 16041723.

[17] "Test: Mosquito Repellents, The Verdict" Choice, The Australian Consumers Association

[18] Mumcuoglu, Kosta Y.; Galun, Rachel; Back, Uri; Miller, Jacqueline; Magdassi, Shlomo (1996). "Repellency of essential oils and their components to the human body louse, Pediculus humanus humanus". *Entomologia Experimentalis et Applicata* **78** (3): 309–14 doi:10.1111/j.1570-7458.1996.tb00795.x.

[19] Mumcuoglu, KY; Magdassi, S; Miller, J; Ben-Ishai, F; Zentner, G; Helbin, V; Friger, M; Kahana, F; Ingber, A (2004). "Repellency of citronella for head lice: Double-blind randomized trial of efficacy and safety". *The Israel Medical Association Journal* **6** (12): 756–9. PMID 15609890.

[20] http://www.dtic.mil/dtic/tr/fulltext/u2/413979.pdf

[21] "U.S. EPA Citronella Factsheet". Retrieved June 9, 2014.

[22] *Re-evaluation of Citronella Oil and Related Active Compounds for Use as Personal Insect Repellents* (PDF). *Responsible Pesticide Use* (Pest Management Regulatory Agency (Canada)). 2004-09-17. ISBN 0-662-38012-6.

[23] "So Then: Who's Afraid of Citronella Oil? Update!" *Cropwatch Newsletter* Vol 2,Issue 1, No. 1

[24] "HSE Biocides Unit responds to The Daily Telegraph article" 13 October 2006

2.17 Copaiba

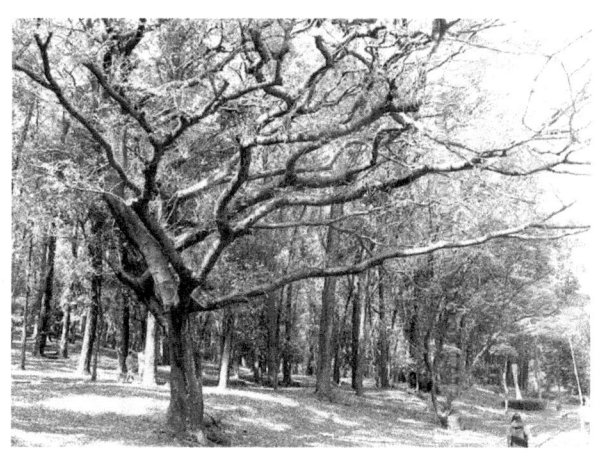

Copaifera langsdorfii in a park in São Paulo Brazil.

Copaiba is a stimulant oleoresin obtained from the trunk of several pinnate-leaved South American leguminous trees (genus *Copaifera*). The thick, transparent exudate varies in color from light gold to dark brown, depending on the ratio of resin to essential oil. Copaiba is used in making varnishes and lacquers.

The balsam may be steam distilled to give *copaiba oil*, a colorless to light yellow liquid with the characteristic odor of the balsam and an aromatic, slightly bitter, pungent taste.

The oil consists primarily of sesquiterpene hydrocarbons; its main component is caryophyllene.[1]

The hydrocarbons in copaiba are terpenes, which are made by plants from isoprene, a "five-carbon-atom building block, so they always contain carbon atoms in multiples of five. Pinene is one of several useful 10-carbon terpenes. It is commonly known as turpentine. Heated up, terpenes break down into methanol (CH_3OH) and other simple compounds useful for fuel and as raw materials in the chemical industry."[2]

Copaiba is also a common name for several species of trees of the legume family native to Tropical Africa and North and South America.

2.17.1 Uses

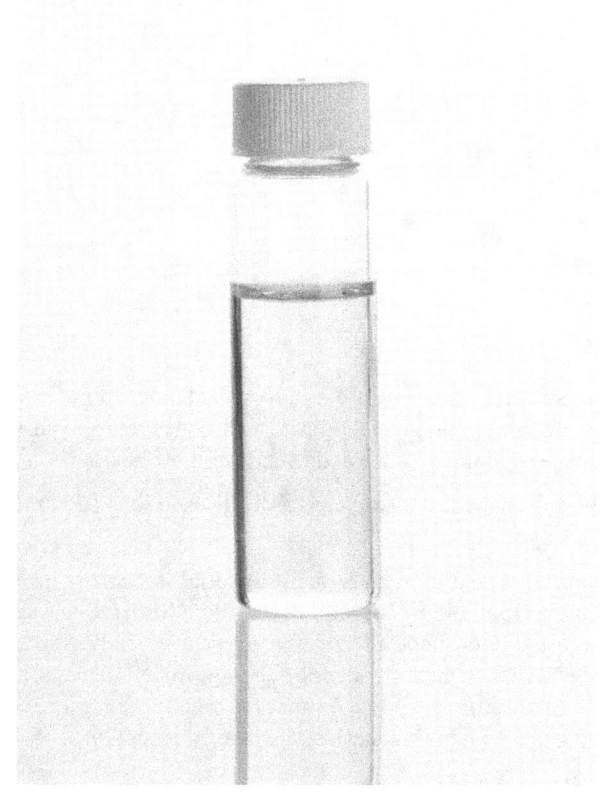

Copaiba (Copaifera reticulata) oleoresin (non-fractionated) in a clear glass vial

Copaiba is particularly interesting as a source of biodiesel, because of the high yield of 12,000 liters per ha. The resin is tapped from standing trees, with an individual tree yielding 40 liters per year.[3] [4]

Copaiba has been used in traditional medicine.

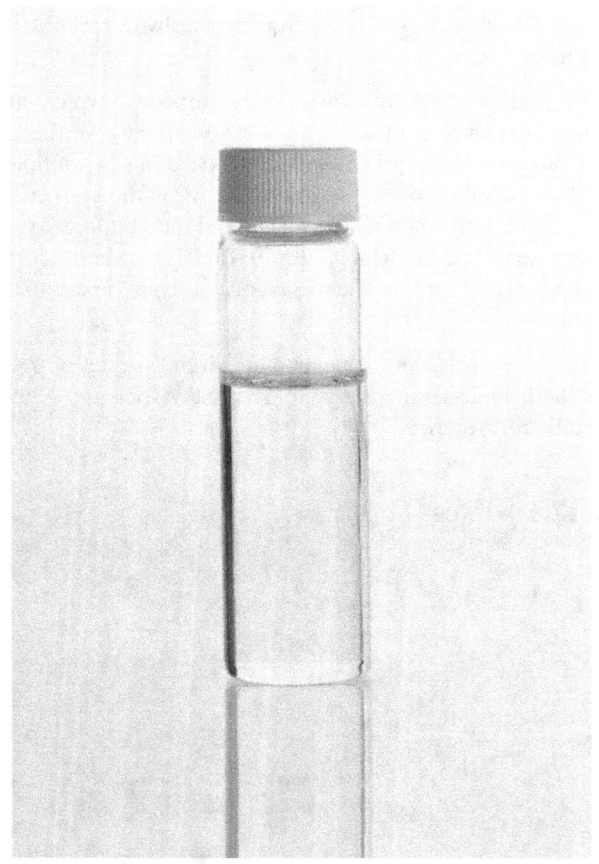

*Copaiba (*Copaifera reticulata*) essential oil (fractionated) in a clear glass vial*

It has a long history of use as a folk medicine. In Panama, the Yaviza people mix the resin with honey and give it to newborns to impart knowledge and ward off hexes.[5]

The balsam and its oil are used as fixatives in soap perfumes and fragrances.[1]

Copaiba is also used as an artist material, especially in oil paint recipes and in ceramic decoration. Mineral painters use a medium made of copaiba, turpentine and lavender to mix with their minerals for adhesion to ceramic vessels before kiln firing. Copaiba makes a good medium for oils and helps with both adhesion and quality of shine.

2.17.2   History

Copaiba oil-resins extracted have been used medicinally dating back to the 16th century by the natives of north and northeastern Brazil. The folk remedies were administered orally or used as an ointment in the treatment of various diseases.[6]

Medicinal

In the 21st century, studies have shown that the beneficial effects of Copaiba are due to its anti-inflammatory, anti-tumor, anti-tetanus, antiseptic and antihemorrhagic properties.[7][8]

In Brazil, studies on the medicinal plants, especially Copaiba oil-resin, are documented in medical literature.[9]

2.17.3   Industry and commerce

Amazon rainforest

The production of Copaiba oil is socially significant to the Amazon because it represents approximately 95% of Brazil's oil-resin production industry. The Annual production of Copaiba oil in the Amazon is estimated to be 500 tons/year.[10] The commercialization of Copaiba as an oil or in capsule form has grown due to demand by traditional and widespread use, and is exported to other countries, including the United States, France, and Germany.[11]

Despite its usage in various pharmacological forms and wide use in folk medicine, Copaiba has not been officially registered as a phytochemical drug. Experiments to assess any cytotoxic and mutagenic potential of Copaiba-derived resin are underway in Brazil to determine safe usage, prior to phytochemical drug development. Under experimental conditions employed in a study on mice, it was concluded that the oil-resin from commercial Copaiba oil-resin showed no genotoxic or mutagenic effects.[12]

2.17.4   References

[1] Karl-Georg Fahlbusch et al. (2007), "Flavors and Fragrances", *Ullmann's Encyclopedia of Industrial Chemistry* (7th ed.), Wiley, p. 96

[2] Don Button. "Diesel Trees". Science Forum. Retrieved 2006-10-14.

[3] "Farmer planning diesel tree biofuel". Sydney Morning Herald. 2006-09-19. Retrieved 2006-10-14.

[4] "New fuel source from trees". Australian Broadcasting Corporation. 2007-04-24. Retrieved 2007-04-26.

[5] Duke, James A., (1982). Handbook of Energy Crops: Copaifera langsdorfii Desf.. From the Purdue Center for New Crops Web site.

[6] Genotoxicity assessment of Copaiba oil and its fractions in Swiss mice; Genetics and Molecular Biology. Mara Ribeiro Almeida, Joana D'Arc Castania Darin, Lívia Cristina Hernandes, Mônica Freiman de Souza Ramos, Lusânia Maria Greggi Antunes, Osvaldo de Freitas; Aug 2, 2012

[7] *Antinociceptive activity of Amazonian Copaiba oils.* Gomes NM1, Rezende CM, Fontes SP, Matheus ME, Fernandes PD

[8] *In vitro evaluation of the genotoxic activity and apoptosis induction of the extracts of roots and leaves from the medicinal plant Coccoloba mollis (Polygonaceae)* Tsuboy MS, Marcarini JC, Luiz RC, Barros IB, Ferreira DT, Ribeiro LR, Mantovani MS. J Med Food. 2010.

[9] *Rupture point analysis of intestinal anastomotic healing in rats under the action of pure Copaíba* (Copaifera langsdorfii) oil. Comelli Júnior E, Skinovski J, Sigwalt MF, Branco AB, Luz SR, Baulé Cde P. Acta Cir Bras. 2010 Aug; 25(4).

[10] *Sustainability of extraction and production of copaiba (Copaifera multijuga Hayne) oleoresin in Manaus, AM, Brazil.* (Medeiros and Vieira, 2008; Brazil, 2011). Medeiros RD, Vieira G. For Ecol Manage. 2008;256:282–288.

[11] *Phytochemical and antioedematogenic studies of commercial copaiba oils available in Brazil.* Phytother Res. 2001 Sep; Zunino L, Calixto JB, Patitucci ML, Pinto AC.

[12] Genetic Molecular Biol. Genotoxicity Study 2012 Jul-Sep; 35(3): 664–672.

2.18 Cymbopogon martinii

Cymbopogon martinii is a species of grass in the lemon grass genus native to India and Indochina but widely cultivated in many places for its aromatic oil. It is best known by the common name **palmarosa**. Other common names include **Indian geranium**, **gingergrass** and **rosha** or **rosha grass**.

2.18.1 Uses

The essential oil of this plant, which contains the active compound geraniol, is valued for its scent and for a number of traditional medicinal and household uses. Palmarosa oil has been shown to be an effective insect repellent when applied to stored grain and beans,[3] an antihelmintic against nematodes,[4] and an antifungal and mosquito repellent.[5]

Palmarosa oil, which has a scent similar to roses, is added to soaps and cosmetics.[5]

2.18.2 References

[1] Kew World Checklist of Selected Plant Families

[2] The International Plant Names Index

[3] Kumar, R.; Srivastava, M.; Dubey, N. K. (2007). "Evaluation of *Cymbopogon martinii* oil extract for control of postharvest insect deterioration in cereals and legumes". *Journal of Food Protection* **70** (1): 172–78.

[4] Kumarar, A. M.; D'souza, P; Agarwal, A; Bokkolla, RM; Balasubramaniam, M et al. (2003). "Geraniol, the putative anthelmintic principle of *Cymbopogon martinii*". *Phytotherapy Research* **17** (8): 957. doi:10.1002/ptr.1267. PMID 13680833.

[5] Duke, J. A. and J. duCellier. (1993). *CRC Handbook of Alternative Cash Crops.* Boca Raton: CRC Press. 214.

2.18.3 External links

- Kew GrassBase Species Profile
- USDA Plants Profile
- List of Resources about *C. martinii*

2.19 Cyperus scariosus

Cyperus scariosus, also known in English as **cypriol** and in Hindi as **Nagarmotha**, is a plant of the Cyperaceae family, that grows wild in the Madhya Pradesh region of India. Nagarmotha (Cyperus rotundus), a cosmopolitan weed, is found in all tropical, subtropical and temperate regions of the world. In India, it is commonly known as Nagarmotha and it belongs to the family Cyperacea. The major chemical components of this herb are essential oils, flavonoids, terpenoids, sesquiterpenes, cyprotene, cyperene, aselinene, rotundene, valencene, cyperol, gurjunene, trans-calamenene, cadalene, cyperotundone, mustakone, isocyperol, acyperone, etc., Research studies have shown that it possesses various pharmacological activities such as diuretic, carminative, emmenagogue, anthelminthic, analgesic, anti-inflammatory, anti-dysenteric, antirheumatic activities. An extensive review of the ancient traditional literature and modern research revealed that the drug has numerous therapeutic actions, several of which have been established scientifically, which may help the researchers to set their minds for approaching the utility, efficacy and potency of nagarmotha.

2.19.1 Uses

It is highly prized in India for its roots and is used in aromatherapy, as a perfume and for many other purposes.

2.19.2 Biological effects

A number of potential pharmacological effects have been studied in animals, but its effects in humans are unknown. The methanol extract of *C. scariosus* leaves has shown pain relieving effects and has reduced the elevated blood glucose levels of hyperglycemic mice.[1] Aqueous-methanolic extract of *Cyperus scariosus* showed hepatoprotective properties in mice.[2] An oil isolated from *Cyperus scariosus* showed anti-inflammatory activity[3] *C. scariosus* causes immunosuppression by inhibiting Th1 cytokines in mice.[4] Nagarmotha (C. rotundus) is a perennial plant and is one of the most invasive weeds known, having spread out to a world-wide distribution in tropical and temperate regions. The plant is mentioned in the ancient ayurvedic medicine Charaka Samhita. Ayurvedic physicians uses the plant, known as musta or musta moola churna, for treating fevers, digestive system disorders, dysmenorrhea and other maladies. Modern alternative medicine recommends using the plant to treat nausea, fever and inflammation; for pain reduction; for muscle relaxation and many other disorders.

2.19.3 Chemical constituents

Steam distillation of the tubers of cypriol yields 0.075–0.080% of an essential oil, the principal content of which is cyperene.

2.19.4 Etymology

- Latin name: Cyperus scariosus

- English name: Umbrella Sedge

- Sanskrit name: Nagaramustaka, Bhadramusta

- Hindi name: Nagarmotha

2.19.5 References

[1] Alam, M. A.; Jahan, R.; Rahman, S.; Das, A. K.; Rahmatullah, M. (January 2011). "Antinociceptive and anti-hyperglycemic activity of methanol leaf extract of *Cyperus scariosus*". *Pakistan Journal of Pharmaceutical Sciences* **24** (1): 53–56. PMID 21190919.

[2] Gilani, A. U.; Janbaz, K. H. (May 1995). "Studies on protective effect of *Cyperus scariosus* extract on acetaminophen and CCl4-induced hepatotoxicity". *General Pharmacology: The Vascular System* **26** (3): 627–631. doi:10.1016/0306-3623(94)00200-7.

[3] Gupta, S. K.; Sharma, R. C.; Aggarwal, O. P.; Arora, R. B. (January 1972). "Anti-inflammatory activity of the oil isolated from *Cyperus scariosus* (R. Br.)". *Indian Journal of Experimental Biology* **10** (1): 41–42. PMID 4638006.

[4] Bhagwat, D.; Kharya, M. D.; Bani, S.; Pandey, A.; Chauhan, P. S.; Kour, K.; Suri, K. A.; Satti, N. K.; Dutt, P. (2009). "*Cyperus scariosus* chloroform fraction inhibits T cell responses in Balb/C mice". *Tropical Journal of Pharmaceutical Research* **8** (5): 399–408. doi:10.4314/tjpr.v8i5.48083.

2.20 Dill oil

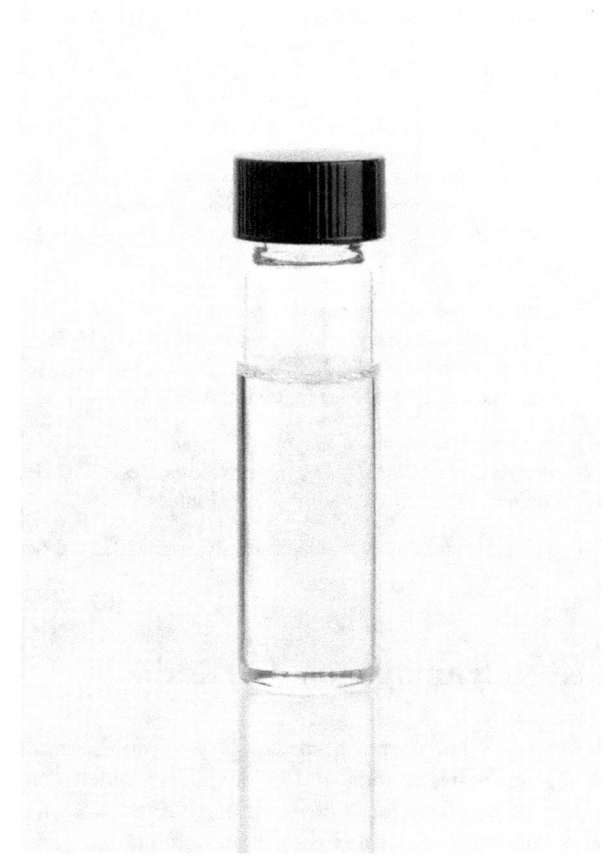

A glass vial containing pure Dill essential oil

Dill oil is an essential oil extracted from the seeds or leaves/stems (dillweed) of the Dill plant. It can be used with water to create *dill water*. Dill (Anethum graveolens) is an annual herb in the celery family Apiaceae. It is the sole species of the genus Anethum.

2.20.1 Origin

Also known as **Indian Dill**, originally from Southwest Asia, Dill is an annual or biennial herb that grows up to 1 meter (3 feet). It has green feathery leaves and umbels of small yellow flowers, followed by tiny compressed seeds.

It was popular with the Egyptians, Greeks and Romans, who called it **"Anethon"** from which the botanical name was derived. The common name comes from the Anglo-Saxon **dylle** or **dylla**, which then changed to dill. The word means **'to lull'** – referring to its soothing properties. In the Middle Ages it was used as a charm against witchcraft.

From 812 onwards, when Charlemagne, Emperor of France, ordered the extensive cultivation of this herb, it has been widely used, especially as a culinary herb.

2.20.2 Properties

Dill oil is known for its grass-like smell and its pale yellow color, with a watery viscosity. Dill oil is used for the relief of flatulence, especially in babies.

2.20.3 Production

Dill oil is extracted by steam distillation, mainly from the seeds, or the whole herb, fresh or partly dried.

2.21 Enfleurage

For the album by Megumi Hayashibara, see Enfleurage (album).

Enfleurage is a process that uses odorless fats that are solid at room temperature to capture the fragrant compounds exuded by plants. The process can be "cold" enfleurage or "hot" enfleurage.

2.21.1 Process

There are two types of processes:

- In **cold enfleurage**, a large framed plate of glass, called a chassis, is smeared with a layer of animal fat, usually lard or tallow (from pork or beef, respectively), and allowed to set. Botanical matter, usually petals or whole flowers, is then placed on the fat and its scent is allowed to diffuse into the fat over the course of 1-3 days. The process is then repeated by replacing the spent botanicals with fresh ones until the fat has reached a desired degree of fragrance saturation. This procedure was developed in southern France in the 19th century for the production of high-grade concentrates.

- In **hot enfleurage**, solid fats are heated and botanical matter is stirred into the fat. Spent botanicals are repeatedly strained from the fat and replaced with fresh material until the fat is saturated with fragrance. This method is considered the oldest known procedure for preserving plant fragrance substances.

In both instances, once the fat is saturated with fragrance, it is then called the "enfleurage pomade". The enfleurage pomade was either sold as it was, or it could be further washed or soaked in ethyl alcohol to draw the fragrant molecules into the alcohol. The alcohol is then separated from the fat and allowed to evaporate, leaving behind the absolute of the botanical matter. The spent fat is usually used to make soaps since it is still relatively fragrant.

2.21.2 Other fragrance extraction methods

See also: Fragrance extraction

The enfleurage fragrance extraction method is by far one of the oldest. It is also highly inefficient and costly but was the sole method of extracting the fragrant compounds in delicate floral botanical such as jasmine and tuberose, which would be destroyed or denatured by the high temperatures required by methods of fragrance extraction such as steam distillation. The method is now superseded by more efficient techniques such as solvent extraction or supercritical fluid extraction using liquid carbon dioxide (CO_2) or similar compressed gases.

2.21.3 See also

2.21.4 References

- Bauer, Kurt; Dorothea Garbe; Horst Surburg (2001). *Common Fragrance and Flavor Materials*. WILEY-VCH. p. 170. ISBN 3-527-30364-2.

2.22 Eucalyptus oil

Eucalyptus oil is the generic name for distilled oil from the leaf of *Eucalyptus*, a genus of the plant family Myrtaceae native to Australia and cultivated worldwide. Eucalyptus oil has a history of wide application, as a pharmaceutical, antiseptic, repellent, flavouring, fragrance and industrial uses. The leaves of selected Eucalyptus species are steam distilled to extract eucalyptus oil.

2.22.1 Types and production

Eucalyptus oils in the trade are categorized into three broad types according to their composition and main end-use: medicinal, perfumery and industrial.[1] The most prevalent is the standard cineole-based "oil of eucalyptus", a colourless mobile liquid (yellow with age) with a penetrating, camphoraceous, woody-sweet scent.[2]

China produces about 75% of the world trade, but most of this is derived from camphor oil fractions rather than be-

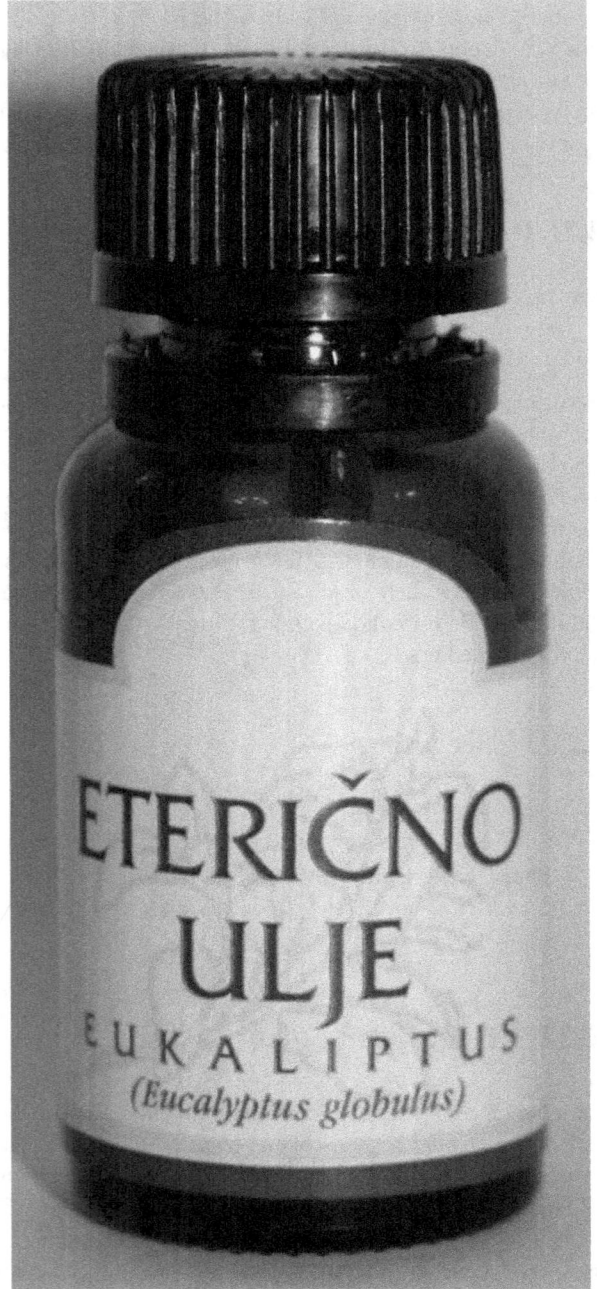

Eucalyptus oil for pharmaceutical use.

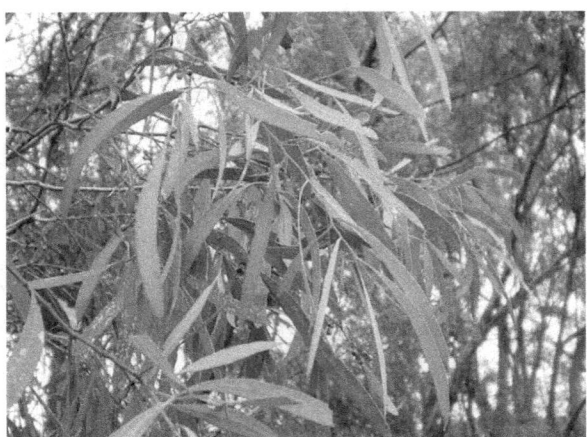

Eucalyptus polybractea *or Blue-leaf Mallee, a species yielding high quality eucalyptus oil*

to the high cineole standard required. Global annual production of eucalyptus oil is estimated at 3,000 tonnes.[4] The eucalyptus genus also produces non-cineole oils, including piperitone, phellandrene, citral, methyl cinnamate and geranyl acetate.

Eucalyptus oil should not be confused with the term "eucalyptol", another name for cineole.

2.22.2 Uses

Medicinal and antiseptic

The cineole-based oil is used as component in pharmaceutical preparations to relieve the symptoms of influenza and colds, in products like cough sweets, lozenges, ointments and inhalants. Eucalyptus oil has antibacterial effects on pathogenic bacteria in the respiratory tract.[5] Inhaled eucalyptus oil vapor is a decongestant and treatment for bronchitis.[6] Cineole controls airway mucus hypersecretion and asthma via anti-inflammatory cytokine inhibition.[7][8] Eucalyptus oil also stimulates immune system response by effects on the phagocytic ability of human monocyte derived macrophages.[9]

Eucalyptus oil also has anti-inflammatory and analgesic qualities as a topically applied liniment ingredient.[10][11]

Eucalyptus oil is also used in personal hygiene products for antimicrobial properties in dental care[12] and soaps. It can also be applied to wounds to prevent infection.

Repellent and biopesticide

Cineole-based eucalyptus oil is used as an insect repellent and biopesticide. In the U.S., eucalyptus oil was first regis-

ing true eucalyptus oil.[3] Significant producers of true eucalyptus oil include South Africa, Portugal, Spain, Brazil, Australia, Chile and Swaziland.

Global production is dominated by *Eucalyptus globulus*. However, *Eucalyptus kochii* and *Eucalyptus polybractea* have the highest cineole content, ranging from 80-95%. The British Pharmacopoeia states that the oil must have a minimum cineole content of 70% if it is pharmaceutical grade. Rectification is used to bring lower grade oils up tered in 1948 as an insecticide and miticide.[13]

Flavouring

Eucalyptus oil is used in flavouring. Cineole-based eucalyptus oil is used as a flavouring at low levels (0.002%) in various products, including baked goods, confectionery, meat products and beverages.[14] Eucalyptus oil has antimicrobial activity against a broad range of foodborne human pathogens and food spoilage microorganisms.[15] Non-cineole peppermint gum, strawberry gum and lemon ironbark are also used as flavouring.

Fragrance

Eucalyptus oil is also used as a fragrance component to impart a fresh and clean aroma in soaps, detergents, lotions and perfumes. It is known for its pungent, intoxicating scent.

Industrial

Research shows that cineole-based eucalyptus oil (5% of mixture) prevents the separation problem with ethanol and petrol fuel blends. Eucalyptus oil also has a respectable octane rating and can be used as a fuel in its own right. However, production costs are currently too high for the oil to be economically viable as a fuel.[16]

Phellandrene- and piperitone-based eucalyptus oils have been used in mining to separate sulfide minerals via flotation.

2.22.3 Safety and toxicity

If consumed internally at low dosage as a flavouring component or in pharmaceutical products at the recommended rate, cineole-based 'oil of eucalyptus' is safe for adults. However, systemic toxicity can result from ingestion or topical application at higher than recommended doses.[17]

The probable lethal dose of pure eucalyptus oil for an adult is in the range of 0.05 mL to 0.5 mL/per kg of body weight.[18] Because of their high body surface area to mass ratio, children are more vulnerable to poisons absorbed transdermally. Severe poisoning has occurred in children after ingestion of 4 mL to 5 mL of eucalyptus oil.[19]

2.22.4 History

Australian Aboriginals use eucalyptus leaf infusions (which contain eucalyptus oil) as a traditional medicine for treating body pains, sinus congestion, fever, and colds.[20][21]

Dennis Considen and John White, surgeons on the First Fleet, distilled eucalyptus oil from *Eucalyptus piperita* found growing on the shores of Port Jackson in 1788 to treat convicts and marines.[22][23][24][25] Eucalyptus oil was subsequently extracted by early colonists, but was not commercially exploited for some time.

Baron Ferdinand von Mueller, Victorian botanist, promoted the qualities of Eucalyptus as a disinfectant in "fever districts", and also encouraged Joseph Bosisto, a Melbourne pharmacist, to investigate the commercial potential of the oil.[26] Bosisto started the commercial eucalyptus oil industry in 1852 near Dandenong, Victoria, Australia. when he set up a distillation plant and extracted the essential oil from the cineole chemotype of *Eucalyptus radiata*. This resulted in the cineole chemotype becoming the generic 'oil of eucalyptus', and "Bosisto's Eucalyptus Oil" still survives as a brand.

French chemist, F.S. Cloez, identified and ascribed the name *eucalyptol* — also known as cineole — to the dominant portion of *E. globulus* oil.[27] By the 1870s oil from *Eucalyptus globulus*, Tasmanian blue gum, was being exported worldwide and eventually dominated world trade, while other higher quality species were also being distilled to a lesser extent. Surgeons were using eucalyptus oil as an antiseptic during surgery by the 1880s.[28]

The Australian eucalyptus oil industry peaked in the 1940s, the main area of production being the central goldfields region of Victoria, particularly Inglewood; then the global establishment of eucalyptus plantations for timber resulted in increased volumes of eucalyptus oil as a plantation by-product. By the 1950s the cost of producing eucalyptus oil in Australia had increased so much that it could not compete against cheaper Spanish and Portuguese oils (closer to European Market therefore less costs). Non-Australian sources now dominate commercial eucalyptus oil supply, although Australia continues to produce high grade oils, mainly from blue mallee (*E. polybractea*) stands.

2.22.5 Species utilised

Commercial cineole-based eucalyptus oils are produced from several species of *Eucalyptus*:

- *Eucalyptus cneorifolia*
- *Eucalyptus dives*
- *Eucalyptus dumosa*
- *Eucalyptus globulus*
- *Eucalyptus goniocalyx*
- *Eucalyptus horistes*

- *Eucalyptus kochii*
- *Eucalyptus leucoxylon*
- *Eucalyptus oleosa*
- *Eucalyptus polybractea*
- *Eucalyptus radiata*
- *Eucalyptus sideroxylon*
- *Eucalyptus smithii*
- *Eucalyptus tereticornis*
- *Eucalyptus viridis*

Non-cineole oil producing species:

- *Eucalyptus dives* - phellandrene variant
- *Eucalyptus dives* - piperitone variant
- *Eucalyptus elata* - piperitone variant
- *Eucalyptus macarthurii* - geranyl acetate
- *Eucalyptus olida* - methyl cinnamate
- *Eucalyptus radiata* - phellandrene variant
- *Eucalyptus staigeriana* - citral, limonene

The former lemon eucalyptus species *Eucalyptus citriodora* is now classified as *Corymbia citriodora*, which produces a citronellal-based oil.

2.22.6 Compendial status

- British Pharmacopoeia[29]

2.22.7 See also

- Essential oil
- Eucalypts, woody plants belonging to three closely related genera: *Eucalyptus*, *Corymbia* and *Angophora*

2.22.8 References

[1] William M. Ciesla. "Types of oil and uses". *Non-wood Forest Products from Temperate Broad-leaved Trees*. Food & Agriculture Org (2002). p. 30.

[2] Lawless, J., *The Illustrated Encyclopedia of Essential Oils*, Element Books 1995 ISBN 1-85230-661-0

[3] Ashurst, P. R (1999-07-31). *Food Flavorings*. ISBN 9780834216211.

[4] FOA

[5] Salari, M. H.; Amine, G.; Shirazi, M. H.; Hafezi, R.; Mohammadypour, M. (2006). "Antibacterial effects of Eucalyptus globulus leaf extract on pathogenic bacteria isolated from specimens of patients with respiratory tract disorders". *Clinical Microbiology and Infection* 12 (2): 194–6. doi:10.1111/j.1469-0691.2005.01284.x. PMID 16441463.

[6] Lu, XQ; Tang, FD; Wang, Y; Zhao, T; Bian, RL (2004). "Effect of Eucalyptus globulus oil on lipopolysaccharide-induced chronic bronchitis and mucin hypersecretion in rats". *Zhongguo Zhong yao za zhi = Zhongguo zhongyao zazhi = China journal of Chinese materia medica* 29 (2): 168–71. PMID 15719688.

[7] Juergens, U.R; Dethlefsen, U; Steinkamp, G; Gillissen, A; Repges, R; Vetter, H (2003). "Anti-inflammatory activity of 1.8-cineol (eucalyptol) in bronchial asthma: A double-blind placebo-controlled trial". *Respiratory Medicine* 97 (3): 250–6. doi:10.1053/rmed.2003.1432. PMID 12645832.

[8] Juergens, Uwe R.; Engelen, Tanja; Racké, Kurt; Stöber, Meinolf; Gillissen, Adrian; Vetter, Hans (2004). "Inhibitory activity of 1,8-cineol (eucalyptol) on cytokine production in cultured human lymphocytes and monocytes". *Pulmonary Pharmacology & Therapeutics* 17 (5): 281–7. doi:10.1016/j.pupt.2004.06.002. PMID 15477123.

[9] Serafino, A; Sinibaldi Vallebona, PS; Andreola, F; Zonfrillo, M; Mercuri, L; Federici, M; Rasi, G; Garaci, E; Pierimarchi, P (2008). "Stimulatory effect of Eucalyptus essential oil on innate cell-mediated immune response". *BMC Immunology* 9: 17. doi:10.1186/1471-2172-9-17. PMC 2374764. PMID 18423004.

[10] Göbel, H; Schmidt, G; Soyka, D (1994). "Effect of peppermint and eucalyptus oil preparations on neurophysiological and experimental algesimetric headache parameters". *Cephalalgia : an international journal of headache* 14 (3): 228–34; discussion 182. doi:10.1046/j.1468-2982.1994.014003228.x. PMID 7954745.

[11] Hong, CZ; Shellock, FG (1991). "Effects of a topically applied counterirritant (Eucalyptamint) on cutaneous blood flow and on skin and muscle temperatures. A placebo-controlled study". *American journal of physical medicine & rehabilitation / Association of Academic Physiatrists* 70 (1): 29–33. doi:10.1097/00002060-199102000-00006. PMID 1994967.

[12] Nagata, Hideki; Inagaki, Yoshika; Tanaka, Muneo; Ojima, Miki; Kataoka, Kosuke; Kubomiwa, Masae; Nishida, Nobuko; Shimizu, Katsumasa; Osawa, Kenji; Shizukuishi, Satoshi (2008). "Effect of Eucalyptus Extract Chewing Gum on Periodontal Health: A Double-Masked, Randomized Trial". *Journal of Periodontology* **79** (8): 1378–85. doi:10.1902/jop.2008.070622. PMID 18672986.

[13] Flower and Vegetable Oils, R.E.D. Facts, EPA

[14] Harborne, J.B., Baxter, H., *Chemical Dictionary of Economic Plants*, ISBN 0-471-49226-4

[15] Zhao, J., Agboola, S., Functional Properties of Australian Bushfoods - A Report for the Rural Industries Research and Development Corporation, *2007, RIRDC Publication No 07/030*

[16] Boland, D.J., Brophy, J.J., and A.P.N. House, *Eucalyptus Leaf Oils*, 1991, p. 8 ISBN 0-909605-69-6

[17] Darben, T; Cominos, B; Lee, CT (1998). "Topical eucalyptus oil poisoning". *The Australasian journal of dermatology* **39** (4): 265–7. doi:10.1111/j.1440-0960.1998.tb01488.x. PMID 9838728.

[18] Hindle, R.C. (1994). "Eucalyptus oil ingestion". *New Zealand Medical Journal*: 185–186.

[19] Foggie, WE (1911). "Eucalyptus Oil Poisoning". *British Medical Journal* **1** (2616): 359–360. doi:10.1136/bmj.1.2616.359. PMC 2332914. PMID 20765463.

[20] Low, T., *Bush Medicine, A Pharmacopeia of Natural Remedies*, Angus & Robertson, p. 85, 1990.

[21] Barr, A., Chapman, J., Smith, N., Beveridge, M., *Traditional Bush Medicines, An Aboriginal Pharmacopoeia*, Greenhouse Publications, pp. 116–117, 1988, ISBN 086436167X

[22] Maiden, J.H., *The Forest Flora of New South Wales*, vol. 4, Government Printer, Sydney, 1922.

[23] Copy of letter received by Dr Anthony Hamilton, from Dennis Consider, 18 November 1788, and sent onto Joseph Banks.

[24] Lassak, E.V., & McCarthy, T., *Australian Medicinal Plants*, Methuen Australia, 1983, p. 15, ISBN 0-454-00438-9.

[25] White, J., *Journal of a Voyage to New South Wales*, 1790

[26] Grieve, M.,(author) & Leyel, C.F., (ed), *A Modern Herbal*, Jonathon Cape, 1931, p. 287.

[27] Boland, D.J., Brophy, J.J., and A.P.N. House, *Eucalyptus Leaf Oils*, 1991, p. 6 ISBN 0-909605-69-6

[28] Maiden, J.H., *The Useful Native Plants of Australia*, pp. 255, 1889

[29] The British Pharmacopoeia Secretariat (2009). "Index, BP 2009" (PDF). Retrieved 10 September 2009.

2.22.9 Further reading

- Boland, D.J., Brophy, J.J., and A.P.N. House, *Eucalyptus Leaf Oils*, 1991, ISBN 0-909605-69-6

- FAO Corporate Document Repository, Flavours and fragrances of plant origin

2.22.10 External links

- Toxicity Eucalyptus oil profile, Chemical Safety Information from Intergovernmental Organizations

- Eucalyptus oil (E. globulus Labillardiere E. fructicetorum F. Von Mueller, E. smithii R.T. Baker) MedlinePlus, U.S. National Library of Medicine, U.S. National Institutes of Health evidence-based monograph prepared by the Natural Standard Research Collaboration

2.23 Fragrance extraction

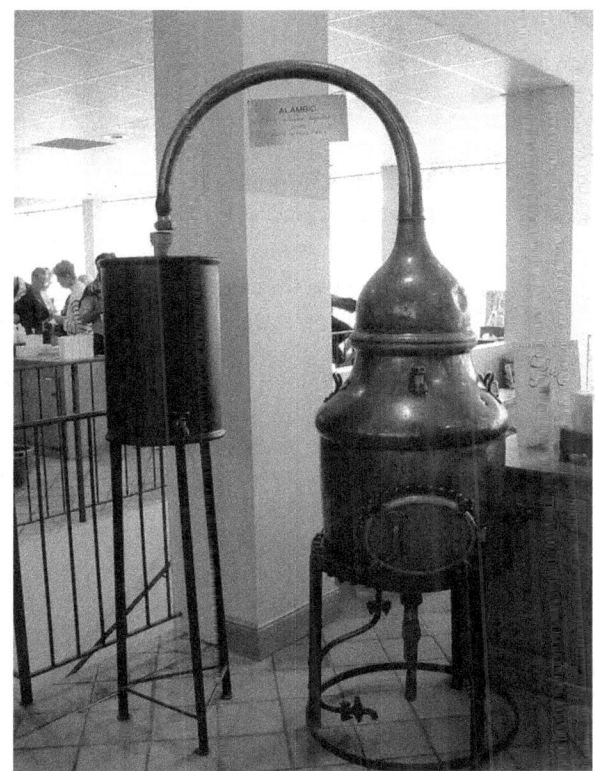

Copper still from 19th to 20th century Grasse, France for steam distillation

Fragrance extraction refers to the extraction of aromatic compounds from raw materials, using methods such as distillation, solvent extraction, expression, or enfleurage. The results of the extracts are either essential oils, absolutes, concretes, or butters, depending on the amount of waxes in the extracted product.

To a certain extent, all of these techniques tend to distort the odour of the aromatic compounds obtained from the raw materials. Heat, chemical solvents, or exposure to oxygen in the extraction process denature the aromatic compounds, either changing their odour character or rendering them odourless.

2.23.1   Maceration/Solvent extraction

See also: Maceration

Certain plant materials contain too little volatile oil to undergo expression, or their chemical components are too delicate and easily denatured by the high heat used in steam distillation. Instead, the oils are extracted using their solvent properties.

Organic solvent extraction

Organic solvent extraction is the most common and most economically important technique for extracting aromatics in the modern perfume industry. Raw materials are submerged and agitated in a solvent that can dissolve the desired aromatic compounds. Commonly used solvents for *maceration/solvent extraction* include hexane, and dimethyl ether.

In organic solvent extraction, aromatic compounds as well as other hydrophobic soluble substances such as wax and pigments are also obtained. The extract is subjected to vacuum processing, which removes the solvent for re-use. The process can last anywhere from hours to months. Fragrant compounds for woody and fibrous plant materials are often obtained in this matter as are all aromatics from animal sources. The technique can also be used to extract odorants that are too volatile for *distillation* or easily denatured by heat. The remaining waxy mass is known as a *concrete*, which is a mixture of essential oil, waxes, resins, and other lipophilic (oil-soluble) plant material, since these solvents effectively remove all hydrophobic compounds in the raw material. The solvent is then removed by a lower temperature distillation process and reclaimed for re-use.

Although highly fragrant, concretes are too viscous - even solid - at room temperature to be useful. This is due to the presence of high-molecular-weight, non-fragrant waxes and resins. Another solvent, often ethyl alcohol, which only dissolves the fragrant low-molecular weight compounds, must be used to extract the fragrant oil from the concrete. The

alcohol is removed by a second distillation, leaving behind the *absolute*. These extracts from plants such as jasmine and rose, are called absolutes.

Due to the low temperatures in this process, the absolute may be more faithful to the original scent of the raw material, which is subjected to high heat during the distillation process.

Supercritical fluid extraction

Supercritical fluid extraction is a relatively new technique for extracting fragrant compounds from a raw material, which often employs Supercritical CO_2 as the extraction solvent. When carbon dioxide is put under high pressure at slightly above room temperature, a supercritical fluid forms (Under normal pressure CO_2 changes directly from a solid to a gas in a process known as sublimation.) Since CO_2 in a non-polar compound has low surface tension and wets easily, it can be used to extract the typically hydrophobic aromatics from the plant material. This process is identical to one of the techniques for making decaffeinated coffee.

In supercritical fluid extraction, high pressure carbon dioxide gas (up to 100 atm.) is used as a solvent. Due to the low heat of process and the relatively unreactive solvent used in the extraction, the fragrant compounds derived often closely resemble the original odour of the raw material. Like solvent extraction, the CO_2 extraction takes place at a low temperature, extracts a wide range of compounds, and leaves the aromatics unaltered by heat, rendering an essence more faithful to the original. Since CO_2 is gas at normal atmospheric pressure, it also leaves no trace of itself in the final product, thus allowing one to get the absolute directly without having to deal with a concrete. It is a low-temperature process, and the solvents are easily removed. Extracts produced using this process are known as *CO_2 extracts*.

Ethanol extraction

Ethanol extraction is a type of solvent extraction used to extract fragrant compounds directly from dry raw materials, as well as the impure oils or concrete resulting from organic solvent extraction, expression, or enfleurage. Ethanol extracts from dry materials are called *tinctures*, while ethanol washes for purifying oils and concretes are called *absolutes*.

The impure substances or oils are mixed with ethanol, which is less hydrophobic than solvents used for organic extraction, dissolves more of the oxidized aromatic constituents (alcohols, aldehydes, etc.), leaving behind the wax, fats, and other generally hydrophobic substances. The alcohol is evaporated under low-pressure, leaving behind absolute. The absolute may be further processed to remove any impurities that are still present from the solvent extraction.

Ethanol extraction is not used to extract fragrance from fresh plant materials; these contain large quantities of water, which would also be extracted into the ethanol.

2.23.2 Distillation

Distillation is a common technique for obtaining aromatic compounds from plants, such as orange blossoms and roses. The raw material is heated and the fragrant compounds are re-collected through condensation of the distilled vapor. Distilled products, whether through steam or dry distillation are known either as *essential oils* or *ottos*.

Today, most common essential oils, such as lavender, peppermint, and eucalyptus, are distilled. Raw plant material, consisting of the flowers, leaves, wood, bark, roots, seeds, or peel, is put into an alembic (distillation apparatus) over water,

Steam distillation

Steam from boiling water is passed through the raw material for 60-105 minutes, which drives out most of their volatile fragrant compounds. The condensate from distillation, which contain both water and the aromatics, is settled in a Florentine flask. This allows for the easy separation of the fragrant oils from the water as the oil will float to the top of the distillate where it is removed, leaving behind the watery distillate. The water collected from the condensate, which retains some of the fragrant compounds and oils from the raw material, is called hydrosol and is sometimes sold for consumer and commercial use. This method is most commonly used for fresh plant materials such as flowers, leaves, and stems. Popular hydrosols are rose water, lavender water, and orange blossom water. Many plant hydrosols have unpleasant smells and are therefore not sold.

Most oils are distilled in a single process. One exception is Ylang-ylang (Cananga odorata), which takes 22 hours to complete distillation. It is fractionally distilled, producing several grades (Ylang-Ylang "extra", I, II, III and "complete," in which the distillation is run from start to finish with no interruption).

Dry/destructive distillation

Also known as *rectification*, the raw materials are directly heated in a still without a carrier solvent such as water. Fragrant compounds that are released from the raw material by the high heat often undergo anhydrous pyrolysis, which results in the formation of different fragrant compounds, and thus different fragrant notes. This method is used to obtain fragrant compounds from fossil amber and fragrant woods (such as birch tar) where an intentional "burned" or "toasted" odour is desired.

Fractionation distillation

Through the use of a fractionation column, different fractions distilled from a material can be selectively excluded to manipulate the scent of the final product. Although the product is more expensive, this is sometimes performed to remove unpleasant or undesirable scents of a material and affords the perfumer more control over their composition process.

2.23.3 Expression

Expression as a method of fragrance extraction where raw materials are pressed, squeezed or compressed and the essential oils are collected. In contemporary times, the only fragrant oils obtained using this method are the peels of fruits in the citrus family. This is due to the large quantity of oil is present in the peels of these fruits as to make this extraction method economically feasible. Citrus peel oils are expressed mechanically, or *cold-pressed*. Due to the large quantities of oil in citrus peel and the relatively low cost to grow and harvest the raw materials, citrus-fruit oils are cheaper than most other essential oils. Lemon or sweet orange oils that are obtained as by-products of the commercial citrus industry are among the cheapest citrus oils.

Expression was mainly used prior to the discovery of distillation, and this is still the case in cultures such as Egypt. Traditional Egyptian practice involves pressing the plant material, then burying it in unglazed ceramic vessels in the desert for a period of months to drive out water. The water has a smaller molecular size, so it diffuses through the ceramic vessels, while the larger essential oils do not The lotus oil in Tutankhamen's tomb, which retained its scent after 3000 years sealed in alabaster vessels, was pressed in this manner.

2.23.4 Enfleurage

Enfleurage is a two-step process during which the odour of aromatic materials is absorbed into wax or fat, then extracted with alcohol. Extraction by enfleurage was commonly used when distillation was not possible because some fragrant compounds denature through high heat. This technique is not commonly used in modern industry, due to both its prohibitive cost and the existence of more efficient and effective extraction methods.

2.23.5   See also

- Enfleurage

- Essential oil

- Perfume

- Rose oil

- Rosemary oil

- Clove oil

2.23.6   References

2.24   Fragrance oil

Fragrance oil(s), also known as **aroma oils**, **aromatic oils**, and **flavor oils**, are blended synthetic aroma compounds or natural essential oils that are diluted with a carrier like propylene glycol, vegetable oil, or mineral oil. To some people, synthetic fragrance oils are less desirable than plant-derived essential oils as components of perfume.

Aromatic oils are used in perfumery, cosmetics, flavoring of food.

Some include (out of a very diverse range):

- Ylang ylang

- Vanilla

- Sandalwood

- Cedar wood

- Mandarin orange

- Cinnamon

- Lemongrass

- Rosehip

- Peppermint

2.24.1   See also

- Perfume

- Essential oil

- Aroma compound

2.25   Herbal distillate

"Aquasol" redirects here. For the medicine, see Aquasol A.
Herbal distillates, also called floral water, hydrosol,

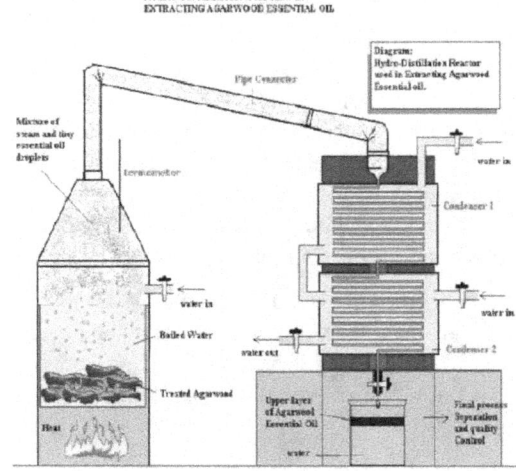

Hydro-Distillation Process in Extracting Of Agarwood Essential Oil.

hydrolate, herbal water and essential water, are aqueous products of distillation. They are colloidal suspensions (hydrosol) of essential oils as well as water-soluble components obtained by steam distillation or hydrodistillation (a variant of steam distillation) from plants/herbs. These herbal distillates have uses as flavorings, medicine and cosmetics (skin care).

Herbal distillates are produced in the same or similar manner as essential oils. However, the essential oil will float to the top of the distillate where it is removed, leaving behind the watery distillate. For this reason perhaps the term *essential water* is more descript. In the past, these essential waters were often considered a byproduct of distillation, but now are considered an important co-product.

The science of distillation is based on the fact that different substances vaporize at different temperatures. Unlike other extraction techniques based on solubility of a compound in either water or oil, distillation will separate components regardless of their solubility. The distillate will contain compounds that vaporize at or below the temperature of distillation. The actual chemical components of distillates have not yet been fully identified, but distillates will contain essential oil compounds as well as organic acids and other water-soluble plant components. Compounds with a higher vaporization point will remain behind and will include many of the water-soluble plant pigments and flavonoids.

Herbal waters contain diluted essential oils. Besides aromatic chemicals, these distillates also contain many more of the plant acids than pure essential oils making them skin friendly. Cosmetics and toiletries makers are finding many uses for herbal distillates. A pH between 5-6 makes them suitable for use as facial toners. They can be used alone as room sprays. Distillates are also used as flavorings and curables.

Because hydrosols are produced at high temperatures and are somewhat acidic, they tend to inhibit bacterial growth but not fungal growth. They are not sterile. They are a fresh product, like milk, and should be kept refrigerated.[1] Small-scale producers of hydrosols must be particularly aware of, and take steps to prevent bacterial contamination.[2]

2.25.1 See also

- Hydrosol

- Hydrodistillation

- Rose water

- Orange flower water

- Witch hazel (astringent)

2.25.2 References

[1] Cindy Jones. "Herbal Waters or Distillates (Hydrosols)". Sagescript Institute. Archived from the original on 2006-10-28. Retrieved 2006-10-23.

[2] Martin Watt. "Hydrosols or Distillation Waters: Their Production, Safety, Efficacy and the Sales Hype".

3. National Association for Holistic Aromatherapy. What are Hydrosols. Accessed 12-5-13

2.25.3 Books

- Firth, Grace. Secrets of the Still. Epm Pubns Inc; First edition (June 1983)

- Price, Len and Price, Shirley. Understanding Hydrolats: The Specific Hydrosols for Aromatherapy: A Guide for Health Professional. Churchill Livingstone 2004

- Rose, Jeanne. 375 Essential Oils & Hydrosols. Frog, Ltd, Berkeley, CA, 1999. ISBN 1-883319-89-7

- Rose, Jeanne. Hydrosols & Aromatic Waters. Institute of Aromatic & Herbal Study, 2007.

2.26 Hydnocarpus wightiana seed oil

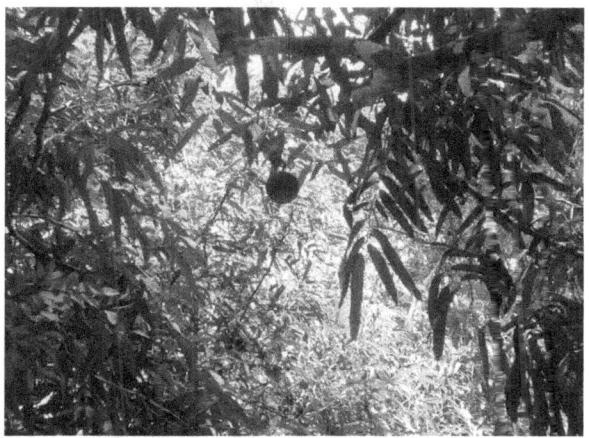

tree

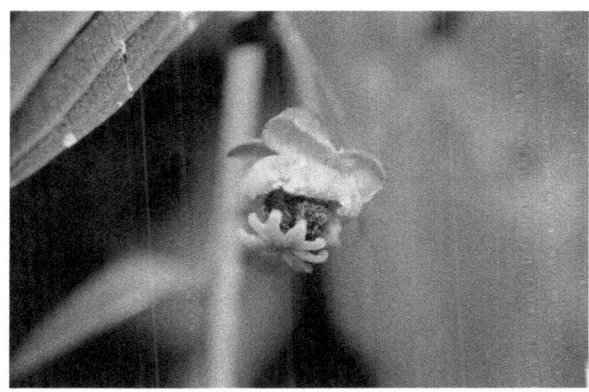

flower

Hydnocarpus wightiana or **Chaulmoogra** is a tree in the Achariaceae family. The oil from its seeds has been widely used in Indian medicine and Chinese traditional medicine for the treatment of leprosy. It entered early Western medicine in the nineteenth century before the era of sulfones and antibiotics for the treatment of several skin diseases and leprosy.[1]

2.26.1 Physical characteristics and composition

The oil is semi-solid at room temperature and does not have a strong odor. Gas–liquid chromatography analysis has shown the oil to contain the following fatty acids - hydnocarpic acid, chaulmoogric acid, gorlic acid, lower cyclic homologues, myristic acid, palmitic acid, stearic

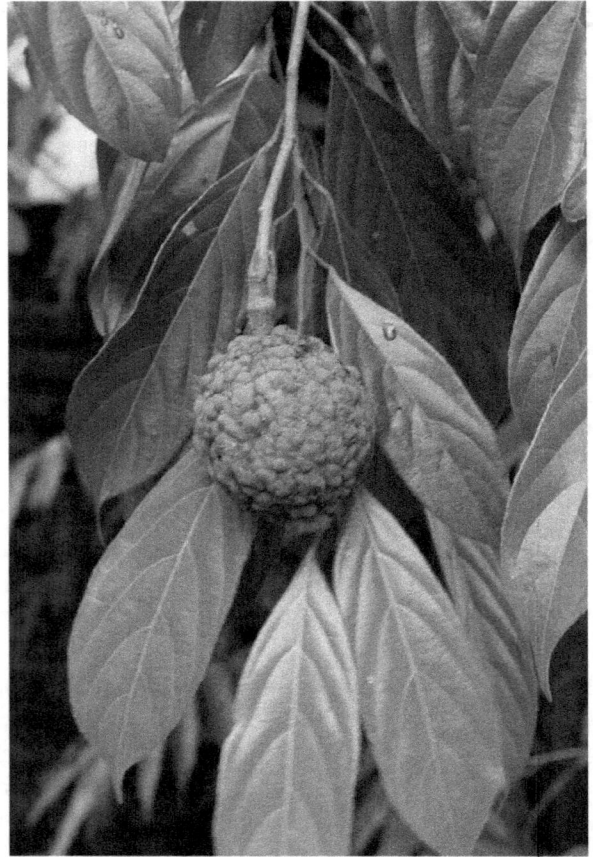

Fruit

acid, palmitoleic acid, oleic acid, linoleic acid and linolenic acid.[2]

2.26.2   Medical use

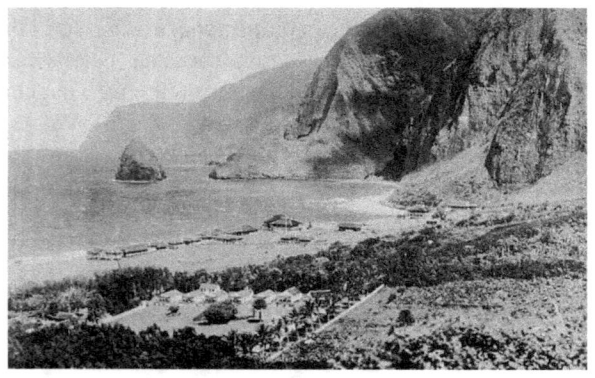

The Molokai island in Hawaii once the "Land of the Living Death," where lepers were treated with remarkable success by the then new chaulmoogra oil. Photo from 1922

The active ingredient that produces antimicrobial activity has been identified as hydnocarpic acid, a lipophilic compound. It acts by being an antagonist of biotin.[3] The oil was used intravenously or intramuscularly in the early part of the twentiety century against leprosy. An ethyl ester of the oil was developed by Alice Ball in 1916 [4] which led to the preparation and marketing of it by Burroughs Wellcome in the early 1920s. This was also used intravenously for leprosy patients often producing local reactions. The oil was also often obtained directly from India by several doctors in Africa, such as the East African Rift. The doctors would locally prepare ethyl esters to treat their patients. In June 1927, Burroughs Wellcome released the commercial preparation, sodium hydnocarpate marketed as Alepol, which produced lesser disagreeable symptoms of pain, swelling, irritating cough and blocking of the veins. In May 1928, doctors reported cure of leprosy in some patients after treatment with alepol [5]

The oil contains 5′-methoxyhydnocarpin, an amphipathic weak acid.[6] Although a minor component in the oil with no antimicrobial activitiy on its own, it plays a role in preventing multidrug resistance among some bacteria such as *Staphylococcus aureus*. It potentiates the action of berberine by preventing its removal from within bacteria thus leading to accumulation of berberine in the cells. Several *berberis* medicinal plants producing berberine also synthesize an inhibitor of the multidrug resistance pump of a human pathogen *Staphylococcus aureus*. Berberine alkaloids, which are cationic antimicrobials produced by a variety of plants, are readily extruded by multidrug resistance pumps. They are constituents of several Native American herbal medicine preparations.[7] By extracting and using hydnocarpic acid only, western medicine could not utilise the action of the other ingredients of the oil which have been now shown to have synergistic antimicrobial activitiy.[7]

In view of its anti-mycobacterial activity, it has also been tried on other conditions caused by mycobacteria such as tuberculous laryngitis.[8]

Collection and preprocessing – processing – extraction

Fruits plucked by climbing up to the tree or using long sticks with sickle tied to it. Fruits are peeled by knife and seed s are washed in water, and dried in sun.Seeds are decorticated by millet,hand hammers or by decoricator. Kernels yields 43% oil in ghani. Also crushed in expeller and rotary.Extracted oil is stored in Zinc barrels and exported[9]

Properties and fatty acid composition

The crude oil is of pale greenish-brown tinged. The oil can be easily into white, watery oil. The oil contains three cyclopentene fatty acids.

Table:fatty acid composition of oil[10]

The oil is used up to 15% in medicated soap .The oil is used internally and externally in leprocy treatment and skin diseases also.

Table of physical properties of oil[11]

Uses of oil

- Employed internally and externally in the treatment of skin diseases, scrofula, rheumatism, eczema, also in leprosy, as a counter-irritant for bruises, sprains, etc., and sometimes applied to open wounds and sores. Also used in veterinary practice. Dose of oil, 5 or 10 to 60 minims. Gynocardia Ointment, I.C.A.[12]

- Chaulmoogra is used in the treatment of skin diseases such as eczema. It is also used for bruises, sprains, sores, wounds, and scrofula. Chaulmoogra is sometimes used in the cosmetics industry to even the pigmentation of the skin.[13]

- Despite serious safety concerns, people put chaulmoogra powder, oil, emulsion, or ointment on the skin to treat skin problems including psoriasis and eczema. Chaulmoogra is given intravenously (by IV) for leprosy. This is not surprising since the first drugs used for treating leprosy used chemicals found in chaulmoogra seeds.[14]

- This oil is thought to possess antibacterial properties and has been used for ages for treating various health conditions, including eczema, skin inflammations, sprains, arthritis and bruises. In addition, chaulmoogra oil may be included as an active ingredient in several lotions, creams, balms, ointment, massage oil, lip balm as well as balm formulations for wound care.[15]

- The oil is used to make soaps with a musk-like odor[9]

See also

- Hydnocarpus wightiana

- trees of India

2.26.3 References

[1] Norton, SA (October 1994). "Useful plants of dermatology. I. Hydnocarpus and chaulmoogra.". *Journal of the American Academy of Dermatology* **31** (4): 683–6. doi:10.1016/s0190-9622(08)81744-6. PMID 8089304.

[2] Sengupta, A.; Gupta, J. K.; Dutta, J.; Ghosh, A. (1 June 1973). 'The component fatty acids of chaulmoogra oil". *Journal of the Science of Food and Agriculture* **24** (6): 669–674. doi:10.1002/jsfa.2740240606. PMID 4737104.

[3] Jacobsen, PL; Levy, L (March 1973). "Mechanism by which hydnocarpic acid inhibits mycobacterial multiplication.". *Antimicrobial agents and chemotherapy* **3** (3): 373–9. doi:10.1128/aac.3.3.373. PMC 444418. PMID 4799554.

[4] Mendheim, Beverly (September 2007). "Lost and Found: Alice Augusta Ball, an Extraordinary Woman of Hawai'i Nei". *Northwest Hawaii Times*. Retrieved 20 May 2013.

[5] Simpkin, Alice (December 1928). "The Treatment of Leprosy". *British Journal of Nursing*: 313–4. Retrieved 22 October 2011.

[6] Ranganathan, KR; Seshadri T R (1974). *Indian Journal of Chemistry* **12**: 993. Missing or empty |title= (help)

[7] Stermitz, F. R. (3 February 2000). "Synergy in a medicinal plant: Antimicrobial action of berberine potentiated by 5'-methoxyhydnocarpin, a multidrug pump inhibitor". *Proceedings of the National Academy of Sciences* **97** (4): 1433–1437. doi:10.1073/pnas.030540597. PMC 26451. PMID 10677479.

[8] Lukens, RM (1922). "CHAULMOOGRA OIL IN THE TREATMENT OF TUBERCULOUS LARYNGITIS". *JAMA* **78** (4): 274–275. doi:10.1001/jama.1922.02640570018009.

[9] SEA HandBook, 2009 by the Solvent Extractors' Association Of India

[10] "The component fatty acids of chaulmoogra oil - Sengupta - 2006 - Journal of the Science of Food and Agriculture - Wiley Online Library". Onlinelibrary.wiley.com. Retrieved 2013-11-21.

[11] *Encyclopaedic Dictionary of Bio-Medecine - Rita Singh - Google Books*. Books.google.co.in. Retrieved 2013-11-21.

[12] "A Modern Herbal | Chaulmoogra". Botanical.com. Retrieved 2013-11-21.

[13] "Butterfly Expressions". Butterfly Expressions. Retrieved 2013-11-21.

[14] "CHAULMOOGRA: Uses, Side Effects, Interactions and Warnings". WebMD. Retrieved 2013-11-21.

[15] "Chaulmoogra". Herbs2000.com. Retrieved 2013-11-21.

External links

- Pubs.acs.org

2.27 Jasmine

This article is about the plant genus. For the given name, see Jasmine (given name). For other uses, see Jasmine (disambiguation).

Jasmine (taxonomic name *Jasminum* /ˈjæsmɪnəm/)[5] is a genus of shrubs and vines in the olive family (Oleaceae). It contains around 200 species native to tropical and warm temperate regions of the Eurasia, Australasia and Oceania. Jasmines are widely cultivated for the characteristic fragrance of their flowers. A number of unrelated plants contain the word "Jasmine" in their common names (see Other plants called "Jasmine").

2.27.1 Description

See also: Glossary of botanical terms

Jasmines can be either deciduous (leaves falling in autumn) or evergreen (green all year round), and can be erect, spreading, or climbing shrubs and vines. Their leaves are borne opposite or alternate. They can be simple, trifoliate, or pinnate. The flowers are typically around 2.5 cm (0.98 in) in diameter. They are white or yellow in color, although in rare instances they can be slightly reddish. The flowers are borne in cymose clusters with a minimum of three flowers, though they can also be solitary on the ends of branchlets. Each flower has about four to nine petals, two locules, and one to four ovules. They have two stamens with very short filaments. The bracts are linear or ovate. The calyx is bell-shaped. They are usually very fragrant. The fruits of jasmines are berries that turn black when ripe.[6][7]

The basic chromosome number of the genus is 13, and most species are diploid (2n=26). However, natural polyploidy exists, particularly in *Jasminum sambac* (2n=39), *Jasminum flexile* (2n=52), *Jasminum mesnyi* (2n=39), and *Jasminum angustifolium* (2n=52).[6]

2.27.2 Distribution and habitat

Jasmines are native to tropical and subtropical regions of Eurasia, Australasia and Oceania, although only one of the 200 species is native to Europe.[8] [9] Their center of diversity is in South Asia and Southeast Asia.[7]

A number of jasmine species have become naturalized in Mediterranean Europe. For example, the so-called Spanish jasmine (*Jasminum grandiflorum*) was originally from Iran and western South Asia, and is now naturalized in the Iberian peninsula.[6]

Jasminum fluminense (which is sometimes known by the inaccurate name "Brazilian Jasmine") and *Jasminum dichotomum* (Gold Coast Jasmine) are invasive species in Hawaii and Florida.[10][11] *Jasminum polyanthum*, also known as White Jasmine, is an invasive weed in Australia.[12]

2.27.3 Taxonomy

Species belonging to genus *Jasminum* are classified under the tribe Jasmineae of the olive family (Oleaceae).[6] *Jasminum* is divided into five sections—*Alternifolia*, *Jasminum*, *Primulina*, *Trifoliolata*, and *Unifoliolata*.[4]

The genus name is derived from the Persian *Yasameen* ("gift from God") through Arabic and Latin.[13][14][15]

Selected Species

Main article: List of Jasminum species
Species include:[16]

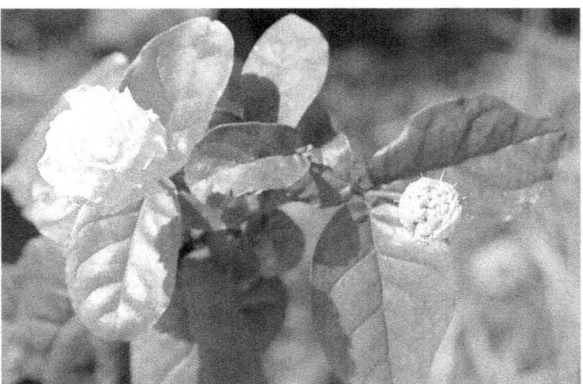

A double-flowered cultivar of Jasminum sambac *in flower with an unopened bud. The flower smells like the tea as it opens.*

- *J. abyssinicum* Hochst. ex DC. – forest jasmine

- *J. adenophyllum* Wall. – bluegrape jasmine, pinwheel jasmine, princess jasmine

- *J. angulare* Vahl

- *J. angustifolium* (L.) Willd.

- *J. auriculatum* Vahl – Indian hasmine, needle-flower jasmine

- *J. azoricum* L.

- *J. beesianum* Forrest & Diels – red jasmine

- *J. dichotomum* Vahl – Gold Coast jasmine

- *J. didymum* G.Forst.

- *J. dispermum* Wall.

- *J. elegans* Knobl.

- *J. elongatum* (P.J.Bergius) Willd.

- *J. floridum* Bunge

- *J. fluminense* Vell.

- *J. fruticans* L.

- *J. grandiflorum* L. – Catalonian jasmine, jasmin odorant, royal jasmine, Spanish jasmine

- *J. humile* L. – Italian jasmine, Italian yellow jasmine

- *J. anceolarium* Roxb.

- *J. mesnyi* Hance – Japanese jasmine, primrose jasmine, yellow jasmine

- *J. multiflorum* (Burm.f.) Andrews – Indian jasmine, star jasmine, winter jasmine

- *J. multipartitum* Hochst. – starry wild jasmine

- *J. nervosum* Lour.

- *J. nobile* C.B.Clarke

- *J. nudiflorum* Lindl. – winter jasmine

- *J. odoratissimum* L. – yellow jasmine

- *J. officinale* L. – common jasmine, jasmine, jessamine, poet's jasmine, summer jasmine, white jasmine

- *J. parkeri* Dunn – dwarf jasmine

- *J. polyanthum* Franch.

- *J. sambac* (L.) Aiton – Arabian jasmine, Sambac jasmine

- *J. simplicifolium* G.Forst.

- *J. sinense* Hemsl.

- *J. subhumile* W.W.Sm.

- *J. subtriplinerve* Blume

- *J. tortuosum* Willd.

- *J. urophyllum* Hemsl.

2.27.4 Cultivation and uses

Widely cultivated for its flowers, jasmine is enjoyed in the garden, as a house plant, and as cut flowers. The flowers are worn by women in their hair in southern and southeast Asia.

Jasmine tea

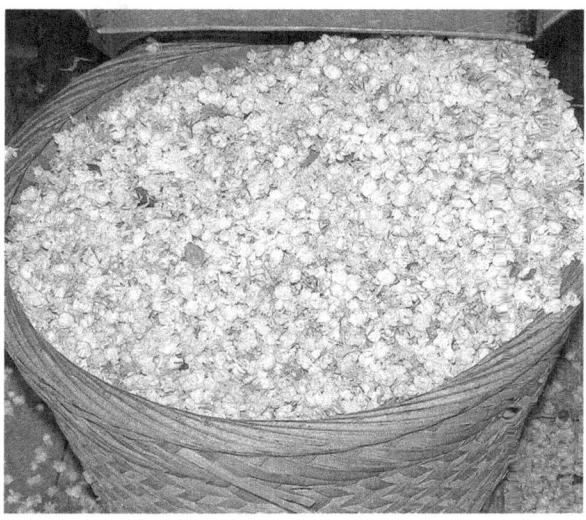

Green tea with jasmine flowers

Jasmine tea is consumed in China, where it is called jasmine-flower tea (茉莉花茶; pinyin: mò lì huā chá). *Jasminum sambac* flowers are also used to make jasmine tea, which often has a base of green tea or white tea but sometimes an Oolong base is used. Flowers and tea are "mated" in machines that control temperature and humidity. It takes four hours or so for the tea to absorb the fragrance and flavour of the jasmine blossoms, and for the highest grades, this process may be repeated as many as seven times. It must be refired to prevent spoilage. The spent flowers may or may not be removed from the final product, as the flowers are completely dry and contain no aroma. Giant fans are used to blow away and remove the petals from the denser tea leaves.

In Okinawa, Japan, jasmine tea is known as *sanpin cha* (さんぴん茶).

Jasmonates

Main article: Jasmonate

Jasmine gave name to the jasmonate plant hormones as methyl jasmonate isolated from the jasmine oil of

Jasminum grandiflorum led to the discovery of the molecular structure of jasmonates.[17]

2.27.5   Cultural importance

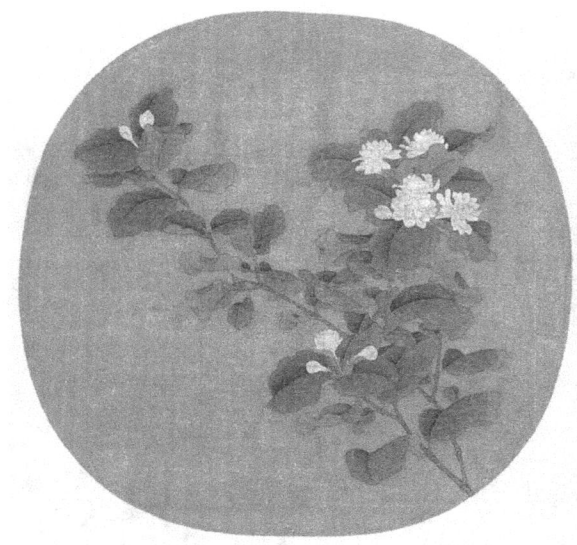

The White Jasmine Branch, *painting of ink and color on silk by Chinese artist Zhao Chang, early 12th century*

Madurai, a city in Tamil Nadu is famous for its Jasmine production. In the western and southern states of India, including Andhra Pradesh, Karnataka, Kerala, Maharashtra and Tamil Nadu, jasmine is cultivated in private homes. These flowers are used in regular worship and for hair ornaments. Jasmine is also cultivated commercially, for both the domestic and industrial uses such as the perfume industry. It is used in rituals like marriages, religious ceremonies and festivals. In the Chandan Yatra of lord Jagannath, the deity is bathed with water flavored in sandalwood paste and jasmine.

Jasmine flower vendors selling ready-made garlands of jasmine, or in the case of the thicker *motiyaa* (in Hindi) or *mograa* (in Marathi) varietal, bunches of jasmine, as well as flowers by weight, are a common sight on city streets in many parts of India. They may be found around entrances to temples, on major thoroughfares, and in major business areas.

A change in presidency in Tunisia in 1987[18][19] and the Tunisian Revolution of 2011 are both called "Jasmine revolutions" in reference to the flower. Jasmine flowers were also used as a symbol during the 2011 Chinese prodemocracy protests in the People's Republic of China.

In Syria, jasmine is the symbolic flower of Damascus, which is called the City of Jasmine. In Thailand, jasmine flowers are used as a symbol for motherhood.

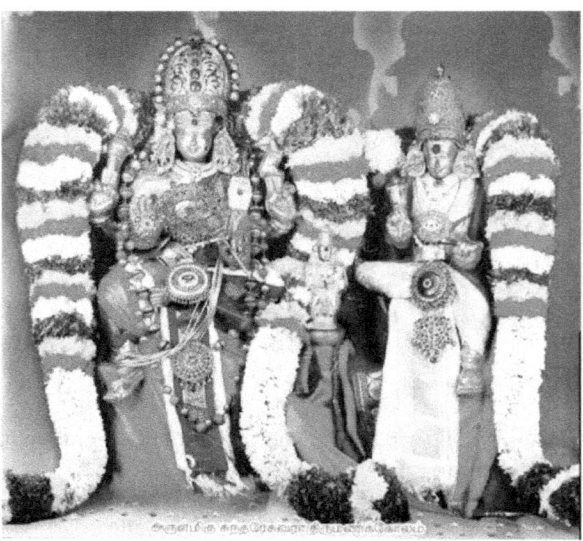

Jasmine used as garland for Meenakshi Sundareswarar, Madurai, Tamil Nadu

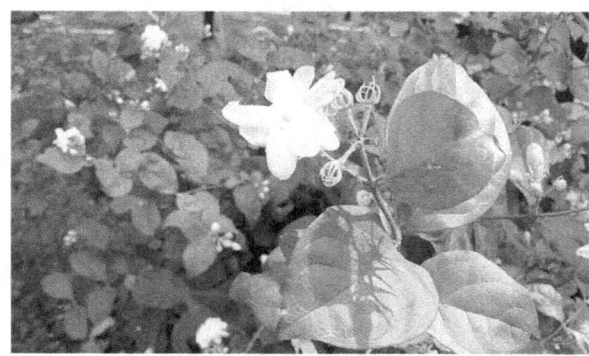

Jasmine flower blooming near Hyderabad, India

"Jasmine" is also a feminine given name in some countries.

Jasmine as a national flower

Several countries and states consider jasmines as a national symbol. They are the following:

- Hawaii: *Jasminum sambac* ("*pikake*") is perhaps the most popular of flowers. It is often strung in leis and is the subject of many songs.

- Indonesia: *Jasminum sambac* is the national flower, adopted in 1990. It goes by the name "*melati putih*" and is the most important flower in wedding ceremonies for ethnic Indonesians, especially in the island of Java.

- Pakistan: *Jasminum officinale* is known as the "*chambeli*" or "*yasmin*", it is the national flower.

- Philippines: *Jasminum sambac* is the national flower. Adopted in 1935, it is known as "sampaguita" in the islands. It is usually strung in garlands which are then used to adorn religious images.

2.27.6 Other plants called "Jasmine"

- Brazilian Jasmine *Mandevilla sanderi*
- Cape Jasmine *Gardenia*,
- Carolina Jasmine *Gelsemium*
- Chilean Jasmine *Mandevilla laxa*
- New Zealand Jasmine *Parsonsia capsularis*
- Night-Blooming Jasmine *Cestrum nocturnum*
- Night-Flowering Jasmine *Nyctanthes arbor-tristis*
- Red Jasmine *Plumeria rubra*
- Star Jasmine, Confederate Jasmine *Trachelospermum*
- Tree Jasmine (disambiguation)
- Jasmine rice, a type of long-grain rice

2.27.7 See also

- Jasmine rice—smells like, but is not related to, Jasmine

2.27.8 References

[1] *"Jasminum"*. *Index Nominum Genericorum*. International Association for Plant Taxonomy. Retrieved 2008-05-03.

[2] "10. Jasminum Linnaeus". *Chinese Plant Names* 15: 307. Retrieved 2008-06-03.

[3] UniProt. "Jasminum". Retrieved 2008-05-03.

[4] USDA, ARS, National Genetic Resources Program. "*Jasminum* L.". *Germplasm Resources Information Network*, National Germplasm Resources Laboratory. Retrieved November 22, 2011.

[5] *Sunset Western Garden Book*, 1995:606–607.

[6] A.K. Singh (2006). *Flower Crops: Cultivation and Management*. New India Publishing. pp. 193–205. ISBN 978-81-89422-35-6.

[7] H. Panda (2005). *Cultivation and Utilization of Aromatic Plants*. National Institute Of Industrial Research. p. 220. ISBN 978-81-7833-027-3.

[8] Ernst Schmidt, Mervyn Lötter, & Warren McCleland (2002). *Trees and shrubs of Mpumalanga and Kruger National Park*. Jacana Media. p. 530. ISBN 978-1-919777-30-6.

[9] *Jasminum* @ EFloras.org.

[10] *"Jasminum fluminense"*. Natural Resources Conservation Service PLANTS Database. USDA.

[11] *"Jasminum dichotomum"*. Natural Resources Conservation Service PLANTS Database. USDA.

[12] "Weeds of the Blue Mountains Bushland - Jasminum polyanthum".

[13] "jasmine, -in, jessamine, -in", OED

[14] "jasmine." Webster's Third New International Dictionary, Unabridged. Merriam-Webster, 2002.

[15] Metcalf, 1999, p. 123.

[16] GRIN. "*Jasminum* information from NPGS/GRIN". *Taxonomy for Plants*. National Germplasm Resources Laboratory, Beltsville, Maryland: USDA, ARS, National Genetic Resources Program. Retrieved October 19, 2012.

[17] Demole E; Lederer, E.; Mercier, D. (1962). "Isolement et détermination de la structure du jasmonate de méthyle, constituant odorant caractéristique de l'essence de jasmin". *Helv Chim Acta* 45 (2): 675–85. doi:10.1002/hlca.19620450233.

[18] Michael, Ayari; Vincent Geisser (2011). "Tunisie : la Révolution des "Nouzouh"* n'a pas l'odeur du jasmin" (in French). Témoignage chrétien. Archived from the original on 2011-03-14. Retrieved 2011-03-14.

[19] "La révolution par le feu et par un clic" (in French). Le Quotidien d'Oran/moofid.com. 2011-02-25. Archived from the original on 2011-03-14. Retrieved 2011-03-14.

2.27.9 Further reading

- *"Jasminum* Linn". *Flora of Pakistan*: 12. Retrieved 2008-06-03.
- Metcalf, Allan A. (1999). *The World in So Many Words*. Houghton Mifflin. ISBN 0-395-95920-9.

2.27.10 External links

- "Jasminum L". Integrated Taxonomic Information System. Retrieved 3 June 2008.
- "Flora Europaea Search Results". *Flora Europaea*. Royal Botanic Garden, Edinburgh. Retrieved 2008-06-03.

- "African Plants Database". South African National Biodiversity Institute, the Conservatoire et Jardin botaniques de la Ville de Genève and Tela Botanica.

- *"Jasminum"*. Natural Resources Conservation Service PLANTS Database. USDA. Retrieved 2008-06-03.

2.28 Juniper berry

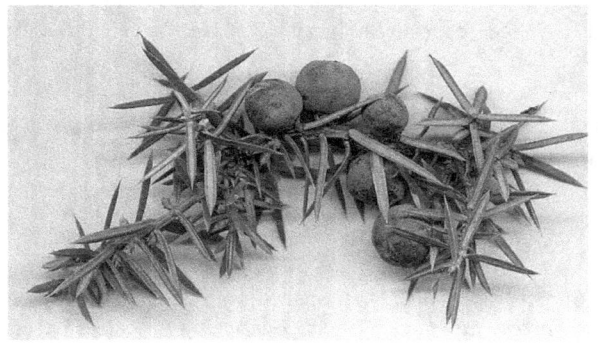

Juniper berries, here still attached to a branch, are actually modified conifer cones.

A **juniper berry** is the female seed cone produced by the various species of junipers. It is not a true berry but a cone with unusually fleshy and merged scales, which give it a berry-like appearance. The cones from a handful of species, especially *Juniperus communis*, are used as a spice, particularly in European cuisine, and also give gin its distinctive flavour. According to one FAO document, juniper berries are the only spice derived from conifers,[1] although tar and inner bark (used as a sweetener in Apache cuisines) from pine trees is sometimes considered a spice as well.

2.28.1 Species

All juniper species grow berries, but some are considered too bitter to eat. In addition to *J. communis*, other edible species include *Juniperus drupacea*,[2][3] *Juniperus phoenicea*,[4] *Juniperus deppeana*, and *Juniperus californica*.[5] Some species, for example *Juniperus sabina*, are toxic and consumption is inadvisable.[6]

2.28.2 Characteristics

Juniperus communis berries vary from four to twelve millimeters in diameter; other species are mostly similar in size, though some are larger, notably *J. drupacea* (20–28 mm). Unlike the separated and woody scales of a typical pine cone, those in a juniper berry remain fleshy and merge

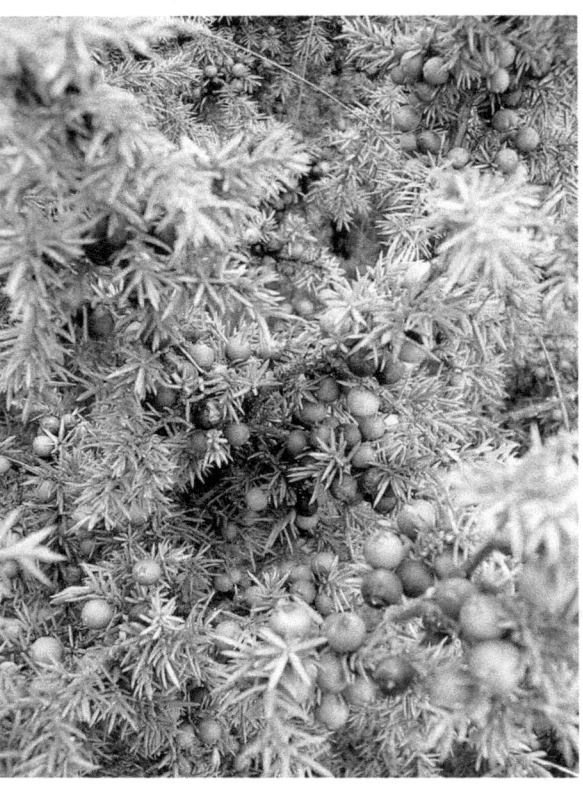

Mature purple and younger green juniper berries can be seen growing alongside one another on the same plant.

into a unified covering surrounding the seeds. The berries are green when young, and mature to a purple-black colour over about 18 months in most species, including *J. communis* (shorter, 8–10 months in a few species, and about 24 months in *J. drupacea*).[2] The mature, dark berries are usually but not exclusively used in cuisine, while gin is flavoured with fully grown but immature green berries.[1]

2.28.3 Uses

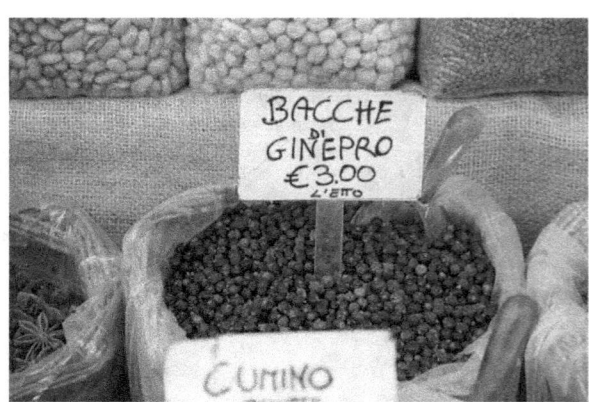

Dried juniper berries at a market in Syracuse, Sicily

The flavor profile of young, green berries is dominated by pinene; as they mature this piney, resinous backdrop is joined by what Harold McGee describes as "green-fresh" and citrus notes.[7] The outer scales of the berries are relatively flavourless, so the berries are almost always at least lightly crushed before being used as a spice. They are used both fresh and dried, but their flavour and odour are at their strongest immediately after harvest and decline during drying and storage.

Juniper berries are used in northern European and particularly Scandinavian cuisine to "impart a sharp, clear flavor"[1] to meat dishes, especially wild birds (including thrush, blackbird, and woodcock) and game meats (including boar and venison).[8] They also season pork, cabbage, and sauerkraut dishes. Traditional recipes for choucroute garnie, an Alsatian dish of sauerkraut and meats, universally include juniper berries.[9] Besides Norwegian and Swedish dishes, juniper berries are also sometimes used in German, Austrian, Czech, Polish and Hungarian cuisine, often with roasts (such as German sauerbraten). Northern Italian cuisine, especially that of the South Tyrol, also incorporates juniper berries.

Juniper, typically *Juniperus communis*, is used to flavor gin, a liquor developed in the 17th century in the Netherlands. The name *gin* itself is derived from either the French *genièvre* or the Dutch *jenever*, which both mean "juniper".[1] Other juniper-flavoured beverages include the Finnish rye-and-juniper beer known as sahti, which is flavored with both juniper berries and branches.[10] The brand Dry Soda produces a juniper-berry soda as part of its lineup. Recently, some American distilleries have begun using 'New World' varieties of juniper such as *Juniperus occidentalis*.[11]

Juniper berry was first intended as a medication since juniper berries are a diuretic and were also thought to be an appetite stimulant and a remedy for rheumatism and arthritis. Native Americans are reported to have used the juniper berry as an appetite suppressant in times of hunger. Juniper berry is being researched as a treatment for diet-controlled diabetes, as it releases insulin from the pancreas, hence alleviating hunger. It is also said to have been used by some tribes as a female contraceptive.

A few North American juniper species produce a seed cone with a sweeter, less resinous flavor than those typically used as a spice. For example, one field guide describes the flesh of the berries of *Juniperus californica* as "dry, mealy, and fibrous but sweet and without resin cells".[12] Such species have been used not just as a seasoning but as a nutritive food by some Native Americans.[13] In addition to medical and culinary purposes, Native Americans have also used the seeds inside juniper berries as beads for jewellery and decoration.[13]

An essential oil extracted from juniper berries is used in aromatherapy and perfumery.[4] The essential oil can be distilled out of berries which have already been used to flavour gin.[1]

2.28.4 History

Juniper berries, including *Juniperus phoenicea* and *Juniperus oxycedrus* have been found in ancient Egyptian tombs at multiple sites. *J. oxycedrus* is not known to grow in Egypt, and neither is *Juniperus excelsa*, which was found along with *J. oxycedrus* in the tomb of Tutankhamun.[14] The berries imported into Egypt may have come from Greece; the Greeks record using juniper berries as a medicine long before mentioning their use in food.[15] The Greeks used the berries in many of their Olympics events because of their belief that the berries increased physical stamina in athletes.[16] The Romans used juniper berries as a cheap domestically produced substitute for the expensive black pepper and long pepper imported from India.[4] It was also used as an adulterant, as reported in Pliny the Elder's *Natural History*: "Pepper is adulterated with juniper berries, which have the property, to a marvellous degree, of assuming the pungency of pepper."[17] Pliny also incorrectly asserted that black pepper grew on trees that were "very similar in appearance to our junipers".

2.28.5 Notes and references

[1] Ciesla, William M (1998). *Non-wood forest products from conifers*. Food and Agriculture Organization of the United Nations. ISBN 92-5-104212-8. Chapter 8: Seeds, Fruits, and Cones. Retrieved July 27, 2006.

[2] Farjon, A. (2005). *A Monograph of Cupressaceae and Sciadopityaceae*. Royal Botanic Gardens, Kew. pp. 223–400. ISBN 1-84246-068-4.

[3] Adams, R. P. (2004). *Junipers of the World: The genus Juniperus*. Trafford. ISBN 1-4120-4250-X.

[4] Dalby, A. (2002). *Dangerous Tastes: The Story of Spices*. University of California Press. p. 33. ISBN 0-520-23674-2.

[5] Peattie, D., & Landacre, P. H. (1991). *A Natural History of Western Trees*. Houghton Mifflin. p. 226. ISBN 0-395-58175-3.

[6] Grieve, M. (1984). *A Modern Herbal*. Penguin. ISBN 0-14-046440-9.

[7] McGee, Harold (2004). *On Food and Cooking (Revised Edition)*. Scribner. p. 410. ISBN 0-684-80001-2.

[8] Montagne, Prosper. *The Concise Larousse Gastronomique*. Octopus. p. 691. ISBN 0-600-60863-8.

[9] Steingarten, Jeffrey (1997). "True Choucroute". *The Man Who Ate Everything*. Vintage Books. p. 244. ISBN 0-375-70202-4. The chapter is an essay first published in 1989.

[10] Jackson, Michael (1995). Sweating up a suitable thirst. Michael Jackson's Beer Hunter. Retrieved 30 July 2006.

[11] Bend Distillery. Cascade Mountain Gin. Bend Distillery. Retrieved 10 Dec 2010.

[12] Peattie, Donald; Paul (1991). *A Natural History of Western Trees*. Houghton Mifflin Field Guides. p. 226. ISBN 0-395-58175-3.

[13] Moerman, Daniel E (1998). *Native American Ethnobotany*. Timber Press. pp. 282–290. ISBN 0-88192-453-9.

[14] Manniche, Lisa (1999). *Sacred Luxuries: Fragrance, Aromatherapy, and Cosmetics in Ancient Egypt*. Cornell University Press. p. 21. ISBN 0-8014-3720-2.

[15] Dalby, Andrew (1997). *Siren Feasts: A History of Food and Gastronomy in Greece*. Routledge. p. 142. ISBN 0-415-15657-2.

[16] James, Lorman. (1997) *Greek Life*. Gregory House: New York. 76-77.

[17] From Bostock and Riley's 1855 translation. Text online.

2.28.6 External links

- Medicinal uses of Juniper in Armenia

2.29 Lavender oil

Lavender oil is an essential oil obtained by distillation from the flower spikes of certain species of lavender. Two forms are distinguished, *lavender flower oil*, a colorless oil, insoluble in water, having a density of 0.885 g/mL; and *lavender spike oil*, a distillate from the herb *Lavandula latifolia*, having density 0.905 g/mL. Like all essential oils, it is not a pure compound; it is a complex mixture of naturally occurring phytochemicals, including linalool and linalyl acetate. Kashmir Lavender oil is famous for being produced from lavender at the foothills of the Himalayas. As of 2011, the biggest lavender oil producer in the world is Bulgaria.[1]

2.29.1 Uses

Lavender oil has long been used in the production of perfume.[2]:184–186

It is used in aromatherapy but there is little evidence that it does anything.[3]

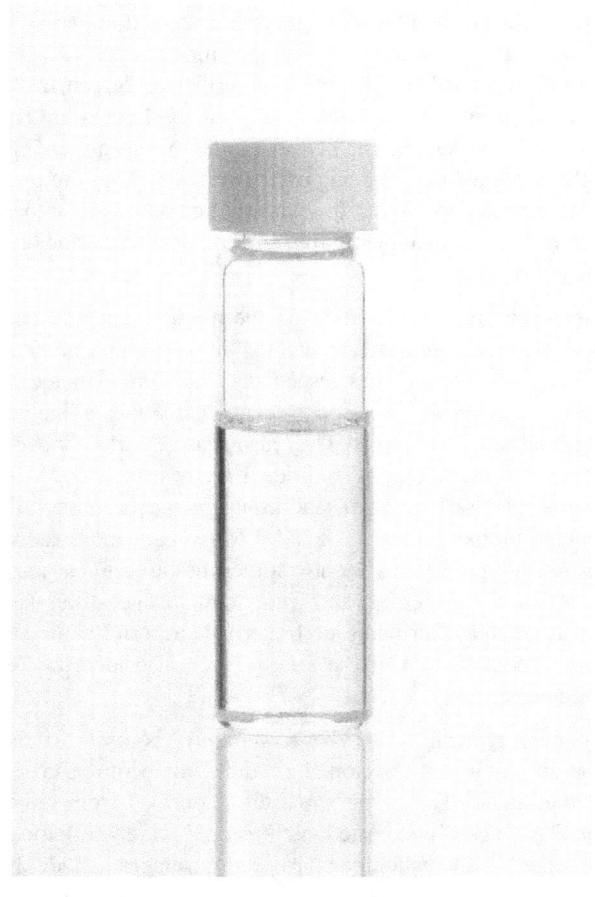

A glass vial of pure essential oil of lavender

Oil of spike lavender was used as a solvent in oil painting, mainly before the use of distilled turpentine became common.[4]

2.29.2 Research

Small clinical studies of Silexan, an oral preparation of lavender oil, have been found it may be useful for alleviating low-level anxiety and sleep disorders.[3][5]

Lavender oil has been implicated in prepubertal gynecomastia, the abnormal development of breasts in pre-adolescent boys.[6]

2.29.3 Composition

The primary components of lavender oil are linalool (51%) and linalyl acetate (35%).[7] Other components include α-pinene, limonene, 1,8-cineole, *cis-* and *trans-*ocimene, 3-octanone, camphor, caryophyllene, terpinen-4-ol and lavendulyl acetate. The composition of lavender essential oil as obtained by chromatography:

2.29.4 References

[1] Bulgarian lavender producers worried about demand drop, China Post, 14 July 2011

[2] N. Groom. New Perfume Handbook. Springer Science & Business Media, 1997 ISBN 9780751404036

[3] National Center for Complementary and Alternative Medicine. Last updated March 2003. Herbs at a Glance: Lavender

[4] "Solvent", pp 605-606 in The Grove Encyclopedia of Materials and Techniques in Art, edited by Gerald W. R. Ward. Oxford University Press, 2008 ISBN 9780195313918

[5] Kasper S (2013). "An orally administered lavandula oil preparation (Silexan) for anxiety disorder and related conditions: an evidence based review". *Int J Psychiatry Clin Pract* (Review). 17 Suppl 1: 15–22. doi:10.3109/13651501.2013.813555. PMID 23808618.

[6] Henley DV, Korach KS (July 2010). "Physiological effects and mechanisms of action of endocrine disrupting chemicals that alter estrogen signaling". *Hormones* 9 (3): 191–205. doi:10.14310/horm.2002.1270. PMID 20688617.

[7] A. Prashar, I. C. Locke, C. S. Evans (2004). Cytotoxicity of lavender oil and its major components to human skin cells. Cell Proliferation 37 (3), 221–229.

2.29.5 See also

- Lavender

- Essential oil

2.30 Lemon oil

This article is about the fruit. For other uses, see Lemon (disambiguation).

The **lemon** (*Citrus × limon*) is a species of small evergreen tree native to Asia.

The tree's ellipsoidal yellow fruit is used for culinary and non-culinary purposes throughout the world, primarily for its juice, which has both culinary and cleaning uses.[1] The pulp and rind (zest) are also used in cooking and baking. The juice of the lemon is about 5% to 6% citric acid, which gives a sour taste. The distinctive sour taste of lemon juice makes it a key ingredient in drinks and foods such as lemonade and lemon meringue pie.

2.30.1 History

See also: Citron § Origin & distribution
The origin of the lemon is unknown, though lemons are

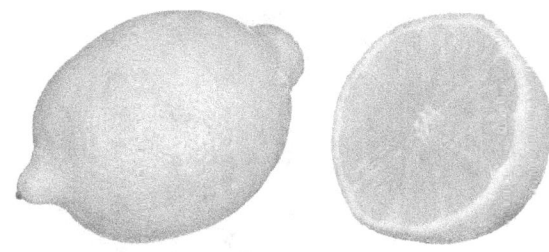

Lemon external and internal surfaces

thought to have first grown in Assam (a region in northeast India), northern Burma or China.[1] A study of the genetic origin of the lemon reported it to be hybrid between bitter orange (sour orange) and citron.[2]

Lemons entered Europe near southern Italy no later than the first century AD, during the time of Ancient Rome.[1] However, they were not widely cultivated. They were later introduced to Persia and then to Iraq and Egypt around 700 AD.[1] The lemon was first recorded in literature in a 10th-century Arabic treatise on farming, and was also used as an ornamental plant in early Islamic gardens.[1] It was distributed widely throughout the Arab world and the Mediterranean region between 1000 and 1150.[1]

The first substantial cultivation of lemons in Europe began in Genoa in the middle of the 15th century. The lemon was later introduced to the Americas in 1493 when Christopher Columbus brought lemon seeds to Hispaniola on his voyages. Spanish conquest throughout the New World helped spread lemon seeds. It was mainly used as an ornamental plant and for medicine.[1] In the 19th century, lemons were increasingly planted in Florida and California.[1]

In 1747, James Lind's experiments on seamen suffering from scurvy involved adding lemon juice to their diets, though vitamin C was not yet known.[1][3]

The origin of the word "lemon" may be Middle Eastern.[1] The word draws from the Old French *limon*, then Italian *limone*, from the Arabic *laymūn* or *līmūn*, and from the Persian *līmūn*, a generic term for citrus fruit, which is a cognate of Sanskrit (*nimbū*, "lime").[4]

2.30.2 Varieties

The 'Bonnie Brae' is oblong, smooth, thin-skinned, and seedless;[5] mostly grown in San Diego County.[6]

The 'Eureka' grows year-round and abundantly. This is the

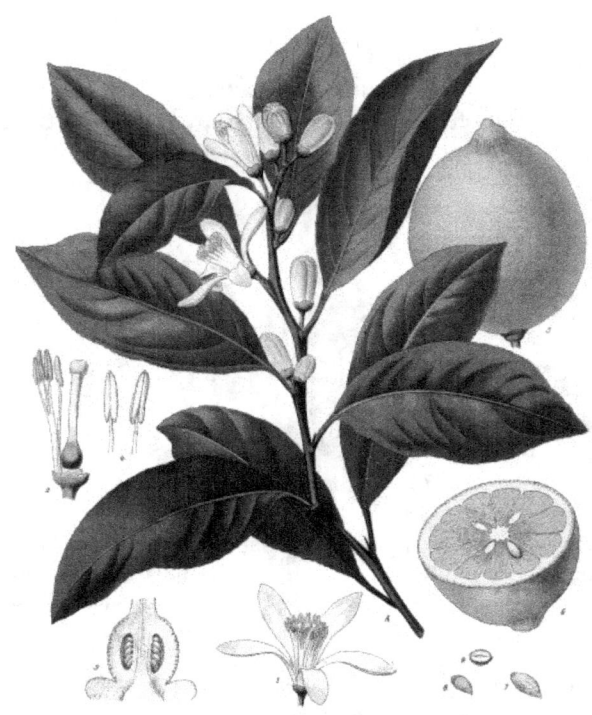

Detailed taxonomic illustration by Franz Eugen Köhler.

2.30.3   Culinary uses

Lemon juice, rind, and zest are used in a wide variety of foods and drinks. Lemon juice is used to make lemonade, soft drinks, and cocktails. It is used in marinades for fish, where its acid neutralizes amines in fish by converting them into nonvolatile ammonium salts, and meat, where the acid partially hydrolyzes tough collagen fibers, tenderizing the meat, but the low pH denatures the proteins, causing them to dry out when cooked. Lemon juice is frequently used in the United Kingdom to add to pancakes, especially on Shrove Tuesday.

Lemon juice is also used as a short-term preservative on certain foods that tend to oxidize and turn brown after being sliced (enzymatic browning), such as apples, bananas, and avocados, where its acid denatures the enzymes.

Lemon juice and rind are used to make marmalade and lemon liqueur. Lemon slices and lemon rind are used as a garnish for food and drinks. Lemon zest, the grated outer rind of the fruit, is used to add flavor to baked goods, puddings, rice, and other dishes.

The leaves of the lemon tree are used to make a tea and for preparing cooked meats and seafoods.

2.30.4   Other uses

Industrial

Lemons were the primary commercial source of citric acid before the development of fermentation-based processes.[12]

As a cleaning agent

The juice of the lemon may be used for cleaning. A halved lemon dipped in salt or baking powder is used to brighten copper cookware. The acid dissolves the tarnish and the abrasives assist the cleaning. As a sanitary kitchen deodorizer the juice can deodorize, remove grease, bleach stains, and disinfect; when mixed with baking soda, it removes stains from plastic food storage containers.[13] The oil of the lemon's peel also has various uses. It is used as a wood cleaner and polish, where its solvent property is employed to dissolve old wax, fingerprints, and grime. Lemon oil and orange oil are also used as a nontoxic insecticide treatment.

A halved lemon is used as a finger moistener for those counting large amounts of bills, such as tellers and cashiers.

common supermarket lemon,[7] also known as 'Four Seasons' (*Quatre Saisons*) because of its ability to produce fruit and flowers together throughout the year. This variety is also available as a plant to domestic customers.[8] There is also a pink-fleshed Eureka lemon, which's outer skin is variegated from green and yellow stripes.[9]

The 'Femminello St. Teresa', or 'Sorrento'[10] is native to Italy. This fruit's zest is high in lemon oils. It is the variety traditionally used in the making of *limoncello*.

The 'Meyer' is a cross between a lemon and possibly an orange or a mandarin, and was named after Frank N. Meyer, who first discovered it in 1908. Thin-skinned and slightly less acidic than the Lisbon and Eureka lemons, Meyer lemons require more care when shipping and are not widely grown on a commercial basis. Meyer lemons have a much thinner rind, and often mature to a yellow-orange color. They are slightly more frost-tolerant than other lemons.

The 'Ponderosa' is more cold-sensitive than true lemons; the fruit are thick-skinned and very large. It is likely a citron-lemon hybrid.

The 'Yen Ben' is an Australasian cultivar.[11]

Medicinal

Lemon oil may be used in aromatherapy. Lemon oil aroma does not influence the human immune system, but may enhance mood.[14] The low pH of juice makes it antibacterial, and in India, the lemon is used in Indian traditional medicines (Siddha medicine and Ayurveda).

Other

One educational science experiment involves attaching electrodes to a lemon and using it as a battery to produce electricity. Although very low power, several lemon batteries can power a small digital watch.[15] These experiments also work with other fruits and vegetables.

Lemon juice is also sometimes used as an acid in educational science experiments.

Lemon juice may be used as a simple invisible ink, developed by heat.

2.30.5 Lemon alternatives

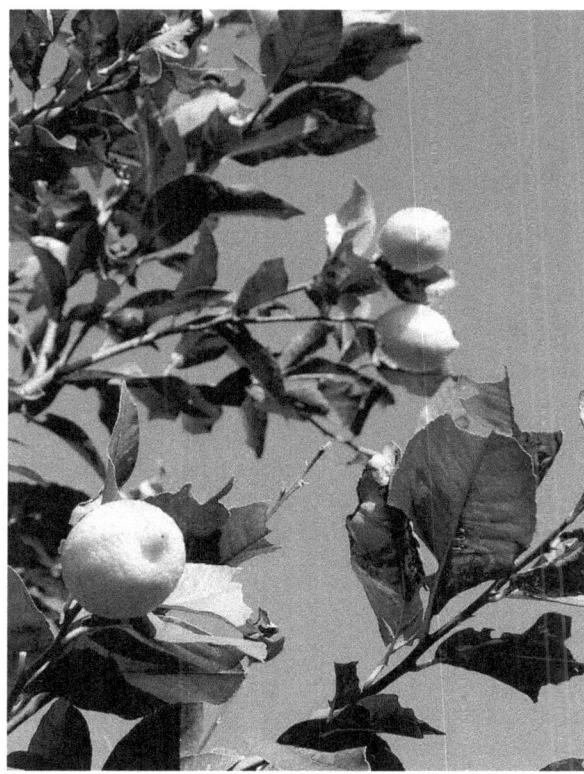

Lemons in growth

Many plants taste or smell similar to lemons.

- Certain cultivars of basil

- *Cymbopogon* (lemongrass)

- Lemon balm, a mint-like herbaceous perennial in the Lamiaceae family

- Two varieties of scented geranium: *Pelargonium crispum* (lemon geranium) and *Pelargonium x melissinum* (lemon balm)

- Lemon myrtle, an Australian bush food, has recently become a popular alternative to lemons.[15] The crushed and dried leaves and edible essential oils have a strong, sweet lemon taste, but contain no citric acid. Lemon myrtle is popular in foods that curdle with lemon juice, such as cheesecake and ice cream.

- Lemon thyme

- Lemon verbena

- Limes, another common sour citrus fruit, used similarly to lemons

- Certain cultivars of mint

- *Magnolia grandiflora* tree flowers

- Several cultivars of hybrid tea roses

2.30.6 Production

As of 2012, the world's top three lemon-producing nations by tonnage were China, India, and Mexico, which together accounted for nearly half (43.5%) of all global production.

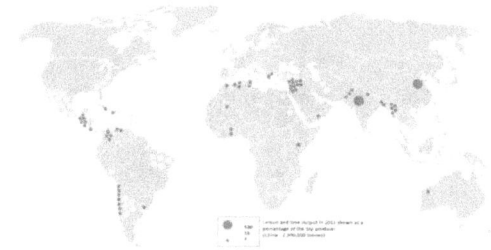

2012 lemon producer countries

2.30.7 Nutritional value and phytochemicals

Lemons are a rich source of vitamin C, providing 64% of the Daily Value in a 100 g serving (table). Other essential nutrients, however, have insignificant content (table).

Lemons contain numerous phytochemicals, including polyphenols and terpenes.[18] As with other citrus fruits, they have significant concentrations of citric acid (about 47 g/l in juice).[19]

2.30.8   Gallery

- Lemon seedling
- Full sized tree
- Green and yellow lemons in growth
- Variegated pink lemon

2.30.9   See also

- List of lemon dishes and beverages

2.30.10   References

[1] Julia F. Morton (1987). "Lemon in Fruits of Warm Climates". Purdue University. pp. 160–168.

[2] Gulsen, O.; M. L. Roose (2001). "Lemons: Diversity and Relationships with Selected *Citrus* Genotypes as Measured with Nuclear Genome Markers". *Journal of the American Society of Horticultural Science* **126**: 309–317.

[3] James Lind (1757). *A treatise on the scurvy. Second edition.* London: A. Millar.

[4] Douglas Harper. "Online Etymology Dictionary".

[5] Spalding, William A. (1885). *The orange: its culture in California.* Riverside, California: Press and Horticulturist Steam Print. p. 88. Retrieved March 2, 2012.

[6] Carque, Otto (2006) [1923]. *Rational Diet: An Advanced Treatise on the Food Question.* Los Angeles, California: Kessinger Publishing. p. 195. ISBN 978-1-4286-4244-7. Retrieved March 2, 2012.

[7] "Complete List of Four Winds Dwarf Citrus Varieties". Fourwindsgrowers.com. Retrieved June 6, 2010.

[8] Buchan, Ursula (January 22, 2005). "Kitchen garden: lemon tree". *The Daily Telegraph* (London). Retrieved January 24, 2014.

[9] Vaiegated pink at the Citrus Variety Collection.

[10] "Taste of a thousand lemons". *Los Angeles Times.* September 8, 2004. Retrieved November 21, 2011.

[11] "New Zealand Citrus". ceventura.ucdavis.edu. Retrieved June 13, 2010.

[12] M. Hofrichter (2010). *Industrial Applications.* Springer. p. 224. ISBN 978-3-642-11458-8.

[13] "6 ingredients for a green, clean home". Shine. Retrieved April 24, 2008.

[14] 9 Ohio State University Research, March 3, 2008 Study is published in the March 2008 issue of the journal *Psychoneuroendocrinology*

[15] "Lemon Power". California Energy Commission. Retrieved December 7, 2014.

[16] Lemon Myrtle

[17] "Production of Lemon and Limes, by Countries". UN Food & Agriculture Organization. 2011. Retrieved January 29, 2015.

[18] Rauf A, Uddin G, Ali J (2014). "Phytochemical analysis and radical scavenging profile of juices of Citrus sinensis, Citrus anrantifolia, and Citrus limonum". *Org Med Chem Lett* **7** (4): 5. doi:10.1186/2191-2858-4-5. PMC 4091952. PMID 25024932.

[19] Penniston KL, Nakada SY, Holmes RP, Assimos DG (2008). "Quantitative Assessment of Citric Acid in Lemon Juice, Lime Juice, and Commercially-Available Fruit Juice Products" (PDF). *Journal of Endourology* **22** (3): 567–570. doi:10.1089/end.2007.0304. PMC 2637791. PMID 18290732.

2.30.11   External links

- Data related to Citrus × limon at Wikispecies

2.31   Monoi oil

Monoï oil[1] is an infused perfume-oil made from soaking the petals of Tahitian gardenias (best known as Tiaré flowers) in coconut oil. Monoï (pronounced Mah-noy) is an ancient Tahitian word meaning "scented oil" in the Reo-Maohi language. Monoï is widely used among French Polynesians as a skin and hair softener. It is also popular in Europe and gaining recognition in the United States.

Today's marketplace is rife with monoi oil imitations. Authentic Tahitian monoi oil follows a strict manufacturing code that oversees the entire process from handpicking the tiare flowers to storage and shipping of the final product. This process has been validated and protected by an Appellation of Origin which was awarded to **Monoi de Tahiti** on April 1, 1992.

2.31.1   History

The date when monoï was first created is unknown; however, its origins can be traced back 2000 years to the Maohi people, the indigenous Polynesians. Early European explorers who travelled to the Polynesian Islands, including James Cook, documented the natives' use of monoi for medicinal, cosmetic and religious purposes. Monoi featured prominently in the lives of these ancient people, from birth until death. It was applied to the bodies of newborns to keep

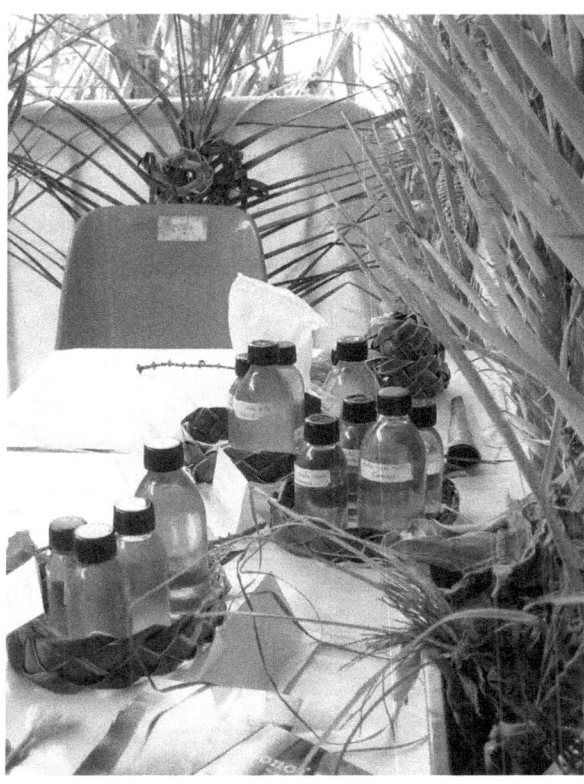

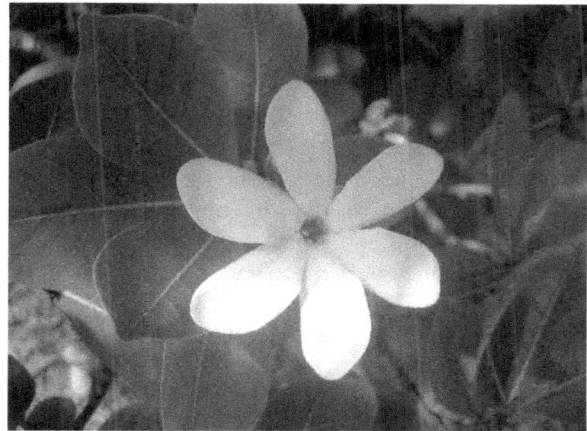

The Tiaré flower.

The Monoi Tiaré Tahiti is a perfume-oil made by infusing the blossoms of Tiaré flowers in coconut oil.

them from dehydrating in hot weather, and from getting chilled in cooler temperatures. When a person died, their body was embalmed and perfumed with manoi to help facilitate their journey into the afterlife.

Monoï was also used in ancient Polynesian religious rites. During ceremonies which took place in the maraes (temples), Maori priests used manoi to anoint sacred objects and purify offerings to their deities.

Maori navigators used manoi to protect their bodies from cold, harsh winds and salt water during long canoe expeditions at sea. (Even today, many divers rub monoi all over their bodies prior to diving for the same purpose.)

In 1942, monoi began to be manufactured commercially.

2.31.2   Ingredients

Tiaré flower

The Tiaré flower (Gardenia tahitensis), from the Rubiaceae family, is Tahiti's national flower. The small white, star-shaped flower grows on 3-foot (0.91 m) high bushes throughout French Polynesia, which features soil of coral origin, and blossoms all year long. Other names for this flower include Tiare Tahiti and Tiare Maohi.

Beyond their contribution to Monoi Tiare Tahiti, tiare flowers are deeply rooted in everyday Polynesian life In traditional medicine, the flower is prepared in a variety of concoctions to alleviate a range of common maladies including the common cold, headaches and sunburn. Many Polynesians enjoy placing a few tiare flowers on a small, water-filled saucer to release the fragrance throughout their "fares" (Polynesian houses). The flower necklaces that are offered to tourists as a welcome gesture are created with tiare flowers, and *vahine* (Polynesian women) customarily wear them behind one ear.

The tiare flowers that are used in Monoi de Tahiti are handpicked at a very particular stage of their growth, specifically when they are still unopened. The flowers are immediately taken to the manufacturing plant and stripped of their pistils. The flower portion is placed in refined coconut oil for a minimum of 15 days. This is known as "enfleurage" (flower soaking), a French term used to designate a specific extraction step. According to specific maceration standards set by the decree of Appellation d'Origine, which each manufacturer must scrupulously follow, a minimum of 15 tiare flowers must be used in every liter of refined coconut oil.

Coconut Oil

Coconut palm trees remain the most utilized Polynesian island tree and cover approximately 150,000 acres (610 km^2) of land. Under favorable conditions, the coconut palm tree grows its first fruits during its 6th year and produces approximately 60 coconuts per year, from its 10th to its 70th year. As the nut begins to form it is completely empty and contains no nutrients. When its size increases, the shell hardens and becomes filled with a transparent liquid that will turn into oil upon full maturity.

When the coconuts fall from the trees, they are gathered to undergo the ancient process of extracting the coconut almonds. The shell is cracked open with an ax. The two coconut halves are left for several hours in the sun, until the almonds have shrunk enough to be removed and broken into small pieces. The fragments are then taken to special flat wooden barracks covered with sliding metal roofs which are popularly known on the Polynesian islands as "*coprah* dryers". The sliding roofs are only used at night and during the rainy season. The *coprah* is left to dry for more than a week until the coconut meat has lost over 90% of its moisture.

Placed into special natural fiber bags, the coconut fragments are shipped to the unique oil mill located on the island of Tahiti where they will be thrown into special machines and ground to a fine coco flour. The flour is then heated up to 125 degrees and finally pressed into raw coconut oil. After that step, the oil will undergo more refining to remove all impurities and obtain the highest possible quality.

Once the refining process is completed the coconut oil is placed into special storage tanks until it is purchased by one of only a handful of Monoi manufacturers. These manufacturers will proceed individually to the final maceration step which is to infuse the oil with Tiare flowers. Monoi de Tahiti must be stored in drums with a food-suitable liner or material. Drums must be lead-sealed when they leave Tahiti and kept away from humidity, light and heat.

2.31.3 Common uses

Recent manufacturer tests verify that monoi oil is rich in methyl salicylate which is a skin-soothing agent. It is a naturally concentrated emollient which penetrates the skin, rehydrates the layers of the epidermis and shields skin against external damages including sun and wind.

Monoi oil is used:

- After a shower or bath to rehydrate skin to its natural healthy look

- Before or after a swim, it provides protection against the effects of sun, wind, sea or pool water

- As a pre-shampoo hot oil treatment, it helps repair and deep condition the hair to a healthy shine.

- During a bath. A few drops in the water reportedly encourages relaxation while keeping skin soft and subtly fragrant.

- As a dark tanning oil

- After being warmed in the palms of the hands, it is suited for massaging sore parts of the body or for warming up a weak body.

- As a pain reliever for sunburn.

2.31.4 References

[1] Monoï Tiaré Tahiti History

2.31.5 External links

- Monoï Institute

- Moana Beauty, Guide to Using Monoi Oil on Hair

2.32 Mustard oil

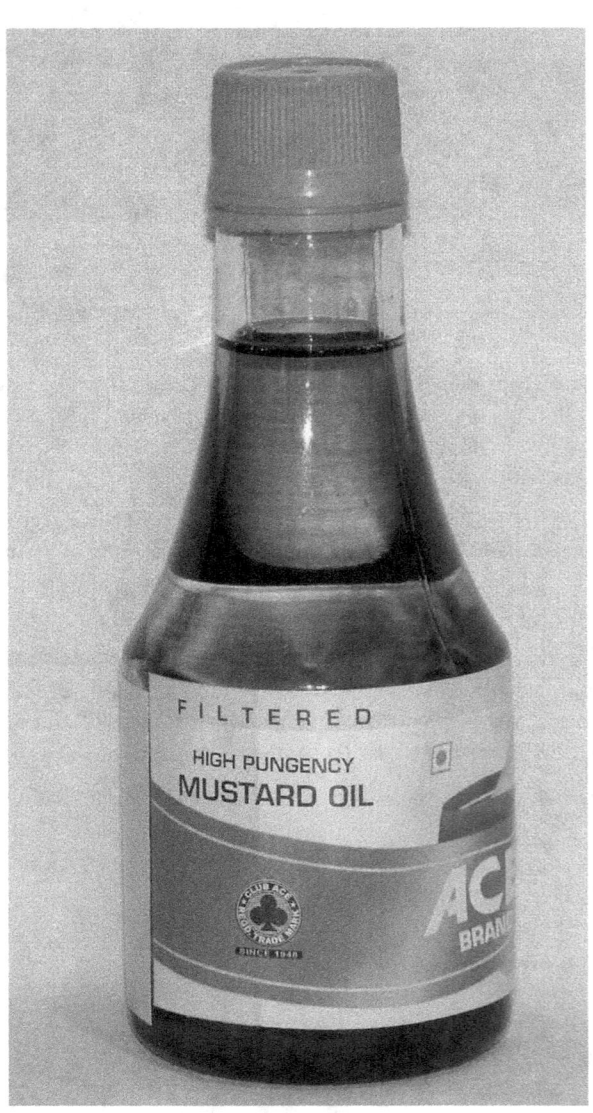

Mustard oil

The term **mustard oil** is used for two different oils that are made from mustard seeds:

- A fatty vegetable oil resulting from pressing the seeds,

- An essential oil resulting from grinding the seeds, mixing them with water, and extracting the resulting volatile oil by distillation.

The pungency of mustard oil is due to the presence of allyl isothiocyanate, an activator of the TRPA1 channel.

2.32.1 Pressed oil

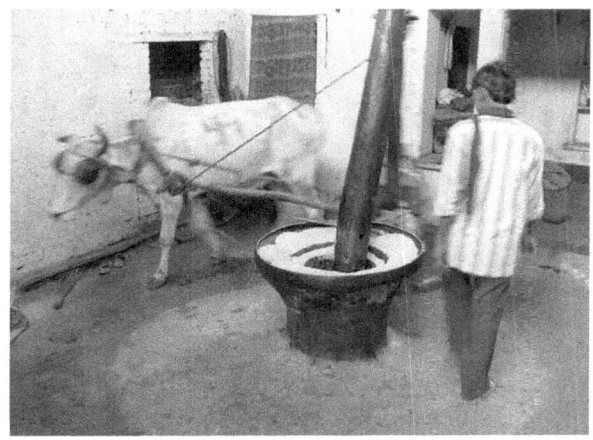

Ox-powered mill grinding mustard seed for oil

This oil has a distinctive pungent taste, characteristic of all plants in the mustard (Brassicaceae) family (for example, cabbage, cauliflower, turnip, radish, horseradish or wasabi). It is often used for cooking in North India, Eastern India, Nepal, Bangladesh and Pakistan. In Bengal, Orissa, Assam and Nepal, it is the traditionally preferred oil for cooking. The oil makes up about 30% of the mustard seeds. It can be produced from black mustard (*Brassica nigra*), brown Indian mustard (*B. juncea*), and white mustard (*B. hirta*).

The characteristic pungent flavour of mustard oil is due to allyl isothiocyanate. Mustard oil has about 60% monounsaturated fatty acids (42% erucic acid and 12% oleic acid); it has about 21% polyunsaturated fats (6% the omega-3 alpha-linolenic acid and 15% the omega-6 linoleic acid), and it has about 12% saturated fats.[1]

Effects on health

Mustard oil has high levels of both alpha-linolenic acid and erucic acid.

Based on studies done on laboratory animals in the early 1970s,[2] erucic acid appears to have toxic effects on the heart at high enough doses.[3] While no negative health effects of any exposure to erucic acid have been documented in humans, publication of those studies led to governments worldwide moving away from oils with high levels of erucic acid,[2] and tolerance levels for human exposure to erucic acid have been established based on the animal studies.[3] Mustard oil is not allowed to be imported or sold in the U.S. for use in cooking, due to its high erucic acid content.[4]

Including oils in the diet that are high in alpha-linolenic acid has been thought to protect the heart and to prevent cardiovascular disease, but recent reviews have cast doubt on this, finding only slightly positive outcomes or even negative outcomes.[5][6][7][8]

Two studies on health effects of mustard oil have been conducted in India, which had conflicting results. One found that mustard oil had no protective effect on the heart, and the authors reckoned that the benefits of alpha-linolenic acid were outweighed by the harm of erucic acid,[9] while another study found that mustard oil had a protective effect, and the authors reckoned that the benefits of alpha-linolenic acid outweighed the harm of erucic acid.[10]

The use of mustard oils in traditional societies for infant massage has been identified by one study as risking damaging skin integrity and permeability.[11] Other studies over larger samples have shown that massaging with mustard oil improved the weight, length, and midarm and midleg circumferences as compared to infants without massage, although sesame oil is a better candidate for this than mustard oil.[12]

Nutritional information

According to the USDA,[13] 1 tbsp of mustard oil contains:

- Calories: 126

- Fat: 14

- Carbohydrates: 0

- Fibers: 0

- Protein: 0

2.32.2 Essential oil

The pungency of the condiment mustard results when ground mustard seeds are mixed with water, vinegar, or other liquid (or even when chewed). Under these conditions, a chemical reaction between the enzyme myrosinase and a glucosinolate known as sinigrin from the seeds of black mustard (*Brassica nigra*) or brown Indian mustard (*Brassica juncea*) produces allyl isothiocyanate. By distillation one can produce a very sharp-tasting essential oil, sometimes called **volatile oil of mustard**, containing more than 92% allyl isothiocyanate. The pungency of allyl isothiocyanate is due to the activation of the TRPA1 ion channel in sensory neurons. White mustard (*Brassica hirta*) does not yield *allyl* isothiocyanate, but a different and milder isothiocyanate.[14]

Allyl isothiocyanate serves the plant as a defense against herbivores. Since it is harmful to the plant itself, it is stored in the harmless form of a glucosinolate, separate from the myrosinase enzyme. Once the herbivore chews the plant, the noxious allyl isothiocyanate is produced. Allyl isothiocyanate is also responsible for the pungent taste of horseradish and wasabi. It can be produced synthetically, sometimes known as **synthetic mustard oil**.[15]

Because of the contained allyl isothiocyanate, this type of mustard oil is toxic and irritates the skin and mucous membranes. In very small amounts, it is often used by the food industry for flavoring. In northern Italy, for instance, it is used in the fruit condiment called *mostarda*. It is also used to repel cats and dogs. It will also denature alcohol, making it unfit for human consumption, thus avoiding the taxes collected on alcoholic beverages.

The CAS number of this type of mustard oil is 8007-40-7, and the CAS number of pure allyl isothiocyanate is 57-06-7.

2.32.3 Use in North Indian, Bangladeshi and Pakistani cultural and artistic activities

Mustard oil was once popular as a cooking oil in northern India and Pakistan and is still the chief ingredient used in Bengali cuisine of Eastern India and Bangladesh. In the second half of the 20th century the popularity of mustard oil receded in Northern India and Pakistan due to the availability of mass-produced vegetable oils. It is still intricately embedded in the culture:

- It is poured on both sides of the threshold when someone important comes home for the first time (e.g. a newly-wedded couple or a son or daughter when returning after a long absence, or succeeding in exams or an election.

- Used as traditional jaggo pot fuel in Punjabi, Bengali and many other weddings in different part of India.

- Used as part of home-made cosmetics during mayian.

- Used as fuel for lighting earthen lamps (diyas) on festive occasions such as Diwali.

- Used in instruments. The residue cake from the mustard oil pressing is mixed with sand, mustard oil and (sometimes) tar. The resulting sticky mixture is then smeared on the inside of Dholak and Dholki membranes to add weight (from underneath) to the bass membrane. This enables the typical Indian drum glissando sound, created by rubbing the heel of the hand over it. This is also known as a (Tel masala) Dholak Masala or oil syahi.

2.32.4 See also

- List of mustard brands

2.32.5 References

[1] Entry for mustard oil in the USDA National Nutrient Database for Standard Reference, Release 22

[2] Amy McInnis, 21 May 2004 The Transformation of Rapeseed Into Canola: A Cinderella Story

[3] Food Standards Australia New Zealand (June 2003) Erucic acid in food : *A Toxicological Review and Risk Assessment*. Technical report series No. 21; Page 4 paragraph 1; ISBN 0-642-34526-0, ISSN 1448-3017

[4] FDA, 18 March 2011 FDA Import Alert 26-04

[5] Pan A et al. α-Linolenic acid and risk of cardiovascular disease: a systematic review and meta-analysis. *Am J Clin Nutr*. 2012 Dec;96(6):1262-73. PMID 23076616

[6] Vedtofte MS et al. The role of essential fatty acids in the control of coronary heart disease. Curr Opin Clin Nutr Metab Care. 2012 Nov;15(6):592-6. PMID 23037902

[7] Salter AM. Dietary fatty acids and cardiovascular disease. Animal. 2013 Mar;7(Suppl 1):163-71. PMID 23031737

[8] Billman GE. The effects of omega-3 polyunsaturated fatty acids on cardiac rhythm: a critical reassessment. Pharmacol Ther. 2013 Oct;140(1):53-80. PMID 23735203

[9] Ghafoorunissa. Requirements of dietary fats to meet nutritional needs & prevent the risk of atherosclerosis--an Indian perspective. Indian J Med Res. 1998 Nov;108:191-202. PMID 9863275

[10] Rastogi T, Reddy KS, Vaz M, et al. (April 2004). "Diet and risk of ischemic heart disease in India". *Am. J. Clin. Nutr.* **79** (4): 582–92. PMID 15051601.

[11] Darmstadt GL, Mao-Qiang M, Chi E, Saha SK, Ziboh VA, Black RE, Santosham M, Elias PM. (2002). Impact of topical oils on the skin barrier: possible implications for neonatal health in developing countries. Acta Paediatr. 91(5):546-54. PMID 12113324

[12] Effects of massage & use of oil on growth, blood flow & sleep pattern in infants, Agarwal KN, Gupta A, Pushkarna R, Bhargava SK, Faridi MM, Prabhu MK, Indian J Med Res. 2000 Dec;112:212-7, PMID 11247199

[13] http://www.nal.usda.gov/fnic/foodcomp/search/

[14] "Mustard". *A Guide to Medicinal and Aromatic Plants.* Center for New Crops and Plant Products, Purdue University. Retrieved 3 January 2009.

[15] "Mustard Oil, Synthetic". JT Baker. Retrieved 3 March 2010.

2.32.6 External links

- Effect of an Indo-Mediterranean diet on progression of coronary artery disease in high risk patients (Indo-Mediterranean Diet Heart Study) a randomised single-blind trial.

- Isolation of Erucic Acid from Mustard Seed Oil by Candida rugosa lipase

- Tanuja Rastogi; Reddy, KS; Vaz, M; Spiegelman, D; Prabhakaran, D; Willett, WC; Stampfer, MJ; Ascherio, A (2004). "Diet and risk of ischemic heart disease in India". *American Journal of Clinical Nutrition* **79** (4): 582–592. PMID 15051601.

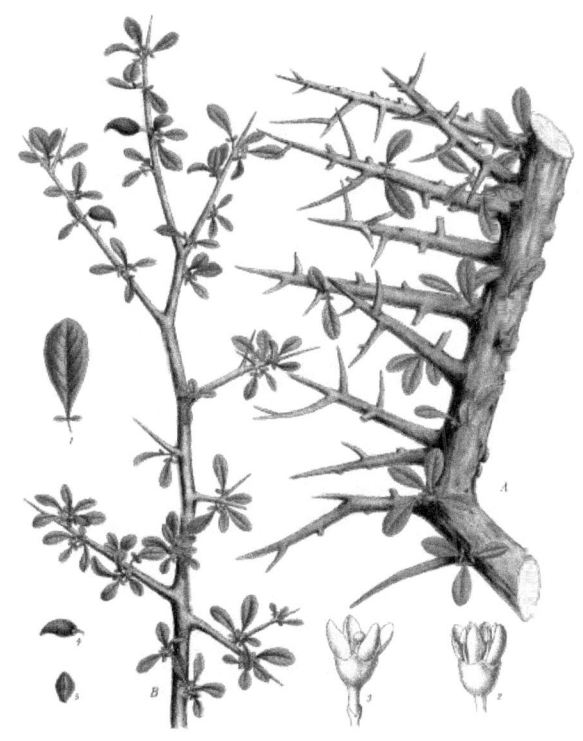

Commiphora myrrha *tree, one of the primary trees from which myrrh is harvested.*

2.33 Myrrh

For the record label, see Myrrh Records.

Myrrh /ˈmɜr/ from the Hebrew '"מור"' (ᶜmor") and Arabic مر (*mur*) is the aromatic resin of a number of small, thorny tree species of the genus *Commiphora*,[1] which is an essential oil termed an *oleoresin*. Myrrh resin is a natural gum. It has been used throughout history as a perfume, incense and medicine. It can also be ingested by mixing it with wine.[2]

When a tree wound penetrates through the bark and into the sapwood, the tree bleeds a resin. Myrrh gum, like frankincense, is such a resin. When people harvest myrrh, they wound the trees repeatedly to bleed them of the gum. Myrrh gum is waxy, and coagulates quickly. After the harvest, the gum becomes hard and glossy. The gum is yellowish, and may be either clear or opaque. It darkens deeply as it ages, and white streaks emerge.[3]

Myrrh gum is commonly harvested from the species *Commiphora myrrha*, which is native to Yemen, Somalia, Eritrea and eastern Ethiopia. Another commonly used name, *Commiphora molmol*,[4] is now considered a synonym of *Commiphora myrrha*.[5] The related *Commiphora*

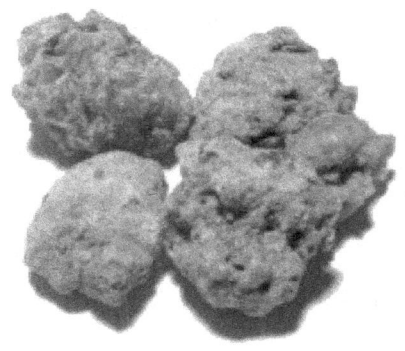

Myrrh is a common resin in the Horn of Africa.

gileadensis, native to Eastern Mediterranean and particularly the Arabian Peninsula,[6] is the biblically referenced Balm of Gilead,[7] also known as Balsam of Mecca. Several other species yield bdellium and Indian myrrh.

The oleo gum resins of a number of other *Commiphora* species are also used as perfumes, medicines (such

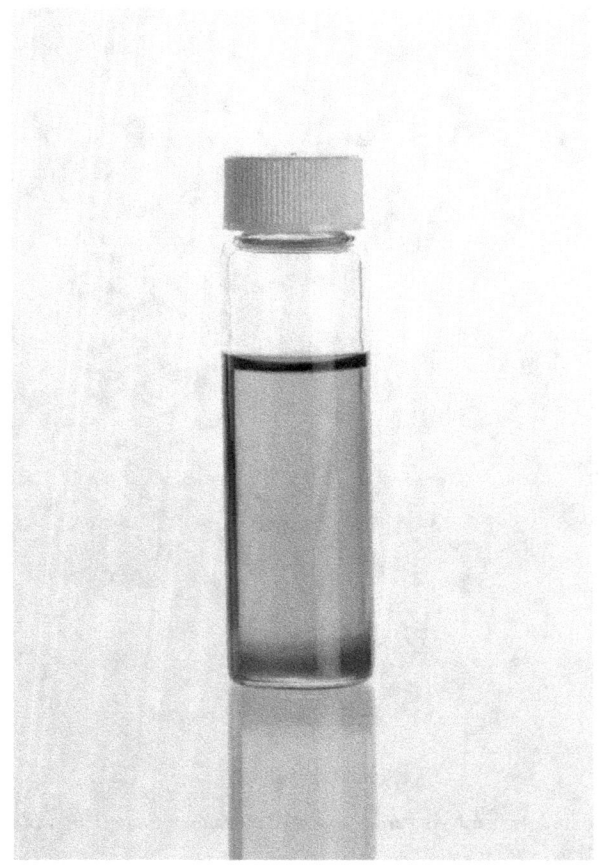

*An essential oil extracted from myrrh (*Commiphora myrrha*)*

as aromatic wound dressings), and incense ingredients. These myrrh-like resins are known as opopanax, balsam, bdellium, guggul and bisabol.

Fragrant "myrrh beads" are made from the crushed seeds of *Detarium microcarpum*, an unrelated West African tree. These beads are traditionally worn by married women in Mali as multiple strands around the hips.

The name "myrrh" is also applied to the potherb *Myrrhis odorata*, otherwise known as "cicely" or "sweet cicely".

Myrrh is mentioned in the Old Testament numerous times as a rare perfume with intoxicating qualities, such as Genesis 37:25 and Exodus 30:23.

Myrrh is also found in the Christian Bible as one of the three gifts the wise men presented to the Christ Child, according to the gospel of Matthew. According to the gospel of Mark, Jesus was offered wine and myrrh before the crucifixion.

2.33.1 Etymology

The word "myrrh" derives from the Aramaic ???????? (*murr*), and Arabic مر (*mur*), meaning "bitter". Its name

entered the English language from the Hebrew Bible, where it is called *mor*, מור, and later as a Semitic loanword[8] was used in the Greek myth of Myrrha, and later in the Septuagint; in the Greek language, the related word μύρον (*mýron*) became a general term for perfume.

2.33.2 Attributed medicinal properties

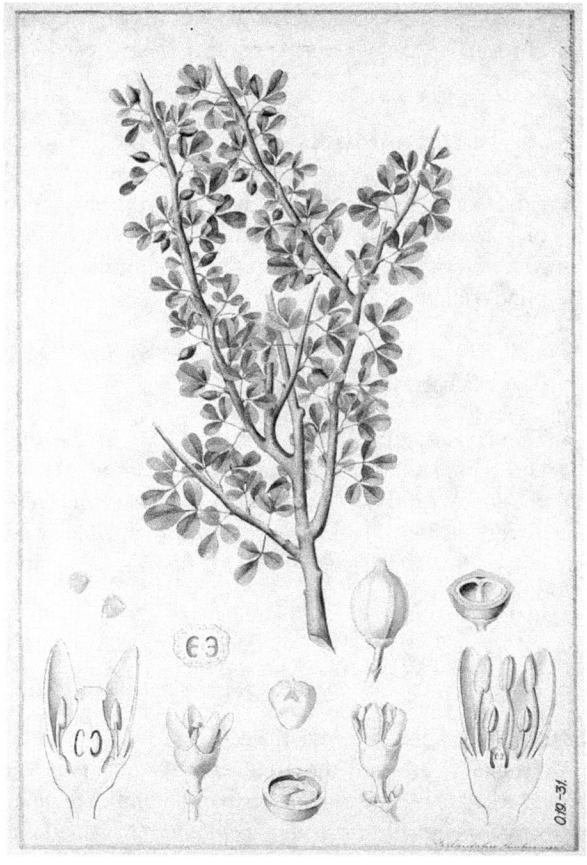

Commiphora gileadensis *(listed as "Balsamodendron ehrenbergianum"*

Conventional medicine

In pharmacy, myrrh is used as an antiseptic in mouthwashes, gargles, and toothpastes[9] Myrrh is currently used in some liniments and healing salves that may be applied to abrasions and other minor skin ailments. Myrrh has also been recommended as an analgesic for toothaches, and can be used in liniment for bruises, aches, and sprains.[10]

Myrrh is a common ingredient of tooth powders. Myrrh and borax in tincture can be used as a mouth-wash. A compound tincture, or horse tincture, using myrrh is used in veterinary practice for healing wounds. Meetiga, the trade-name of Arabian Myrrh, is more brittle and gummy than that of the Somalian variety and does not have the latter's white markings. Liquid Myrrh, or Stacte, spoken of by Pliny, also an ingredient of Jewish holy incense, was formerly obtainable and greatly valued but cannot now be identified in today's markets. Myrrh gum is used for indigestion, ulcers, colds, cough, asthma, lung congestion, arthritis pain, and cancer.[11]

> "As part of a larger search for anticancer compounds from plants, the researchers obtained extracts from a particular species of myrrh plant (*Commiphora myrrha*) and tested it against a human breast tumor cell line (MCF-7) known to be resistant to anticancer drugs. Research data indicated that the extract killed all of the cancer cells in laboratory dishes.".[12]

Traditional Chinese medicine

In traditional Chinese medicine, myrrh is classified as bitter and spicy, with a neutral temperature. It is said to have special efficacy on the heart, liver, and spleen meridians, as well as "blood-moving" powers to purge stagnant blood from the uterus. It is therefore recommended for rheumatic, arthritic, and circulatory problems, and for amenorrhea, dysmenorrhea, menopause, and uterine tumors.

Myrrh's uses are similar to those of frankincense, with which it is often combined in decoctions, liniments and incense. When used in concert, myrrh is "blood-moving" while frankincense moves the *Qi*, making it more useful for arthritic conditions.

It is combined with such herbs as notoginseng, safflower petals, angelica sinensis, cinnamon, and salvia miltiorrhiza, usually in alcohol, and used both internally and externally.[13]

Ayurvedic medicine

Myrrh is used more frequently in Ayurveda and Unani medicine, which ascribe tonic and rejuvenative properties to the resin. It (*daindhava*) is utilized in many specially processed *rasayana* formulas in Ayurveda. However, non-*rasayana* myrrh is contraindicated when kidney dysfunction or stomach pain is apparent, or for women who are pregnant or have excessive uterine bleeding.

A related species, called *guggul* in Ayurvedic medicine, is considered one of the best substances for the treatment of circulatory problems, nervous system disorders and rheumatic complaints.[14][15]

Mechanisms of action

In an attempt to determine the cause of its effectiveness, researchers examined the individual ingredients of a herbal formula used traditionally by Kuwaiti diabetics to lower blood glucose. Myrrh and aloe gums effectively improved glucose tolerance in both normal and diabetic rats.[16]

Myrrh was shown to produce analgesic effects on mice which were subjected to pain. Researchers at the University of Florence showed that sesquiterpenes furanoeudesma-1,3-diene and curzarene in the myrrh affect opioid receptors in the mouse's brain which influence pain perception.[17][18]

Mirazid, an Egyptian drug made from myrrh, has been investigated as an oral treatment of parasitic ailments, including fascioliasis and schistosomiasis.[19]

Myrrh has been shown to lower LDL cholesterol (bad cholesterol) levels, as well as to increase the HDL cholesterol (good cholesterol) in various tests on humans done in the past few decades. A 2009 laboratory test showed this same effect on albino rats.[20]

In studies done on mice, myrrh has been shown to have significant inhibiting effects on certain types of cancer. The active constituents of myrrh accredited with this property are sesquiterpenes. These tests were done using the myrrh species *Commiphora molmol*, and were also found to inhibit tumor growth.[21]

2.33.3 Religious ritual

Myrrh was used by the ancient Egyptians, along with natron, for the embalming of mummies.[22]

Myrrh was an ingredient of Ketoret, the consecrated incense used in the First and Second Temples at Jerusalem, as described in the Hebrew Bible and Talmud. An offering was made of the Ketoret on a special incense altar, and was an important component of the Temple service. Myrrh is also listed as an ingredient in the holy anointing oil used to anoint the Tabernacle, high priests and kings.

Oil of myrrh is used in the book of Esther (2:12) in a purification ritual for the new queen to King Ahasuerus:

> "Now when every maid's turn was come to go in to king Ahasuerus, after that she had been twelve months, according to the manner of the women, (for so were the days of their purifications accomplished, to wit, six months with oil of myrrh, and six months with sweet odors, and with other things for the purifying of the women;)[23]

Myrrh was traded by camel caravans overland from areas

of production in southern Arabia by the Nabataeans to their capital city of Petra, from which it was distributed throughout the Mediterranean region.[7]

According to the book of Matthew 2:11, gold, frankincense and myrrh were among the gifts to Jesus by the Biblical Magi "from the East." Because of its mention in New Testament, myrrh is an incense offered during Christian liturgical celebrations (see Thurible). Liquid myrrh is sometimes added to egg tempera in the making of icons.

Matthew records that as Jesus went to the cross, they gave him vinegar to drink mingled with gall: and when he had tasted thereof, he would not drink (Matthew 27:34). Mark described the drink as wine mingled with myrrh (Mark 15:23).

Myrrh is mixed with frankincense and sometimes more scents and is used in almost every service of the Eastern Orthodox, Oriental Orthodox, traditional Roman Catholic and Anglican/Episcopal Churches.

Myrrh is also used to prepare the sacramental chrism used by many churches of both Eastern and Western rites. In the Middle East, the Eastern Orthodox Church traditionally uses oil scented with myrrh (and other fragrances) to perform the sacrament of chrismation, which is commonly referred to as "receiving the Chrism".

In the bible myrrh is mentioned 156 times.[24]

According to the Encyclopedia of Islamic Herbal Medicine, "The Messenger of Allah stated, 'Fumigate your houses with al-shih, murr, and sa'tar.'" The author claims that this use of the word "murr" refers specifically to Commiphora myrrha.[25]

2.33.4 Ancient myrrh

Modern myrrh has long been commented on as coming from a different source to that held in high regard by the ancients, having been superior in some way. Pedanius Dioscorides described the myrrh of the first century AD as most likely to refer to a *"species of mimosa"*, describing it *"like the Egyptian thorn"*. He describes its appearance and leaf structure as *"pinnate-winged"*. The ancient type of myrrh conjectured was noted for possessing a far more delightful odor than the modern. It was noted in 1837 that *"The time, perhaps, is not far distant, when, through the spirit of research, the true myrrh-tree will be found".[26]*

2.33.5 See also

- Bdellium
- Chrism
- Frankincense
- Naturalis Historia
- Pliny the Elder

2.33.6 Footnotes

[1] Rice, Patty C., *Amber: Golden Gem of the Ages*, Author House, Bloomington, 2006 p.321

[2] Wondill Froman (30 November 2005). *Biblical Facts About Wine: Is It a Sin to Drink Wine?*. AuthorHouse. pp. 307–. ISBN 978-1-4184-0964-7. Retrieved 15 November 2012.

[3] Caspar Neumann, William Lewis, *The chemical works of Caspar Neumann, M.D.*,2nd Ed., Vol 3, London, 1773 p.55

[4] Newnes, G., ed., *Chambers's encyclopædia*, Volume 9, 1959

[5] *The Plant List*. 2013. Version 1.1. Published on the Internet: http://www.theplantlist.org/. Accessed on February 24, 2014.

[6] Anthony G. Miller, Thomas A. Cope, J. A. Nyberg *Flora of the Arabian Peninsula and Socotra*, Volume 1, Edinburgh University Press, 1996, p.20

[7] Gibson (2011), p. 160.

[8] Klein, Ernest, *A Comprehensive Etymological Dictionary of the Hebrew Language for Readers of English*, The University of Haifa, Carta, Jerusalem, p.380

[9] "Species Information". www.worldagroforestrycentre.org. Archived from the original on September 30, 2011. Retrieved 2009-01-15.

[10] "ICS-UNIDO – MAPs". www.ics.trieste.it. Retrieved 2009-01-16.

[11] Al Faraj, S (2005). "Antagonism of the anticoagulant effect of warfarin caused by the use of Commiphora molmol as a herbal medication: A case report". *Annals of tropical medicine and parasitology* **99** (2): 219–20. doi:10.1179/136485905X17434. PMID 15814041.

[12] American Chemical Society (2001, December 5). "Gift Of The Magi" Bears Anti-Cancer Agents, Researchers Suggest. ScienceDaily. Retrieved April 12, 2013, from http://www.sciencedaily.com/releases/2001/12/011205070038.htm

[13] Michael Tierra. "The Emmenagogues"

[14] Michael Moore *Materia Medica*

[15] Alan Tillotson "Myrrh"

[16] Al-Awadi, FM; Gumaa, KA (1987). "Studies on the activity of individual plants of an antidiabetic plant mixture". *Acta diabetologica latina* **24** (1): 37–41. doi:10.1007/BF02732051. PMID 3618079.

[17] Dolara, Piero; Luceri, Cristina; Ghelardini, Carla; Monserrat, Claudia; Aiolli, Silvia; Luceri, Francesca; Lodovici, Maura; Menichetti, Stefano; Romanelli, Maria Novella (1996). "Analgesic effects of myrrh". *Nature* **379** (6560): 29. doi:10.1038/379029a0. PMID 8538737.

[18] Dolara P, Luceri C, Ghelardini C, et al. Analgesic effects of myrrh. Nature 1996; 379:29. Summary

[19] See, for example, Soliman, OE; El-Arman, M; Abdul-Samie, ER; El-Nemr, HI; Massoud, A (2004). "Evaluation of myrrh (Mirazid) therapy in fascioliasis and intestinal schistosomiasis in children: Immunological and parasitological study". *Journal of the Egyptian Society of Parasitology* **34** (3): 941–66. PMID 15587320.

[20] Amoudi, Nadia Saleh Al (2009). "Hypocholesterolemic effect of some plants and their blend as studied on albino rats". *International Journal of Food Safety, Nutrition and Public Health* **2** (2): 176. doi:10.1504/IJFSNPH.2009.029283.

[21] Morrow. John A. "Encyclopedia of Islamic Herbal Medicine". Jefferson, N.C.: McFarland, 2011, p. 146.

[22] Fritze, Ronald H. "New worlds: The great voyages of discovery 1400-1600". Sutton Publishing Limited, 2002, p. 25.

[23] http://www.kingjamesbibleonline.org/1611_Esther-2-12/ KJV Esther 2:12

[24] http://www.experience-essential-oils.com/ benefits-of-myrrh.html

[25] Morrow, Joh A. "Encyclopedia of Islamic Herbal Medicine". Jefferson, N.C.: McFarland, 2011, p. 145.

[26] *The visitor or monthly instructor*. Religious Tract Society. 1837. pp. 35–. Retrieved 9 May 2013.

2.33.7 References

• Gibson, Dan (2011). *Qur'anic Geography: A Survey and Evaluation of the Geographical References in the Qur'an with Suggested Solutions for Various Problems and Issues*. Independent Scholars Press, Canada. ISBN 978-0-9733642-8-6.

2.33.8 Further reading

• Massoud A, El Sisi S, Salama O, Massoud A (2001). "Preliminary study of therapeutic efficacy of a new fasciolicidal drug derived from *Commiphora molmol* (myrrh)". *Am J Trop Med Hyg* **65** (2): 96–99. PMID 11508399.

• Dalby, Andrew (2000). *Dangerous Tastes: the story of spices*. London: British Museum Press. ISBN 0-7141-2720-5. (US ISBN 0-520-22789-1), pp. 107–122.

• Dalby, Andrew (2003). *Food in the ancient world from A to Z*. London, New York: Routledge. ISBN 0-415-23259-7., pp. 226–227, with additions

• Monfieur Pomet (1709). "Abyssine Myrrh)". *History of Drugs*. Abyssine Myrrh

• *The One Earth Herbal Sourcebook: Everything You Need to Know About Chinese, Western, and Ayurvedic Herbal Treatments* by Ph.D., A.H.G., D.Ay, Alan Keith Tillotson, O.M.D., L.Ac., Nai-shing Hu Tillotson, and M.D., Robert Abel Jr.

• Abdul-Ghani, RA; Loutfy, N; Hassan, A (2009). "Myrrh and trematodoses in Egypt: An overview of safety, efficacy and effectiveness profiles". *Parasitology international* **58** (3): 210–4. doi:10.1016/j.parint.2009.04.006. PMID 19446652. (A good review on its antiparasitic activities) .

2.33.9 External links

• History of Myrrh and Frankincense (www.imonline. org)

• Myrrh article by James A. Duke (www. herbcompanion.com)

2.34 Myrtol standardized

Myrtol standardized is an essential oil derived from *Pinus* spp (pine), *Citrus aurantifolia* (lime) and *Eucalyptus globulus*[1] and most commonly found in various herbal-based remedies for sinus problems.

Myrtol standardized is a phytotherapeutic extract (distillate) consisting mainly of three monoterpenes: (+)-α-pinene, d-limonene and 1,8-cineole (as known as *Eucalyptol*, but not be confused with Eucalyptus oil).[2] For example, in one product (Gelomyrtol forte) the ratio between distillates of Eucalyptol (eucalyptus oil extract), D-limonene (lemon peel extract), and an essential oil mixture of Myrtle and lemon, is (66:32:1:1). This can be somewhat confusing since the first two ingredients are part of the second two.

One systematic review of herbal medicines used for the treatment of rhinosinusitis concluded that the data from clinical study is insufficient to verify the effectiveness of Myrtol.[1] A comprehensive multi-centre, randomised, double-blind, placebo-controlled clinical trial measuring the efficacy of Myrtol for treating acute bronchitis concluded that Myrtol is a statistically significantly superior to placebo in treating acute bronchitis.[3]

2.34.1 References

[1] Guo, R; Canter, PH; Ernst, E (2006). "Herbal medicines for the treatment of rhinosinusitis: A systematic review". *Otolaryngology--head and neck surgery : official journal of American Academy of Otolaryngology-Head and Neck Surgery* **135** (4): 496–506. doi:10.1016/j.otohns.2006.06.1254. PMID 17011407.

[2] Matthys, H; De Mey, C; Carls, C; Ryś, A; Geib, A; Wittig, T (2000). "Efficacy and tolerability of myrtol standardized in acute bronchitis. A multi-centre, randomised, double-blind, placebo-controlled parallel group clinical trial vs. Cefuroxime and ambroxol". *Arzneimittel-Forschung* **50** (8): 700–11. doi:10.1055/s-0031-1300276. PMID 10994153.

[3] Matthys, H; De Mey, C; Carls, C; Ryś, A; Geib, A; Wittig, T (2000). "Efficacy and tolerability of myrtol standardized in acute bronchitis. A multi-centre, randomised, double-blind, placebo-controlled parallel group clinical trial vs. Cefuroxime and ambroxol". *Arzneimittel-Forschung* **50** (8): 700–11. doi:10.1055/s-0031-1300276. PMID 10994153.

2.35 Neroli

For Brian Eno Album, see Neroli (album).

Neroli oil is an essential oil produced from the blossom

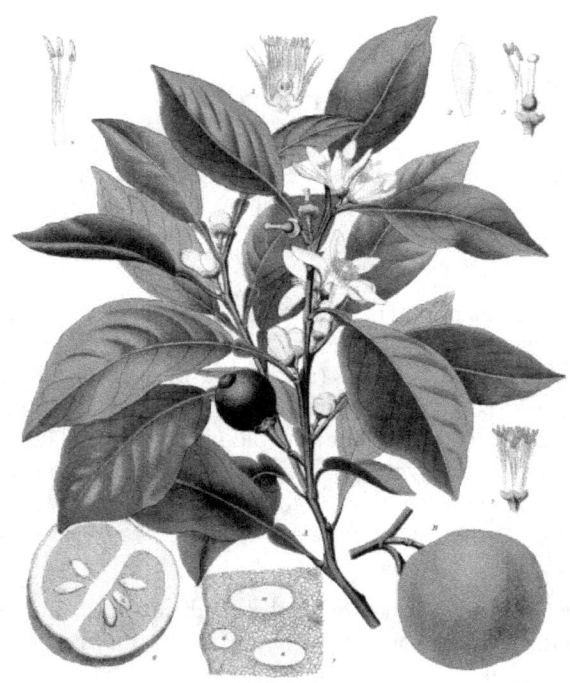

Bitter orange foliage, blossoms and fruit

of the bitter orange tree (*Citrus aurantium subsp. amara* or *Bigaradia*). Its scent is sweet, honeyed and somewhat

metallic with green and spicy facets. Orange blossom is also extracted from the same blossom and both extracts are extensively used in perfumery. Orange blossom can be described as smelling sweeter, warmer and more floral than neroli. The difference between how neroli and orange blossom smell and why they are referred to with different names, is a result of the process of extraction that is used to obtain the oil from the blooms. Neroli is extracted by steam distillation and orange blossom is extracted via a process of enfleurage.

2.35.1 Production

The blossoms are gathered, usually by hand, in late April to early May. The oil is extracted by careful steam distillation.

2.35.2 History

By the end of the 17th century, Anne Marie Orsini, duchess of Bracciano and princess of Nerola, Italy, introduced the essence of bitter orange tree as a fashionable fragrance by using it to perfume her gloves and her bath. Since then, the term "neroli" has been used to describe this essence. Neroli has a refreshing and distinctive, spicy aroma with sweet and flowery notes.

2.35.3 Use

It is one of the most widely used floral oils in perfumery. It is a nontoxic, nonirritant, nonsensitizing, nonphototoxic substance. It blends well with any citrus oil, various floral absolutes, and most of the synthetic components available on the market. Neroli oil is a classic element in fragrance design and one of the most commonly used in the industry.

It also has a limited use in flavorings. Neroli oil is reportedly one of the ingredients in the closely guarded secret recipe for the Coca-Cola soft drink.[1] It is a flavoring ingredient of open source cola recipes,[2] although some variants consider it as optional, owing to the high cost.[3]

2.35.4 See also

- Nerol

- Orange oil

- Orange flower water

- Petitgrain oil

- Citrus aurantium

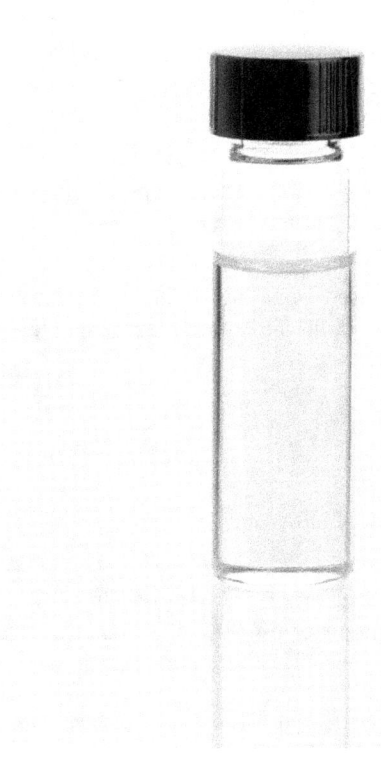

*Neroli (*Citrus aurantium*) essential oil in a clear glass vial*

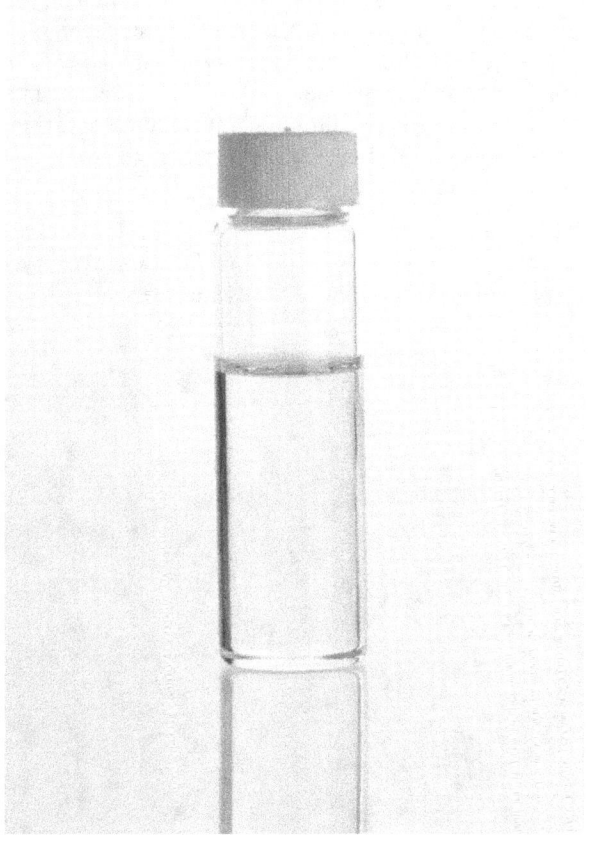

*Nutmeg (*Myristica fragrans*) essential oil*

2.35.5 References

[1] "This American Life, episode#437, Original Recipe". Retrieved 2011-02-15.

[2] "OpenCola Softdrink". Retrieved 2009-05-06.

[3] "Cube-Cola Recipe". Cube Cinema, Bristol. 25 October 2008.

2.35.6 External links

- Entry in the British Pharmaceutical Codex from 1911

2.36 Nutmeg oil

Nutmeg oil is a volatile essential oil from nutmeg (*Myristica fragrans*) containing borneol and eugenol.

2.36.1 General uses

The essential oil is obtained by the steam distillation of ground nutmeg and is used heavily in the perfumery and pharmaceutical industries. The oil is colorless or light yellow and smells and tastes of nutmeg. It contains numerous components of interest to the oleochemical industry, and is used as a natural food flavouring in baked goods, syrups (e.g. Coca Cola), beverages, sweets etc. It replaces ground nutmeg as it leaves no particles in the food. The essential oil is also used in the cosmetic and pharmaceutical industries for instance in tooth paste and as a major ingredient in some cough syrups. In traditional medicine nutmeg and nutmeg oil were used for illnesses related to the nervous and digestive systems . The oil contains myristicin and elemicin which are suspected to be responsible for the hallucinogenic properties of nutmeg oil.

2.36.2 External uses

Externally, the oil is used for rheumatic pain and, like clove oil, can be applied as an emergency treatment to dull toothache. In France, it is given in drop doses in honey for digestive upsets and used for bad breath. Some recommend using one or two drops on a cotton swab, and apply to the gums around an aching tooth until dental treatment can be obtained; or three to five drops on a sugar lump or in a teaspoon of honey for nausea, gastroenteritis, chronic diarrhea, and indigestion.

Alternatively, a massage oil can be created for muscular pains associated with rheumatism or overexertion. It can also be combined with thyme or rosemary essential oils.

2.36.3   See also

- Nutmeg

- Essential oils

2.37   Oil of clove

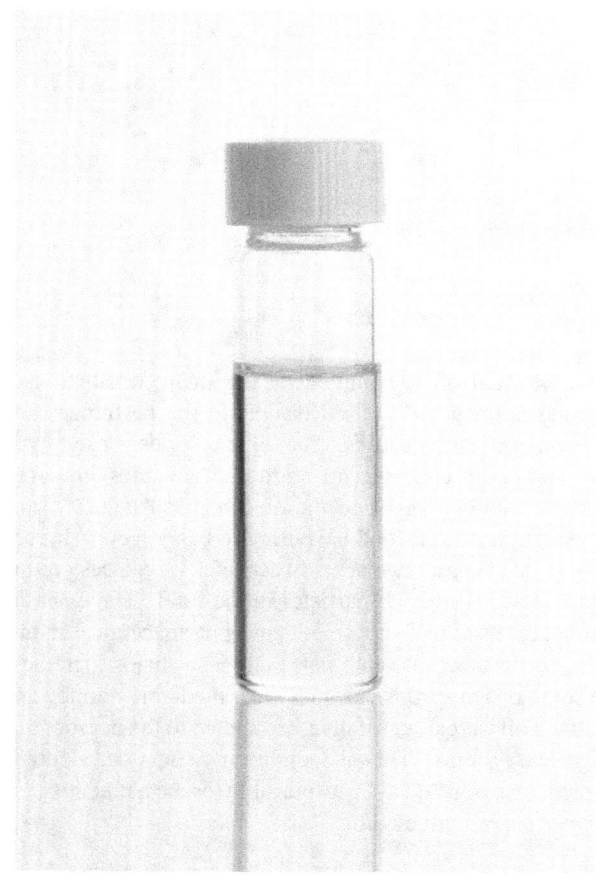

*Clove (*Syzygium aromaticum*) essential oil in clear glass vial*

Oil of clove, also known as **clove oil**, is an essential oil extracted from the clove plant, *Syzygium aromaticum*. It has

the CAS number 8000-34-8.

Clove oil is a natural analgaesic and antiseptic, used primarily in dentistry for its main ingredient eugenol. It can also be purchased in pharmacies over the counter as a home remedy for dental pain relief, mainly toothache. It is also often found in the aromatherapy section of health food stores, and is used in the flavoring of some medicines. Madagascar and Indonesia are the main producers of clove oil.[1]

Clove oil is used widely in microscopical preparation, as it is miscible with Canada balsam, and has a similar refractive index to glass (1.53).

Oil of clove is also used as an ingredient in cat deterrent sprays, coupled with garlic oil, sodium lauryl sulfate, and other ingredients.

2.37.1   Types

There are three types of clove oil:[1]

- **Bud oil** is derived from the flower-buds of *S. aromaticum*. It consists of 60–90% eugenol, eugenyl acetate, caryophyllene and other minor constituents.

- **Leaf oil** is derived from the leaves of *S. aromaticum*. It consists of 82–88% eugenol with little or no eugenyl acetate, and minor constituents.

- **Stem oil** is derived from the twigs of *S. aromaticum*. It consists of 90–95% eugenol, with other minor constituents.

2.37.2   Efficacy

According to the U.S. Food and Drug Administration (FDA):[2]

> Clove oil and eugenol, one of the chemicals it contains, have long been used topically for toothache, but the FDA has reclassified eugenol, downgrading its effectiveness rating. The FDA now believes there isn't enough evidence to rate eugenol as effective for toothache pain.

In a 2006 study conducted by Kuwait University, researchers concluded that a clove preparation was equally effective as a benzocaine gel when administered as a topical anesthetic for intraoral injections.[3][4]

In Australia, after major flooding throughout Queensland, clove oil mixed with water was used as a spray to kill mold.

2.37.3 Toxicity

Taking in large amounts of cloves or clove oil may cause nausea, vomiting, abdominal pain, diarrhea, burns in the mouth and throat, sore throat, seizures, difficulty breathing, rapid heartbeat, sleepiness, intestinal bleeding, and liver or kidney failure.[4] More serious effects have been reported in young children, even with small doses.[4]

Severe reactions may occur in people with allergy to cloves (about 1.5% of the population).[4]

2.37.4 Regulation

Clove cigarettes, once somewhat popular in the United States, are now prohibited due to health hazards [4]

In Germany, *Commission E* permits the sale and administration of clove oil as a medicinal herb.[4][5]

2.37.5 References

[1] Lawless, J. (1995). *The Illustrated Encyclopaedia of Essential Oils*. ISBN 1-85230-661-0.

[2] "Clove". *MedlinePlus*. NIH.

[3] Alqareer, A.; Alyahya, A.; Andersson, L. (2006). "The effect of clove and benzocaine versus placebo as topical anesthetics". *Journal of Dentistry* 34 (10): 747–50. doi:10.1016/j.jdent.2006.01.009. PMID 16530911.

[4] "Cloves". American Cancer Society. Retrieved 2012-05-06.

[5] Rister, R.; Klein, S.; Riggins, C. (1998-03-15). *The Complete German Commission E Monographs: Therapeutic Guide to Herbal Medicines* (1st ed.). American Botanical Council. p. 112. ISBN 978-0-9655555-0-0.

2.38 Oil of guaiac

Oil of guaiac is a fragrance ingredient used in soap and perfumery. It comes from the palo santo tree (*Bulnesia sarmientoi*).

Oil of guaiac is produced through steam distillation of a mixture of wood and sawdust from palo santo. It is sometimes incorrectly called guaiac wood concrete. It is a yellow to greenish yellow semi-solid mass which melts around 40–50 °C. Once melted, it can be cooled back to room temperature yet remain liquid for a long time. Oil of guaiac has a soft roselike odour, similar to the odour of Hybrid Tea roses or violets. Because of this similarity, it has sometimes been used as an adulterant for rose oil.

Oil of guaiac is primarily composed of 42-72% guaiol, bulnesol, δ-bulnesene, β-bulnesene, α-guaiene, guaioxide and β-patchoulene. It is considered non-irritating, non-sensitizing, and non phototoxic to human skin.

Oil of guaiac was also a pre-Renaissance remedy to syphilis.

2.38.1 See also

- Guaiacum

2.38.2 References

- D.L.J. Opdyke, 1974, Food Cosmet. Toxicol., 12 (Suppl.), 905

2.39 Olbas Oil

Olbas oil is a remedy, of Swiss origin,[1] for congestion in the chest and nose, some hayfever relief (in certain cases) and also for muscle ache via massage.[2] It is made from a mixture of several different essential oils.[3]

2.39.1 Available as

There are several trademarked olbas oil products available[4]

- Olbas Oil
- Olbas for children
- Olbas inhaler
- Olbas Pastilles
- Olbas Menthol Lozenges
- Olbas bath

2.39.2 Active ingredients

Active ingredients are listed as;[5]

- Cajuput Oil
- Clove Oil
- Eucalyptus Oil
- Juniperberry Oil
- Levomenthol

- Methyl salicylate

- Peppermint oil

2.39.3   References

[1] Penn Herb Company

[2] Chemist Direct

[3] Olbas UK – About

[4] Olbas UK – Products

[5] Boots – Olbas

2.40   Orange oil

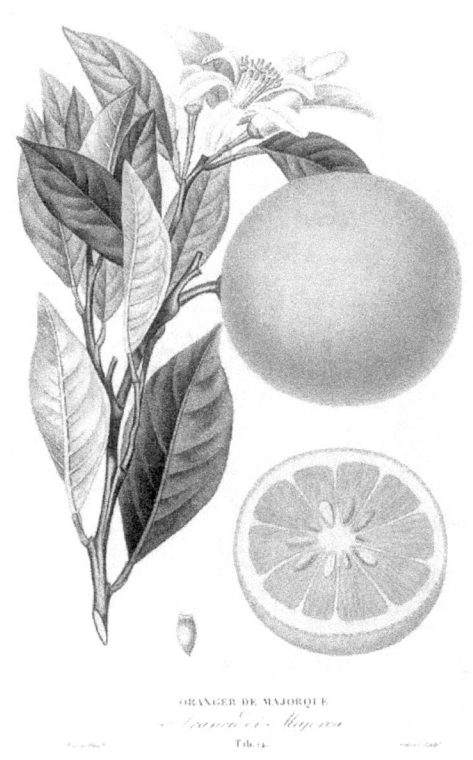

Citrus sinensis *(L.) Histoire et culture des orangers A. Risso et A. Poiteau. - Paris Henri Plon, Editeur, 1872*

Orange oil is an essential oil produced by cells within the rind of an orange fruit (*Citrus sinensis* fruit). In contrast to most essential oils, it is extracted as a by-product of orange juice production by centrifugation, producing a cold-pressed oil.[1] It is composed of mostly (greater than 90%) d-limonene,[2] and is often used in place of pure d-limonene. D-limonene can be extracted from the oil by distillation.

2.40.1   Limonene

Limonene gives citrus fruit their familiar aroma, and is therefore used in perfume and household cleaners for its fragrance. It is also an effective, environmentally friendly, and relatively safe solvent, which makes it an active ingredient of choice in many applications, such as, adhesive and stain removers, cleaners of various sorts, and strippers. Limonene is also highly useful in agriculture.

2.40.2   Composition

The compounds inside an orange oil varies with each different oil extraction. Composition variety happens as a result of regional and seasonal changes as well as the method used for extraction. Several hundred compounds have been identified with gas chromatograph-mass spectrometry. Most of the substances in the oil belong to the terpene group with limonene being the dominant one. Long chain aliphatic hydrocarbon alcohols and aldehydes like 1-octanol and octanal are second important group of substances.

The presence of sinensetin explains the orange color.[7]

2.40.3   Hazards

The limonene which is the main component of the oil is a mild irritant, as it dissolves protective skin oils. Limonene and its oxidation products are skin irritants, and limonene-1,2-oxide (formed by aerial oxidation) is a known skin sensitizer. Most reported cases of irritation have involved long-term industrial exposure to the pure compound, e.g. during degreasing or the preparation of paints. However a study of patients presenting dermatitis showed that 3% were sensitized to limonene.

Limonene has been observed to cause cancer in male rats, by reacting with α2u-globulin, which is not produced by female rats. There is no evidence for carcinogenicity or genotoxicity in humans. The IARC classifies *d*-limonene under Class 3: *not classifiable as to its carcinogenicity to humans.*[8]

Limonene is also flammable.[9]

2.40.4 Biological pest control

Orange oil can be used in biological pest control green pesticides. It can kill an ant, as well as a whole colony of ants. Orange oil also erases an ant's scent-pheromone trail indicators and disrupt re-infestation activities in ants.[10] Their use in organic farming is becoming increasingly important because of their non-toxic nature.[11] They are commonly used in kitchens to safely repel ants.

Orange oil is also known to be useful to control or exterminate termites of the Drywood (Kalotermitidae) variety.

2.40.5 See also

- Neroli
- Petitgrain
- Orange oil tires

2.40.6 References

[1] Dominic W. S. Wong (1989). *Mechanism and theory in food chemistry*. Springer. p. 253. ISBN 0-442-20753-0.

[2] K. Bauer, D. Garbe, and H. Surburg, "Common Fragrance and Flavor Materials", 4th Ed, Wiley VCH, 2001, ISBN 3-527-30364-2. 189.

[3] A. Verzera, A. Trozzi, G. Dugo, G. Di Bella, A. Cotroneo (2004). "Biological lemon and sweet orange essential oil composition". *Flavour and Fragrance Journal* **19** (6): 544–548. doi:10.1002/ffj.1348.

[4] J. Pino *, M. Sánchez, R. Sánchez, E. Roncal (2006). "Chemical composition of orange oil concentrates". *Nahrung / Food* **36** (6): 539–542. doi:10.1002/food.19920360604.

[5] J. D. Vora , R. F. Matthews , P. G. Crandall , R. Cook (1983). "Preparation and Chemical Composition of Orange Oil Concentrates". *Journal of Food Science* **48** (4): 1197–1199. doi:10.1111/j.1365-2621.1983.tb09190.x.

[6] R. L. Colman, E. D. Lund, M. G. Moshonas (1969). "Composition of Orange Essence Oil". *Journal of Food Science* **34** (6): 610–611. doi:10.1111/j.1365-2621.1969.tb12102.x.

[7] Steinke, K., Jose, E., Sicker, D., Siehl, H.-U., Zeller, K.-P. and Berger, S. (2013), Sinensetin. Chemie in unserer Zeit, 47: 158–163. doi:10.1002/ciuz.201300627

[8] "Limonene" MyTamanuOil.com

[9] "Safety data (MSDS) for limonene". Fisher Scientific UK. Retrieved 2015-04-22.

[10] "A Review of "Organic" and Other Alternative Methods for Fire Ant Control" (PDF).

[11] "The Orange Oil".

2.40.7 External links

- The Effect of Citrus Oils on Fruit Flies

2.41 Orris oil

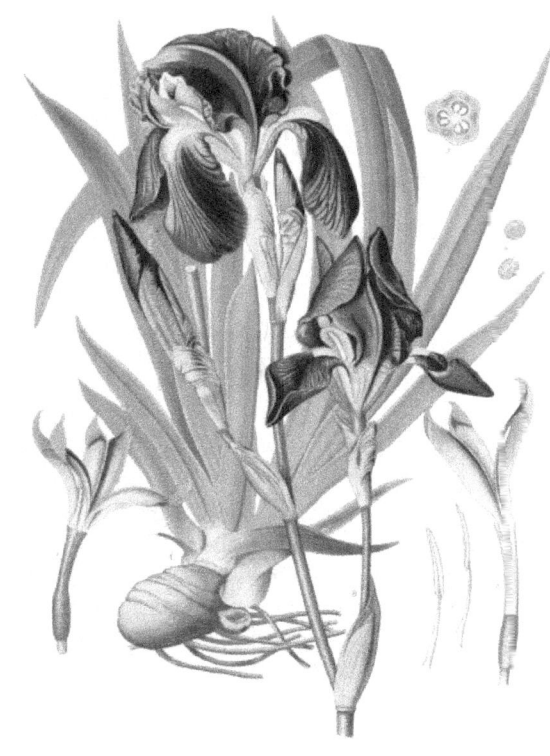

An illustration of the Iris germanica

Orris oil (**orris butter** or **Beurre d'Iris**) is an essential oil derived from irises, particularly *Iris germanica*.[1] It is sometimes used as a flavoring agent and as an ingredient in perfume production. It can also have uses in body lotions.

2.41.1 Storage and use

The rhizomes (roots) must be stored in a cool, dry location for three years to develop the scent.[1] The fresh rhizomes are almost odorless.

The distilled oil solidifies in the receiver as a wax-like and cream-colored mass known as orris concrete. It is solid because of the high content of myristic acid (85%), a white sterin-like substance.[1]

Orris concrete melts when it reaches around body temperature. It has a woody, fatty-oily, yet distinctly violet-like odor: sweet floral, warm & tenacious with a fruity under-tone. Orris concrete is used in perfumery (as such) when the presence of myristic acid is not prohibitive, e.g.: in soap perfumes where the weak acid only acts as a fixative. Also note, the methyl and ethyl esters of myristic acid are often used for blending in violet type perfume bases. Because of the high costs involved in producing orris concrete it limits its application to a certain degree. Yet even small amounts of this exquisite material lends to very fine effects in various perfume types other than the old fashioned violet.

2.41.2 References

[1] Harborne, Jeffrey B.; Baxter, Herbert (2001-08-30). *Chemical Dictionary of Economic Plants*. John Wiley & Sons. p. 85. ISBN 9780471492269. Retrieved 2014-09-22.

2.42 Palmarosa Oil

2.42.1 Description

The botanical name for the source of **palmarosa oil** is *Cymbopogon martinii*, which belongs to the grass family *Poaceae* (Graminae).[1][2] This grass grows fairly tall, ranging from (1.3–3 meters) in height with a pale green colour and a strong thin stem. This crop grows slowly, taking 3 months to flower; once it has flowered, it can be harvested. It received the name palmarosa from the sweet-smelling floral rose aroma it gives off.[3] It is widely used for rose smelling perfumes and cosmetics around the world.[4] It is also known to help repel mosquitoes and flavour tobacco products. It has been added into medicinal solutions for stiff joints, bilious complaints, skin disease, and aromatherapy.[5]

2.42.2 Where/how the product is grown, raised, processed

Palmarosa is wildly grown in wetlands in provinces of India, including Nepal.[6] The Palmarosa oil is extracted from the stem of the grass by distillation of dried leaves.[7] Once the stems and leaves have been distilled for two to three hours, to separate the oil from the palmarose, then the leftover distilled grass is turned into organic matter and becomes manure or is composted.[8]

2.42.3 Growing conditions

The most efficient way to grow palmarosa is in a nursery with lots of irrigation and soil pH of 7-8.[9] Two or three days before planting, it is best to overwhelm the soil with water to increase soil moisture above 60% when planting the seeds. This moisture increases the germination of the seed and increases weed control in the nursery beds as well. It is also recommended to flood the soil once a month to maintain a high moisture level in the soil. Irrigation in a nursery is most important for the first 40 days. Palmarosa grass grows well in sandy texture soil with low nitrogen, sufficient phosphorus and potassium. Weeds are a problem and keeping them out of the nursery beds will increase the yield. Manual weeding must be done often and involves a well-trained eye to uncover the weeds.[10] Also, palmarosa is often intercropped to help suppress the weeds, thus increasing yields and the land efficiency. Mostly farmers intercrop with pigeon pea, also millet and sorghum work well with row or strip intercropping because palmarosa can be harvested three to four times a year.[11][12]

2.42.4 Labour cost and issues

It is mainly used in the perfumery industry not just for the pleasant smell but also as a source of high-grade geranial.[13] The geranial level received from the palmarosa oil is not always the same—it depends on three factors: first being how the diphosphate is removed from the geranyl diphosphate (GPP); second the process of converting geranial into the form of geranyl acetate; and lastly the process of converting geranyl acetate into the geranial. If these steps are done incorrectly the level of geranial will be low along with the profits.[14]

2.42.5 Inputs required

A nursery is needed or there will be poor growth yields, that may not bring any profit to the farmer and potentially the farmer could have an economical loss. This requirement increases the startup cost for farmers which some farmers are unable to pay.[15] If not grown in a nursery this will increase the weeding labour inputs by over 70% and decrease the yield. Farmers will be spending more time weeding the plots and will receive a smaller return then if they had a nursery.[16]

2.42.6 Health or nutritional informant

Palmarosa oil is also known as an antifungal that fights against Aspergillus niger, commonly known as black mold, Chaetomium globosum also known as moldy soil and Penicillium funiculosum, which is a plant pathogen.[17]

2.42.7 References

[1] Prashar, A., Hili, P., Veness, R. & Evans, C. (2003). Antimicrobial action of palmarosa oil (Cymbopogon martinii) on Saccharomyces cerevisiae. *Phytochemistry*, 63(5), 569-575. Retrieved November 18, 2014, from http://www.sciencedirect.com/science/article/pii/S0031942203002267#

[2] Rajeswara Rao, B., Kaul, P., Syamasundar, K., & Ramesh, S. (2005). Chemical profiles of primary and secondary essential oils of palmarosa (Cymbopogon martinii (Roxb.) Wats var. motia Burk.). *IIndustrical Crops and Products*, 21(1), 121-127. Retrieved November 12, 2014, from http://journals2.scholarsportal.info.subzero.lib.uoguelph.ca/details/09266690/v21i0001/121_cpopaspmwvmb.xml

[3] Rajeswara Rao, B., Rajput, D., & Patel, R. (2014). Improving Yield and Quality of Palmarosa [Cymbopogon martinii (Roxb.) Wats. Var. Motia Burk.] with Sulfur Fertilization. *Journal of Plant Nutrition*. Retrieved November 12, 2014, from http://www.tandfonline.com.subzero.lib.uoguelph.ca/doi/pdf/10.1080/01904167.2014.957395

[4] Mallavarapu, G., Rajeswara Rao, B., Kaul, P., Ramesh, S., & Bhattacharya, A. (1998). Volatile constituents of the essential oils of the seeds and the herb of palmarosa (Cymbopogon martinii (Roxb.) Wats. var. motia Burk.). *Journal of Plant Nutrition*, 13, 167-169. Retrieved November 12, 2014, from http://journals1.scholarsportal.info.subzero.lib.uoguelph.ca/details/08825734/v13i0003/167_vcoteopmwvmb.xml

[5] Rajeswara Rao, B., Kaul, P., Syamasundar, K., & Ramesh, S. (2005). Chemical profiles of primary and secondary essential oils of palmarosa (Cymbopogon martinii (Roxb.) Wats var. motia Burk.). *IIndustrial Crops and Products*, 21(1), 121-127. Retrieved November 12, 2014, from http://journals2.scholarsportal.info.subzero.lib.uoguelph.ca/details/09266690/v21i0001/121_cpopaspmwvmb.xml

[6] Guenther, E. (1952). Recent developments in essential oil production. *Economic Botany*, 6(4), 355-378. Retrieved November 15, 2014, from http://resolver.scholarsportal.info.subzero.lib.uoguelph.ca/resolve/001

[7] Kumaran, A., D'Souza, P., Agarwal, A., Bokkolla, R., & Balasubramaniam, M. (2003). Geraniol, the putative anthelmintic principle of Cymbopogon martinii. *Phytotherapy Research*, 17(8), 957-957. Retrieved November 17, 20014, from http://onlinelibrary.wiley.com.subzero.lib.uoguelph.ca/doi/10.1002/ptr.1267/abstract

[8] Rajeswara Rao, B., Kaul, P., Syamasundar, K., & Ramesh, S. (2005). Chemical profiles of primary and secondary essential oils of palmarosa (Cymbopogon martinii (Roxb.) Wats var. motia Burk.). *IIndustrial Crops and Products*, 21(1), 121-127. Retrieved November 12, 2014, from http://journals2.scholarsportal.info.subzero.lib.uoguelph.ca/details/09266690/v21i0001/121_cpopaspmwvmo.xml

[9] Maheshwari, P., & Tandon, S. (1959). Agriculture and economic development in India. *Economic Botany*, 13(3), 205-242. Retrieved November 12, 2014, from http://resolver.scholarsportal.info.subzero.lib.uoguelph.ca/resolve/001

[10] Singh, A., Singh, M., & Singh, D. (1997). Pre-plant weed control for a palmarosa (Cymbopogon martinii) nursery. *International Journal of Pest Management*, 43(1), 45-48. Retrieved November 13, 2014, from http://content.ebscohost.com.subzero.lib.uoguelph.ca/ContentServer.asp?T=P&P=AN&K=7616697&S=R&D=aph&EbscoContent=dGJyMMvl7ESep7U4zOX0OLCmr0yep65Srqi4S7WWxWXS&ContentCustomer=dGJyMPGut0mwrbFPuePfgeyx44Dt6fIA

[11] Maheshwari, P., & Tandon, S. (1959). Agriculture and economic development in India. *Economic Botany* 13(3), 205-242. Retrieved November 12, 2014, from http://resolver.scholarsportal.info.subzero.lib.uoguelph.ca/resolve/001

[12] Rajeswara Rao, B., Kaul, P., Syamasundar, K., & Ramesh, S. (2005). Chemical profiles of primary and secondary essential oils of palmarosa (Cymbopogon martinii (Roxb.) Wats var. motia Burk.). *IIndustrial Crops and Products*, 21(1), 121-127. Retrieved November 12, 2014, from http://journals2.scholarsportal.info.subzero.lib.uoguelph.ca/details/09266690/v21i0001/121_cpopaspmwvmb.xml

[13] Prashar, A., Hili, P., Veness, R., & Evans, C. (2003). Antimicrobial action of palmarosa oil (Cymbopogon martinii) on Saccharomyces cerevisiae. *Phytochemistry*, 63(5), 569-575. Retrieved November 18, 2014, from http://www.sciencedirect.com.subzero.lib.uoguelph.ca/science/article/pii/S0031942203002267#

[14] Dubey, V., Bhalla, R., & Luthra, R. (2003). An esterase is involved in geraniol production during palmarosa inflorescence development. *Phytochemistry*, 63(3), 257-264. Retrieved November 13, 2014, from http://www.sciencedirect.com.subzero.lib.uoguelph.ca/science/article/pii/S0031942203001146#

[15] Maheshwari, P., & Tandon, S. (1959). Agriculture and economic development in India. *Economic Botany*, 13(3), 205-242. Retrieved November 12, 2014, from http://resolver.scholarsportal.info.subzero.lib.uoguelph.ca/resolve/001

[16] Singh, A., Singh, M., & Singh, D. (1997). Pre-plant weed control for a palmarosa (Cymbopogon martinii) nursery. *International Journal of Pest Management*, 43(1), 45-48. Retrieved November 13, 2014, from http://content.ebscohost.com.subzero.lib.uoguelph.ca/ContentServer.asp?T=P&P=AN&K=7616697&S=R&D=aph&EbscoContent=dGJyMMvl7ESep7U4zOX0OLCmr0yep65Srqi4S7WWxWXS&ContentCustomer=dGJyMPGut0mwrbFPuePfgeyx44Dt6fIA

[17] Prashar, A., Hili, P., Veness, R., & Evans, C. (2003). Antimicrobial action of palmarosa oil (Cymbopogon martinii) on Saccharomyces cerevisiae. *Phytochemistry*, 63(5), 569-575. Retrieved November 18, 2014, from http://www.sciencedirect.com.subzero.lib.uoguelph.ca/science/article/pii/S0031942203002267#

2.43 Patchouli

Patchouli (*Pogostemon cablin* (Blanco) Benth; also **patchouly** or **pachouli**) is a species of plant from the genus *Pogostemon*. It is a bushy herb of the mint family, with erect stems, reaching two or three feet (about 0.75 metre) in height and bearing small, pale pink-white flowers. The plant is native to tropical regions of Asia, and is now extensively cultivated in China, Indonesia, India, Malaysia, Mauritius, Taiwan, the Philippines, Thailand, and Vietnam.

2.43.1 Perfume

The heavy and strong scent of patchouli has been used for centuries in perfumes and, more recently, in incense, insect repellents, and alternative medicines. The word derives from the Tamil *patchai* (Tamil: பச்சை) (green), *ellai* (Tamil: இலை) (leaf).[1] In Assamese it is known as *xukloti*.

Pogostemon cablin, P. commosum, P. hortensis, P. heyneasus and *P. plectranthoides* are all cultivated for their essential oil, known as patchouli oil.

2.43.2 Cultivation

Patchouli grows well in warm to tropical climates. It thrives in hot weather but not direct sunlight. If the plant withers due to lack of water, it will recover well and quickly after rain or watering. The seed-producing flowers are very fragrant and blossom in late fall. The tiny seeds may be harvested for planting, but they are very delicate and easily crushed. Cuttings from the mother plant can also be rooted in water to produce additional plants.

2.43.3 Extraction of essential oil

Extraction of patchouli's essential oil is by steam distillation of the leaves, requiring rupture of its cell walls by steam scalding, light fermentation, or drying.

Leaves may be harvested several times a year and, when dried, may be exported for distillation. Some sources claim a highest quality oil is usually produced from fresh leaves distilled close to where they are harvested;[2] others that baling the dried leaves and fermenting them for a period of time is best.[3]

Aroma profile

- Germacrene-B[4]
- Patchoulol[5][6][7]

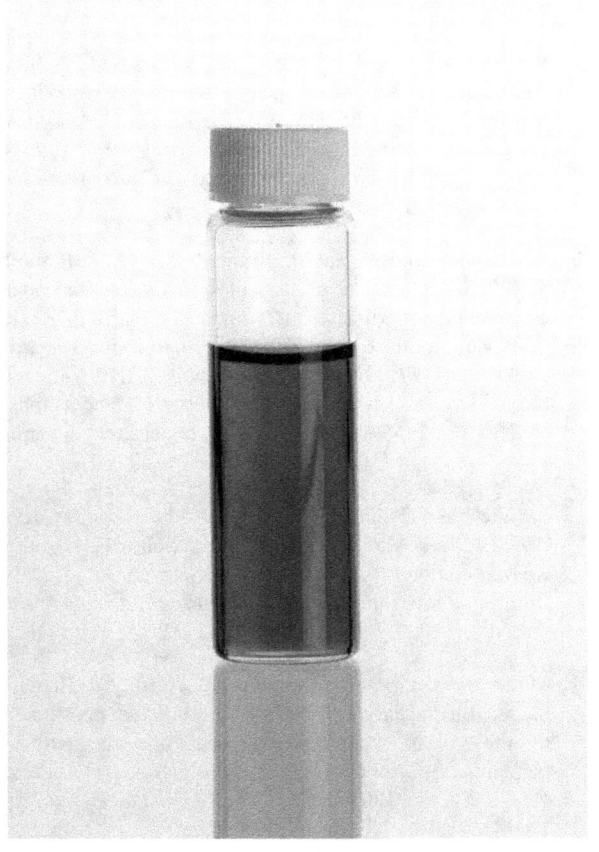

Patchouli (Pogostemon cablin*) essential oil*

- Norpatchoulenol[7]

2.43.4 Uses

Perfume

Patchouli is used widely in modern perfumery,[8] by individuals who create their own scents,[9] and in modern scented industrial products such as paper towels, laundry detergents, and air fresheners. Two important components of its essential oil are patchoulol and norpatchoulenol.[10]

Insect repellent

One study suggests that patchouli oil may serve as an all-purpose insect repellent.[11] More specifically, the patchouli plant is claimed to be a potent repellent against the *Formosan subterranean termite*.[4]

During the 18th and 19th century, silk traders from China traveling to the Middle East packed their silk cloth with dried patchouli leaves to prevent moths from laying their eggs on the cloth. It has also been proven to effectively prevent female moths from adhering to males. Many historians speculate that this association with opulent Eastern goods is why patchouli was considered by Europeans of that era to be a luxurious scent. It is said that patchouli was used in the linen chests of Queen Victoria in this way.

Incense

Patchouli is an important ingredient in East Asian incense. Both patchouli oil and incense underwent a surge in popularity in the 1960s and 1970s in the US and Europe, mainly as a result of the hippie movement of those decades.[12]

Culinary

Patchouli leaves have been used to make an herbal tea. In some cultures, patchouli leaves are eaten as a vegetable.

Toys

In 1985 Mattel used patchouli oil in the plastic used to produce the action figure Stinkor in the Masters of the Universe line of toys.[13]

2.43.5   References

[1] "Patchouli". Online Etymology Dictionary. Retrieved 10 December 2011.

[2] Grieve, Maude (1995) *A Modern Herbal* . 2007

[3] Leung A, Foster S *Encyclopedia of common natural ingredients used in food, drugs and cosmetics* John Wiley and Sons 1996

[4] Hasegawa, Yoshihiro; Tajima, Katsuhiko; Toi, Nao; Sugimura, Yukio; et al. (1992). "An additional constituent occurring in the oil from a patchouli cultivar". *Flavour and Fragrance Journal* **7** (6): 333–335. doi:10.1002/ffj.2730070608.

[5] Weyerstahl, Peter; Gansau, Christian; Marschall, Helga; et al. (1993). "Structure-odour correlation. Part XVIII. Partial structures of patchoulol with bicyclo[2.2.2]octane skeleton". *Flavour and Fragrance Journal* **8** (6): 297–306. doi:10.1002/ffj.2730080603.

[6] Hybertson, Brooks M. (2007). "Solubility of the sesquiterpene alcohol patchoulol in supercritical carbon dioxide". *Journal of Chemical Engineering Data* **52** (1): 235–238. doi:10.1021/je060358w. PMC 2677825. PMID 19424449.

[7] Nikiforov, Alexej *et. al*; Jirovetz, Leopold; Buchbauer, Gerhard; Raverdino, Vittorio (1988). "GC-FTIR and GC-MS in odour analysis of essential oils". *Microchimica Acta* **95** (1 – 6): 193–198. doi:10.1007/BF01349751.

[8] Ballentine, Sandra (5 November 2010). "Vain Glorious | Sex in a Bottle". Tmagazine.blogs.nytimes.com. Retrieved 10 December 2011.

[9] http://www.wisegeek.com/what-is-patchouli.htm

[10] http://www.wisegeek.com/what-is-patchouli.htm

[11] Trongtokit, Yuwadee; Rongsriyam, Yupha; Komalamisra, Narumon; Apiwathnasorn, Chamnarn (2005). "Comparative repellency of 38 essential oils against mosquito bites". *Phytotherapy Research* **19** (4): 303–309. doi:10.1002/ptr.1637. PMID 16041723.

[12] Foster, Steven; Johnson, Rebecca L. (2006). *Desk Reference to Nature's Medicine*. Washington, D.C.: National Geographic Society. p. 282. ISBN 978-0-7922-3666-5.

[13] Stinkor: Masters of the Universe

2.44   Pelargonium graveolens

"Rose geranium" redirects here. For another plant called by this name, see Pelargonium capitatum.

Pelargonium graveolens is an uncommon *Pelargonium* species native to the Cape Provinces and the Northern Provinces of South Africa, Zimbabwe and Mozambique [1] It is in the subgenus *Pelargonium* along with *Pelargonium crispum* and *Pelargonium tomentosum*.

2.44.1   Etymology

Pelargonium comes from the Greek *pelargos* which means stork. Another name for pelargoniums is stork's-bills due to the shape of their fruit. The specific epithet *graveolens* refers to the strong-smelling leaves.

2.44.2   Description

Pelargonium graveolens is an erect, multi-branched shrub, that grows up to 1.5 m and has a spread of 1 m. The leaves are deeply incised leaves are velvety and soft to the touch (due to glandular hairs). The flowers vary from pale pink to almost white and the plant flowers from August to January. The leaves may be strongly rose-scented, although the leaf shape and scent vary. Some plants are very strongly scented and others have little or no scent. Some leaves are deeply incised and others less so, being slightly lobed like *P. capitatum*.

2.44.3 Common names and synonyms

Common names include rose geranium,[1][2] sweet scented geranium,[3] old fashion rose geranium,[2] and rose-scent geranium.[1]

Pelargonium graveolens is also known by taxonomic synonyms *Geranium terebinthinaceum* Cav.   and *Pelargonium terebinthinaceum* (Cav.) Desf.[1] "Rose geranium" is sometimes used to refer to *Pelargonium incrassatum* (Andrews) Sims or its synonym *Pelargonium roseum* (Andrews) DC. – the herbal name.[4] Commercial vendors often list the source of geranium or rose geranium essential oil as *Pelargonium graveolens*, regardless of its botanical name.

2.44.4 Cultivars and hybrids

Many plants are cultivated under the species name "*Pelargonium graveolens*" but differ from wild specimens as they are of hybrid origin[1] (probably a cross between *P. graveolens*, *P. capitatum* and/or *P. radens*). There are many cultivars of *P. graveolens* and they have a wide variety of scents, including rose, citrus, mint and cinnamon as well as various fruits. Cultivars and hybrids include:

- *P.* 'Graveolens' (or *Pelargonium graveolens* hort.) - A rose-scented cultivar of *P. graveolens*. Possibly a hybrid between *P. graveolens* and *P. radens* or *P. capitatum*. This cultivar is often incorrectly labeled as *Pelargonium graveolens* (the species). The main difference between the species and this cultivar is the dissection of the leaf. The species had about 5 lobes but the cultivar has about 10.

- *P.* 'Citrosum' - A lemony, citronella-scented cultivar of *P. graveolens*, similar to *P.* 'Graveolens'. It is meant to repel mosquitos and rumour has it that it was made by genetically bonding genes from the citronella grass but this is highly unlikely.

- *P.* 'Cinnamon Rose' - A cinnamon-scented variety of *P. graveolens*.

- *P.* 'Dr Westerland' - A lemony rose-scented cultivar of *P. graveolens*, similar to *P.* 'Graveolens'.

- *P.* 'Graveolens Bontrosai' - A genetically challenged form of *P. graveolens*. The leaves are smaller and curl back on themselves and the flowers often don't open fully. Known as *P.* 'Colocho' in the US.

- *P.* 'Grey Lady Plymouth' - A lemony rose-scented cultivar of *P. graveolens*. Similar to *P.* 'Lady Plymouth'. The leaves are grey - green in colour and beautifully contrast of scented pelargonium varieties.

- *P.* 'Lady Plymouth' - A minty lemony rose-scented cultivar of *P. graveolens*. A very popular variety with a definite mint scent. Possibly a *P. radens* hybrid.

- *P.* 'Lara Starshine' - A lemony rose-scented cultivar of *P. graveolens*, similar to *P.* 'Graveolens' but with more lemony scented leaves and reddish pink flowers. Bred by Australian Plantsman Cliff Blackman.

- *P.* 'Lucaeflora' - A rose-scented variety of *P. graveolens*, much more similar to the species that most other cultivars and varieties of *P. graveolens*.

- *P.* × *melissinum* - The lemon balm pelargonium (lemon balm - *Melissa officinalis*). This is a hybrid between *P. crispum* and *P. graveolens*.

- *P.* 'Mint Rose' - A minty rose-scented cultivar of *P. graveolens*. Similar to *P.* 'Lady Plymouth' but without the variegation of the leaves and lemony undertones.

- *P.* 'Secret Love' - An unusual eucalyptus-scented variety of *P. graveolens* with pretty pale pink flowers.

- *P.* 'Van Leeni' - A lemony rose-scented cultivar of *P. graveolens*, similar to *P.* 'Graveolens' and *P.* 'Dr Westerland'.

2.44.5 Uses

Both the true species and the cultivated plant may be called **rose geranium** – pelargoniums are often called geraniums, as they fall within the plant family Geraniaceae, and were previously classified in the same genus. The common *P.* 'Graveolens' or *P.* 'Rosat' has great importance in the perfume industry. It is cultivated on a large scale and its foliage is distilled for its scent. *Pelargonium* distillates and absolutes, commonly known as "geranium oil", are sold for aromatherapy and massage therapy applications. They are also sometimes used to supplement or adulterate more expensive rose oils. The essential oil is an ingredient in a "natural" haemorrhoid treatment.[5] As a flavoring, the flowers and leaves are used in cakes, jams, jellies, ice creams, sorbets, salads, sugars,[6] and teas. In addition, it is used as a flavoring agent in some pipe tobaccos, being one of the characteristic "Lakeland scents."

2.44.6 Chemical constituents of geranium oil

A modern analysis listed the presence of over 50 organic compounds in the essential oil of *P. graveolens* from an Australian source.[7] Analyses of Indian geranium oils indicated a similar phytochemical profile, and showed that the major

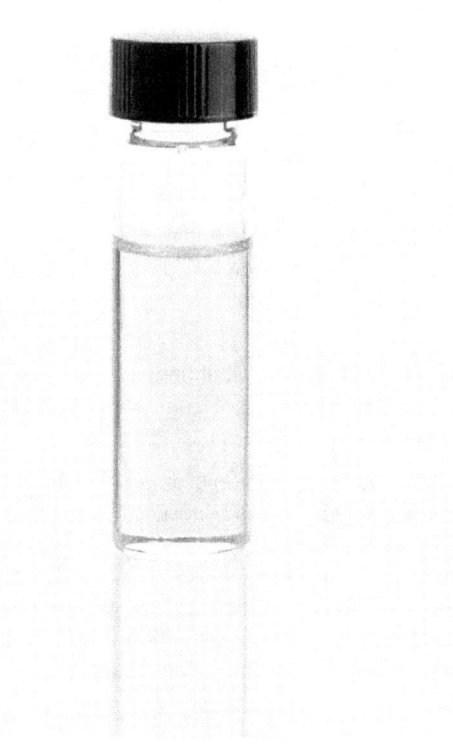

Geranium (Pelargonium 'Graveolens') essential oil in a clear glass vial

constituents (in terms of % composition) were citronellol + nerol and geraniol.[8][9]

2.44.7 Gallery

- The flower cluster of cultivated *P.* 'Graveolens'
- A bee on a flower cluster of cultivated *P.* 'Graveolens'
- At Ryton Organic Gardens, near Rugby, Warwickshire.
- *Pelargonium* 'Graveolens' leaf
- An adult *Pelargonium* 'Mint Rose' at Ryton Organic Gardens, near Rugby, Warwickshire

2.44.8 See also

- Essential oil
- Pelargonium

2.44.9 References

[1] USDA ARS NPGS. "Pelargonium graveolens information from NPGS/GRIN". United States Department of Agriculture (USDA), Agricultural Research Service (ARS), National Plant Germplasm System (NPGS). Accessed June 23, 2007.

[2] "Pelargonium graveolens". *Plants For A Future.* Accessed June 23, 2007.

[3] USDA NCRS. "PLANTS Profile for Pelargonium graveolens (sweet scented geranium)". *United States Department of Agriculture (USDA), Natural Resources Conservation Service (NCRS), PLANTS Database.* Accessed June 23, 2007.

[4] "Pelargonium incrassatum". *Plants For A Future.* Accessed June 23, 2007.

[5] http://www.amoils.com/h-hemorrhoids-ingredients.html, http://www.amoils.com/hemorrhoids.html

[6] Encyclopedia of Spices

[7] R. A. Shellie and P. J. Marriott (2003). "Comprehensive two-dimensional gas chromatography-mass spectrometry analysis of Pelargonium graveolens essential oil using rapid scanning quadrupole mass spectrometry." *Analyst* **128** 879-883.

[8] N. Jain, K. K. Aggarwal, K. V. Syamasundar, S. K. Srivastava and S. Kumar (2001). "Essential oil composition of geranium (Pelargonium sp.) from the plains of Northern India." *Flavour and Fragrance J.* **16** 44–46.

[9] R. Gupta, G. R. Mallavarapu, S. Banerjee and S. Kumar (2001). "Characteristics of an isomenthone-rich somaclonal mutant isolated in a geraniol-rich rose-scented geranium accession of Pelargonium graveolens." *Flavour and Fragrance J.* **16** 319–324.

2.44.10 External links

- Plantzafrica
- Scented Geraniums Nursery

2.45 Petitgrain

Petitgrain is an essential oil that is extracted from the leaves and green twigs of the bitter orange tree (*Citrus aurantium* ssp. *amara*) via steam distillation.

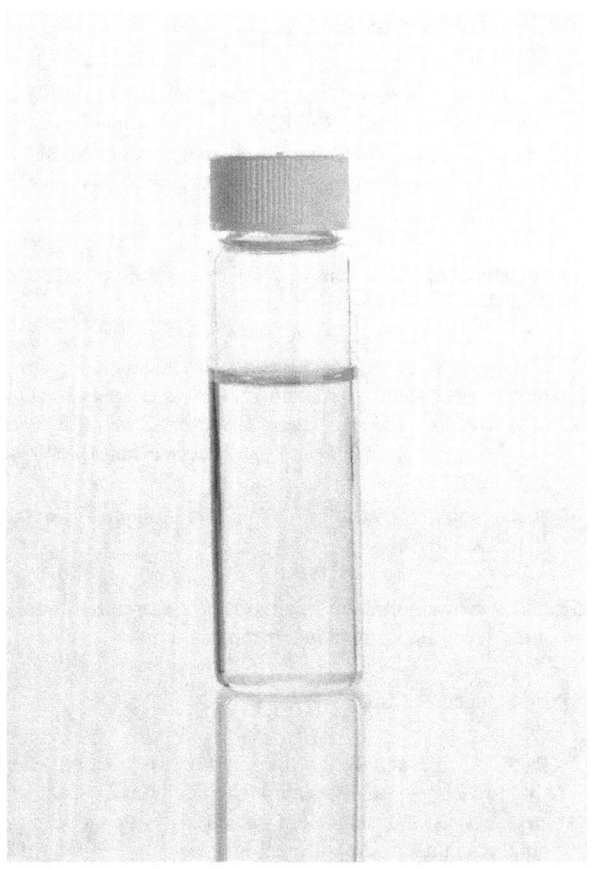

Petitgrain (Citrus aurantium *ssp.* amara*) essential oil in a clear glass vial*

2.45.1 Production

Its main regions of production are Paraguay and France, with the former's product being of higher odour tenacity. Petitgrain oil (fr. little grain) gains its name from the fact that it used to be extracted from the small unripe oranges of the plant. The oil has a greenish woody orange smell that is widely used in perfumery and found in colognes. Though distilled from the same botanical species as neroli and bitter orange, Petitgrain Essential Oil possesses its own characteristically unique aroma. Petitgrain Essential Oil is distilled from the leaves and sometimes the twigs and branches of the tree whereas neroli essential oil is distilled from the blossoms and Orange Essential Oil is typically cold pressed from the rinds of the fruits.

2.45.2 Chemical composition

The main constituents of petitgrain oil are geraniol, geranyl acetate, linalool, linalyl acetate, myrcene, nerol, neryl acetate, and terpineol.

2.45.3 Use

In perfumery and aromatherapy as fresh-scented essential oils.

2.45.4 References

2.46 Pine oil

Not to be confused with Pine nut oil.
For the byproduct of wood pulp production sometimes called pine oil, see tall oil.

Pine oil is an essential oil obtained by the steam distillation of needles, twigs and cones from a variety of species of pine, particularly *Pinus sylvestris*.

It is used in aromatherapy, as a scent in bath oils, as a cleaning product, and as a lubricant in small and expensive clockwork instruments. It is naturally deodorizing, and antibacterial. It may also be used varyingly as a disinfectant, massage oil and an antiseptic. It is also used as an effective organic herbicide where its action is to modify the waxy cuticle of plants, resulting in desiccation.[2]

Pine oil is distinguished from other products from pine, such as turpentine, the low-boiling fraction from the distillation of pine sap, and rosin, the thick tar remaining after turpentine is distilled.

Chemically, pine oil consists mainly of cyclic terpene alcohols.[1] It may also contain terpene hydrocarbons, ethers, and esters. The exact composition depends on various factors, such as the variety of pine from which it is produced and the parts of the tree used.

2.46.1 Properties as a disinfectant

Pine oil is a phenolic disinfectant that is mildly antiseptic.[3] Pine oil disinfectants are relatively inexpensive and widely available. They are effective against *Brevibacterium ammoniagenes*, the fungi *Candida albicans*, *Enterobacter aerogenes*, *Escherichia coli*, Gram-negative enteric bacteria, household germs, Gram-negative household germs such as those causing salmonellosis, herpes simplex types 1 and 2, influenza type A, influenza virus type A/Brazil, influenza virus type A2/Japan, intestinal bacteria, *Klebsiella pneumoniae*, odor-causing bacteria, mold, mildew, *Pseudomonas aeruginosa*, *Salmonella choleraesuis*, *Salmonella typhi*, *Salmonella typhosa*, *Serratia marcescens*, *Shigella sonnei*, *Staphylococcus aureus*, *Streptococcus faecalis*, *Streptococcus pyogenes*, and *Trichophyton mentagrophytes*.[4]

It will kill the causative agents of typhoid, gastroenteritis (some agents), rabies, enteric fever, cholera, several forms of meningitis, whooping cough, gonorrhea and several types of dysentery.[5] It is not effective against spore related illnesses, such as tetanus or anthrax, or against non-enveloped viruses such as poliovirus, rhinovirus, hepatitis B or hepatitis C.[5]

2.46.2 Froth flotation

Industrially, pine oil is used as collector in metal extraction from ores.[1] For example, in copper extraction pine oil is used to soak all copper sulfide ores for froth flotation. Therefore, it is important in the industry for the froth flotation process.

2.46.3 Safety

Pine oil has a relatively low human toxicity level, a low corrosion level and limited persistence; however, it irritates the skin and mucous membranes and has been known to cause breathing problems.[3] Large doses may cause central nervous system depression.[1]

2.46.4 References

[1] *Merck Index*, 11th Edition, **7416**. p. 1182

[2] http://www.abc.net.au/gardening/stories/s963151.htm

[3] PDRhealth

[4] http://www.epa.gov/pesticides/reregistration/REDs/ pineoil_red.pdf

[5] Detailed Information On Chemical Disinfectants University of Arizona Veterinary Diagnostic Laboratory, accessed June 26, 2007.

2.47 Rose oil

Rose oil (**rose otto, attar of rose, attar of roses** or **rose essence**) is the essential oil extracted from the petals of various types of rose. *Rose ottos* are extracted through steam distillation, while *rose absolutes* are obtained through solvent extraction or supercritical carbon dioxide extraction, with the absolute being used more commonly in perfumery. Even with their high price and the advent of organic synthesis, rose oils are still perhaps the most widely used essential oil in perfumery.

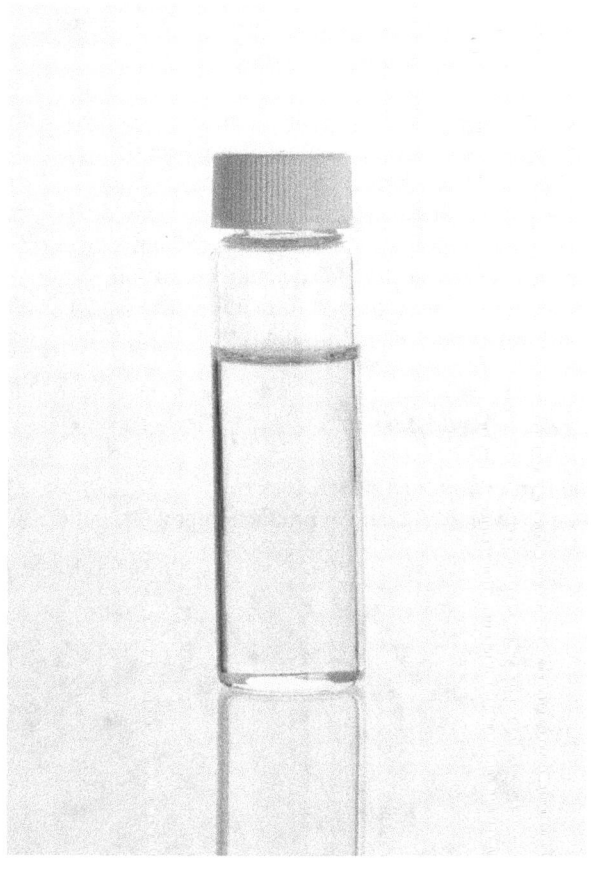

*Rose (*Rosa damascena*) essential oil in clear glass vial*

2.47.1 Components

Two major species of rose are cultivated for the production of rose oil:[1]

- *Rosa damascena*, the damask rose, which is widely grown in Syria, Bulgaria, Turkey, Russia, Pakistan, India, Uzbekistan, Iran and China

- *Rosa centifolia*, the cabbage rose, which is more commonly grown in Morocco, France and Egypt

Bulgaria produces about 70% of all rose oil in the world.[2] Other significant producers are Morocco, Iran and Turkey.

The most common chemical compounds present in rose oil are:

citronellol, geraniol, nerol, linalool, phenyl ethyl alcohol, farnesol, stearoptene, α-pinene, β-pinene, α-terpinene, limonene, p-cymene, camphene, β-caryophyllene, neral, citronellyl acetate, geranyl acetate, neryl acetate, eugenol, methyl eugenol, rose oxide, α-damascenone, β-damascenone, benzaldehyde, benzyl alcohol, rhodinyl acetate and phenyl ethyl formate.[3]

The key flavor compounds that contribute to the distinctive scent of rose oil, however, are beta-damascenone, beta-damascone, beta-ionone, and rose oxide. Beta-damascenone presence and quantity is considered as the marker for the quality of rose oil. Even though these compounds exist in less than 1% quantity of rose oil, they make up for slightly more than 90% of the odor content due to their low odor detection thresholds.[4]

2.47.2   Production

Main article: Extraction (fragrance)
Due to the labor-intensive production process and the low

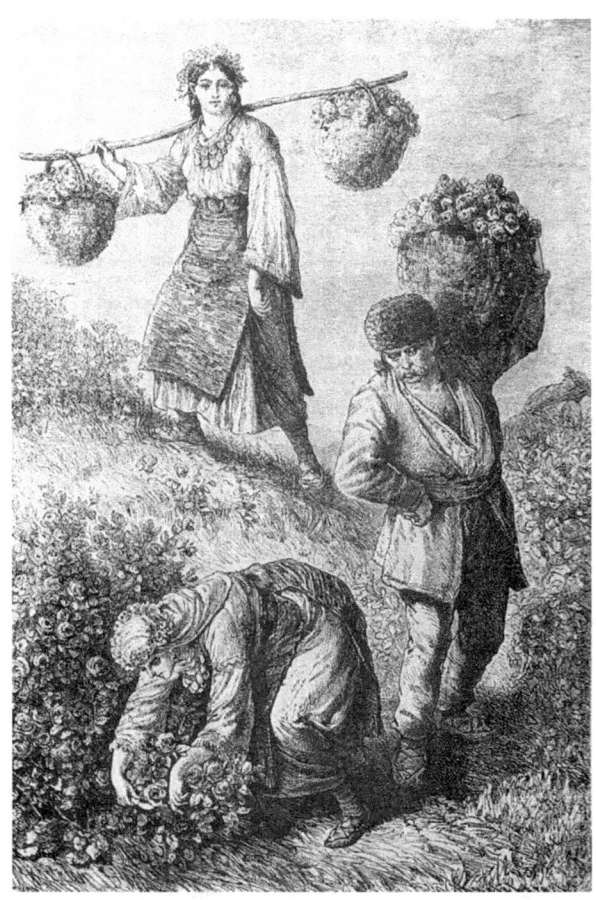

Rose-picking in the Rose Valley near the town of Kazanlak in Bulgaria, 1870s, engraving by Austro-Hungarian traveller Felix Philipp Kanitz

content of oil in the rose blooms, rose oil commands a very high price. Harvesting of flowers is done by hand in the morning before sunrise and material is distilled the same day.

There are three main methods of extracting the oil from the plant material:

- Steam distillation, which produces an oil called *rose otto* or *attar of roses*.

- Solvent extraction, which results in an oil called *rose absolute*.

- Supercritical carbon dioxide extraction, yielding an essential oil that may be marketed as either an *absolute* or as a CO_2 *extract*.

Distillation

In the process of distillation, large stills, traditionally of copper, are filled with roses and water. The still is fired for 60–105 minutes. The vaporized water and rose oil exit the still and enter a condensing apparatus and are then collected in a flask. This distillation yields a very concentrated oil, direct oil, which makes up about 20% of the final product. The water which condenses along with the oil is drained off and redistilled, cohobation, in order to obtain the water-soluble fractions of the rose oil such as phenethyl alcohol which are a vital component of the aroma and which make up the large bulk, 80%, of the oil. The two oils are combined and make the final rose otto.

Rose otto is usually dark olive-green in color and will form white crystals at normal room temperature which disappear when the oil is gently warmed. It will tend to become more viscous at lower temperatures due to this crystallization of some of its components.

The essence has a very strong odor, but is pleasant when diluted and used for perfume. Attar of roses was once made in India, Persia, Syria, and the Ottoman Empire. The Rose Valley in Bulgaria, near the town of Kazanlak, is among the major producers of attar of roses in the world.[5] In India, Kannauj is an important city of fabrication of Rose Attar, Kannauj is nicknamed "The Grasse of East" or "The Grasse of Orient". Grasse (in France) is an important city of fabrication of rose fragance. Due to the heat required for distillation, some of the compounds extracted from the rose undergo denaturing or chemical breakdown. As such, rose otto does not smell very similar to "fresh" roses.

The hydrosol portion of the distillate is known as *rosewater*. This inexpensive by-product is used widely as a food flavoring as well as in skin care.

Solvent extraction

In the solvent extraction method, the flowers are agitated in a vat with a solvent such as hexane, which draws out the aromatic compounds as well as other soluble substances such as wax and pigments. The extract is subjected to vacuum processing which removes the solvent for re-use. The remaining waxy mass is known as a *concrete*. The concrete is then mixed with alcohol which dissolves the aromatic constituents, leaving behind the wax and other substances. The alcohol is low-pressure evaporated, leaving behind the finished absolute. The absolute may be further processed to remove any impurities that are still present from the solvent extraction.

Rose absolute is a deep reddish brown with no crystals. Due to the low temperatures in this process, the absolute may be more faithful to the scent of the fresh rose than the ottor.

Carbon dioxide extraction

A third process, supercritical carbon dioxide extraction, combines the best aspects of the other two methods. When carbon dioxide is put under at least 72.9 atm (73.900 mb) of pressure and at a temperature of at least 31.1 °C (88.0 °F) (the critical point), it becomes a supercritical fluid with the permeation properties of a gas and the solvation properties of a liquid. (Under normal pressure CO_2 changes directly from a solid to a gas in a process known as sublimation.) The supercritical fluid CO_2 extracts the aromatics from the plant material.

Like solvent extraction, the CO_2 extraction takes place at a low temperature, extracts a wide range of compounds rendering an essence more faithful to the original, and leaves the aromatics unaltered by heat. Because CO_2 is gas at normal atmospheric pressure, it leaves no trace of itself in the final product. The equipment for CO_2 extraction is expensive, which is reflected in the price of the essential oils obtained from the process.

2.47.3 Adulteration

It takes many pounds of rose petals to distill one ounce of essential oil. Depending on extraction method and plant species, the average yield can range from 1:1,500 to 1:10,000.[6] To mitigate the cost, some dishonest dealers will dilute rose oil with geranium (*Pelargonium graveolens*) or palmarosa (*Cymbopogon martinii*) essential oils, both of which are rich in geraniol, the main constituent of rose oil. Some of these "rose oils" are up to 90% geranium or palmarosa to 10% rose. This is referred to as *extending* the rose fragrance. This may be done to compensate for chemotype, e.g. Bulgarian distilled rose oil is naturally low in phenylethanol, and Ukrainian or Russian rose oil is naturally high in phenylethanol. Pure rose oil should not be used directly on the skin, as it can cause allergic reactions such as red skin and spots.

2.47.4 References

[1] Hass, Nancy (September 24, 2015). "Francis Kurkdjian and Fabien Ducher, Changing History in a Bottle". *The New York Times (Style Magazine)*. ISSN 0362-4331. Retrieved 2015-10-26.

[2] Bulgaria - U.S. Central Command Factbook

[3] , Chemical composition of rose oil.

[4] Leffingwell, John C. (1999). "Rose (Rosa damascena)". *Aroma from Carotenoids*. Leffingwell & Associates. Retrieved 2006-06-08.

[5] This article incorporates text from a publication now in the public domain: Wood, James, ed. (1907). "article name needed". *The Nuttall Encyclopædia*. London and New York: Frederick Warne.

[6] *The Chemistry of Essential Oils and Artificial Perfumes.* 1921.

2.47.5 External links

The dictionary definition of rose oil at Wiktionary

2.48 Rosewood oil

Rosewood oil is a valuable essential oil, especially in perfumery. It contains the substance linalool, which has a number of uses.

The oil is extracted from the wood of Aniba rosaeodora. When it arrives at the distillery, the wood is chipped, and then steam distilled. Each tree yields about 1% oil by weight of wood. After a history of massive over-harvesting, and species depletion, efforts are underway to cultivate Aniba rosaeodora, and to develop techniques for extracting the essential oil from leaves.

Because many unrelated woods are called "Rosewood", some confusion has arisen about the origin of "Rosewood oil". Members of the genus Dalbergia (e.g. "Brazilian Rosewood"-Dalbergia nigra, and "Indian Rosewood"- Dalbergia latifolia) have never been a source of "Rosewood oil".

2.48.1 See also

- Rosewood

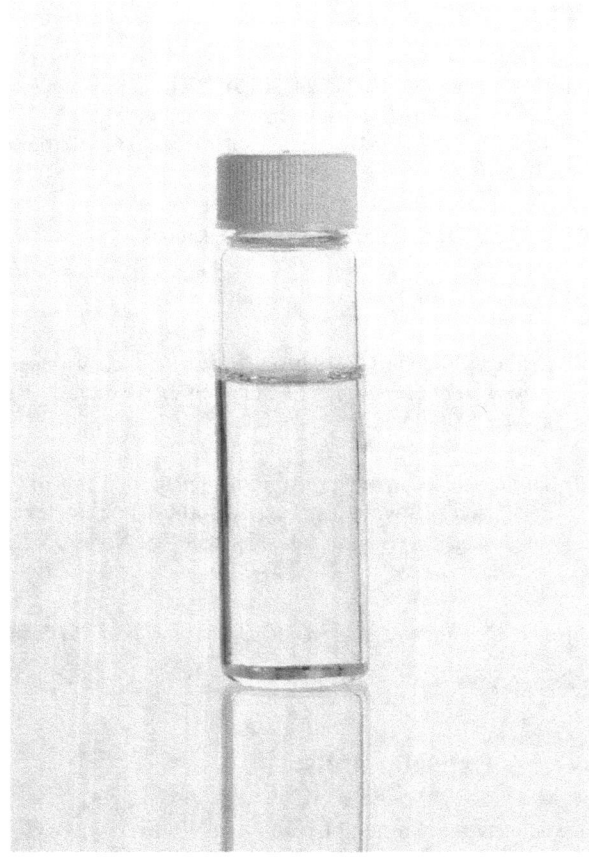

*Rosewood (*Aniba rosaeodora*) essential oil in a clear glass vial*

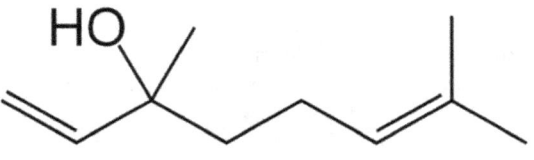

Structure of linalool, a substance extracted from A. rosaeodora

2.48.2   References

2.49   Sage oil

Sage oil is the essential oil made from the culinary herb sage, *Salvia officinalis*. In addition to its valuable flavoring characteristics, sage oil can contain as much as 50% thujone by weight. The exact amount varies based on the time in the season and which part of the plant is tested.[1] Thujone is traditionally regarded as one of the active ingredients in absinthe, distinguishing it from "less controversial" alcoholic beverages.

Sage oil has been suggested to boost short-term memory

performance in many using it as a dietary supplement.[2][3] Sage oils can be toxic and may trigger miscarriages, as well as "cause dizziness, rapid heartbeat, and provoke epileptic seizures".[4]

2.49.1   References

[1] Nigel B. Perry, Rosemary E. Anderson, Nerida J. Brennan, Malcolm H. Douglas, Anna J. Heaney, Jennifer A. McGimpsey, and Bruce M. Smallfield (1999). "Essential Oils from Dalmatian Sage (Salvia officinalis L.): Variations among Individuals, Plant Parts, Seasons, and Sites". *J. Agric. Food Chem.* **47** (5): 2045–2054. doi:10.1021/jf981170m. PMID 10552494.

[2] Melissa Hantman (Nov 11, 2003). "Spicing Up Your Memory". *Psychology Today*.

[3] Kennedy, D. O.; Dodd, F. L.; Robertson, B. C.; Okello, E. J.; Reay, J. L.; Scholey, A. B.; Haskell, C. F. (11 October 2010). "Monoterpenoid extract of sage (Salvia lavandulaefolia) with cholinesterase inhibiting properties improves cognitive performance and mood in healthy adults". *Journal of Psychopharmacology* **25** (8): 1088–1100. doi:10.1177/0269881110385594.

[4] http://www.thefreelibrary.com/Sage+advice:+aroma+ and+flavor+from+the+garden:+they're+as+decorative+.. .-a0162785550

2.50   Salvia sclarea

Salvia sclarea, **clary**, or **clary sage**, is a biennial or short-lived herbaceous perennial in the genus *Salvia*. It is native to the northern Mediterranean, along with some areas in north Africa and Central Asia. The plant has a lengthy history as a medicinal herb, and is currently grown for its essential oil.[1]

2.50.1   Description

S. sclarea reaches 3 to 4 ft (0.91 to 1.22 m) in height, with thick square stems that are covered in hairs. The leaves are approximately 1 ft (0.30 m) long at the base, .5 ft (0.15 m) long higher on the plant. The upper leaf surface is rugose, and covered with glandular hairs. The flowers are in verticils, with 2-6 flowers in each verticil, and are held in large colorful bracts that range in color from pale mauve to lilac or white to pink with a pink mark on the edge. The lilac or pale blue corolla is approximately 1 in (2.5 cm), with the lips held wide open.[1] The cultivar *S. sclarea* 'Turkestanica' bears pink stems, petiolate leaves, and white, pink-flecked blossoms on spikes to 30 inches tall (75 cm).[2]

2.50.2 History

Descriptions of medicinal use of the plant goes back to the writings of Theophrastus (4th century BCE), Dioscorides (1st century CE), and Pliny the Elder (1st century CE).

2.50.3 Uses

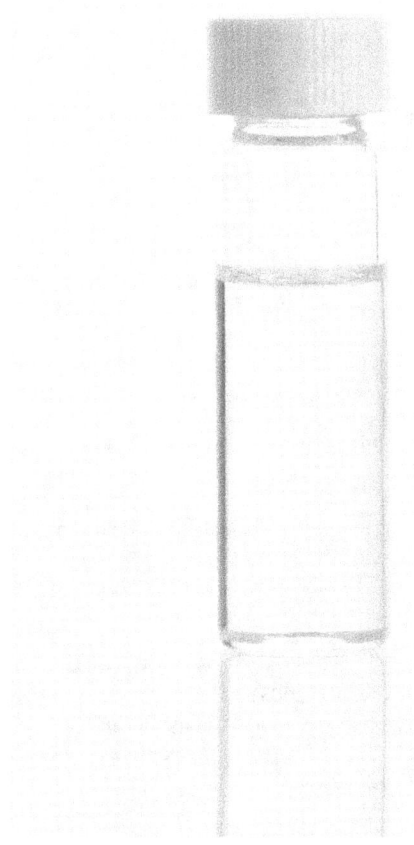

*Clary sage (*Salvia sclarea*) essential oil*

Clary seeds have a mucilaginous coat, which is why some old herbals recommended placing a seed into the eye of someone with a foreign object in it so that it could adhere to the object and make it easy to remove. This practice is noted by Nicholas Culpeper in his *Complete Herbal* (1653), who referred to the plant as "clear-eye".[3]

The distilled essential oil is used widely in perfumes and as a muscatel flavoring for vermouths, wines, and liqueurs.[1] It is also used in aromatherapy for relieving anxiety and fear, menstrual-related problems such as PMS and cramping, and helping with insomnia.[4]

2.50.4 Gallery

- Plants of *Salvia sclarea*
- Plant of *Salvia sclarea*
- Clusters of clary flowers
- Close-up
- Close-up
-
- Leaves

2.50.5 References

[1] Clebsch, Betsy; Barner, Carol D. (2003). *The New Book of Salvias*. Timber Press. p. 261. ISBN 978-0-88192-560-9.

[2] Mark Griffiths. *Index of Garden Plants, 2nd American Edition*. (Portland, Oregon: Timber Press, 1995; ISBN 0-88192-246-3).

[3] *The Complete Herbal* at Bibliomania, with link to entry for Clary, or More Properly Clear-Eye.

[4] Kintzios, Spiridon E. (2000). *Sage: The Genus Salvia* CRC Press. p. 20. ISBN 978-90-5823-005-8.

2.50.6 External links

- German: *Wikipedia: Muskatellersalbei*
-
- *Salvia sclarea* in Plantarium Database - A Photo Guide.

2.51 Sandalwood oil

Sandalwood oil is an essential oil obtained from the steam distillation of chips and billets cut from the heartwood of the sandalwood (*Santalum album*) tree. Sandalwood oil is used in perfumes, cosmetics, and sacred unguents.[1]

2.51.1 Main constituents

Sandalwood oil contains more than 90% sesquiterpenic alcohols of which 50-60% is the tricyclic α-santalol. β-Santalol comprises 20-25%.[2][3]

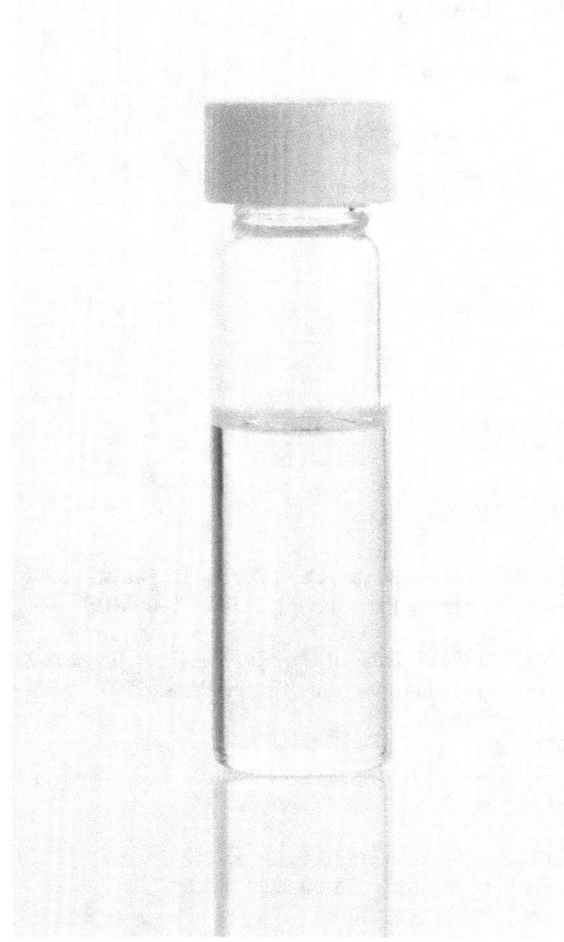

A glass vial containing pure Sandalwood Essential Oil

2.51.2 Traditional uses

Sandalwood essential oil is used in Ayurvedic medicine for the treatment of both somatic and mental disorders.[4] A study investigating the effects of inhalation of East Indian sandalwood oil and its main compound, α-santalol, on human physiological parameters found that the compounds elevated pulse rate, skin conductance, and systolic blood pressure.[4]

Sandalwood oil and α-santalol have been associated with chemopreventive activity in animal models of carcinogenesis.[5][6][7]

2.51.3 Synthetic equivalents

There are several synthetic odorants with odour similar to sandalwood oil, used as lower-cost alternatives for perfumes, emollients, and skin cleaning agents. Two of these, Sandalore and Brahmanol, have been found to be agonists of the cutaneous olfactory receptor OR2AT4, with potential therapeutic benefits for wound healing. Natural sandalwood oil, and other synthetic sandalwood odorants, did not have the same effect. [8][9]

2.51.4 See also

- Isobornyl cyclohexanol, a synthetic sandalwood oil

2.51.5 References

[1] Kapoor LD (2001). *Handbook of Ayurvedic Medicinal Plants.* Herbal Reference Library Series **2**. Boca Raton, FL: CRC Press. ISBN 9780849329296.

[2] Krotz A, Helmchen G (1994). "Total Syntheses, Optical Rotations and Fragrance Properties of Sandalwood Constituents: (−)-(Z)- and (−)-(E)-β-Santalol and Their Enantiomers, *ent*-β-Santalene". *Liebigs Ann Chem* **1994** (6): 601–609. doi:10.1002/jlac.199419940610.

[3] Sandalwood Essential Oil, http://scienceofacne.com/sandalwood-essential-oil/

[4] Heuberger, E; Hongratanaworakit, T; Buchbauer, G (2006). "East Indian Sandalwood and alpha-santalol odor increase physiological and self-rated arousal in humans". *Planta Medica* **72** (9): 792–800. doi:10.1055/s-2006-941544. PMID 16783696.

[5] Dwivedi C, Ahang Y (1999). "Sandalwood oil prevents skin tumour development in CD1 mice". *Eur J Cancer Prev* **8** (5): 449–455. doi:10.1097/00008469-199910000-00011. PMID 10548401.

[6] Dwivedi C, Guan X, Harmsen WL, Voss AL, Goetz-Parten DE, Koopman EM et al. (2003). "Chemopreventive effects of alpha-santalol on skin tumor development in CD-1 and SENCAR mice". *Cancer Epidemiol Biomarkers Prev* **12** (2): 151–156. PMID 12582025.

[7] Benencia F, Courreges MC (1999). "Antiviral activity of sandalwood oil against *Herpes simplex* viruses-1 and −2". *Phytomedicine* **6** (2): 119–123. doi:10.1016/S0944-7113(99)80046-4.

[8] A Synthetic Sandalwood Odorant Induces Wound-Healing Processes in Human Keratinocytes via the Olfactory Receptor OR2AT4, Daniela Busse1, Philipp Kudella1, Nana-Maria Grüning, Günter Gisselmann1, Sonja Ständer, Thomas Luger, Frank Jacobsen, Lars Steinsträßer, Ralf Paus, Paraskevi Gkogkolou, Markus Böhm, Hanns Hatt and Heike Benecke, Journal of Investigative Dermatology (2014) 134, 2823–2832; doi:10.1038/jid.2014.273; published online 7 August 2014

[9] New Scientist magazine,Skin's ability to 'smell' seems to help it heal itself, 8 July 2014

2.52 Santalum album

Santalum album or **Indian sandalwood** is a small tropical tree, and is the most commonly known source of sandalwood. This species has historically been cultivated, processed and traded since ancient times. Certain cultures place great significance on its fragrant and medicinal qualities. The high value of the species has caused its past exploitation, to the point where the wild population is vulnerable to extinction. Indian sandalwood still commands high prices for its essential oil, but due to lack of sizable trees it is no longer used for fine woodworking as before. The plant is widely cultivated and long lived, although harvest is viable after 40 years. Etymologically it is derived from Sanskrit Chandanam > Sandanam > Sandalum > Sandal.[2]

2.52.1 Description

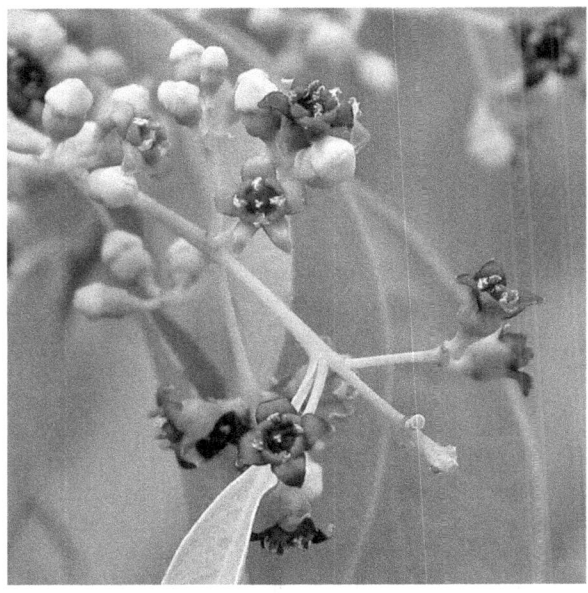

Flowers in Hyderabad, India.

The height of the evergreen tree is between 4 and 9 metres. They may live to one hundred years of age. The tree is variable in habit, usually upright to sprawling, and may intertwine with other species. The plant parasitises the roots of other tree species, with a haustorium adaptation on its own roots, but without major detriment to its hosts. An individual will form a non-obligate relationship with a number of other plants. Up to 300 species (including its own) can host the tree's development - supplying macronutrients phosphorus, nitrogen and potassium, and shade - especially during early phases of development. It may propagate itself through wood suckering during its early development, establishing small stands. The reddish or brown bark can be almost black and is smooth in young trees, becoming cracked with a red reveal. The heartwood is pale green to white as the common name indicates. The leaves are thin, opposite and ovate to lanceolate in shape. Glabrous surface is shiny and bright green, with a glaucous pale reverse. Fruit is produced after three years, viable seeds after five. These seeds are distributed by birds.

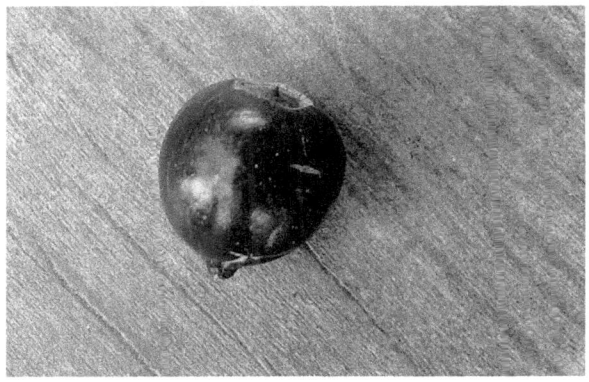

A ripen fruit of Santalum album from Panchkhal Valley, Nepal.

2.52.2 Nomenclature

See also: Sandalwood

The nomenclature for other "sandalwoods" and the taxonomy of the genus are derived from this species' historical and widespread use. *Santalum album* is included in the family Santalaceae, and is commonly known as white or East Indian sandalwood.[3] The name, *Santalum ovatum*, used by Robert Brown in *Prodromus Florae Novae Hollandiae* (1810) was described as a synonym of this species by Alex George in 1984.[4] The epithet *album* refers to the 'white' of the heartwood.

The species was the first to be known as sandalwood. Other species in the genus *Santalum*, such as the Australian *S. spicatum*, are also referred to as true sandalwoods, to distinguish them from trees with similar-smelling wood or oil.

2.52.3 Distribution

It is a hemiparasitic tree, native to semi-arid areas of the Indian subcontinent. It is now planted in India, China, Sri Lanka, Indonesia, Malaysia, the Philippines and Northern Australia.

2.52.4 Habitat

S. album occurs from coastal dry forests up to 700 m elevation. It normally grows in sandy or stony red soils, but a wide range of soil types are inhabited. This habitat has a temperature range from 0 to 38 °C and annual rainfall between 500 and 3000 mm.

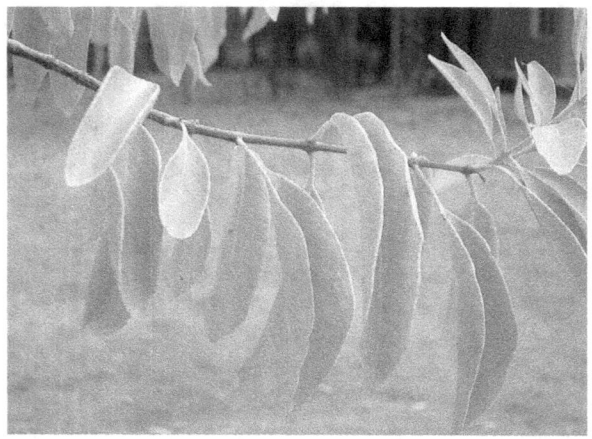

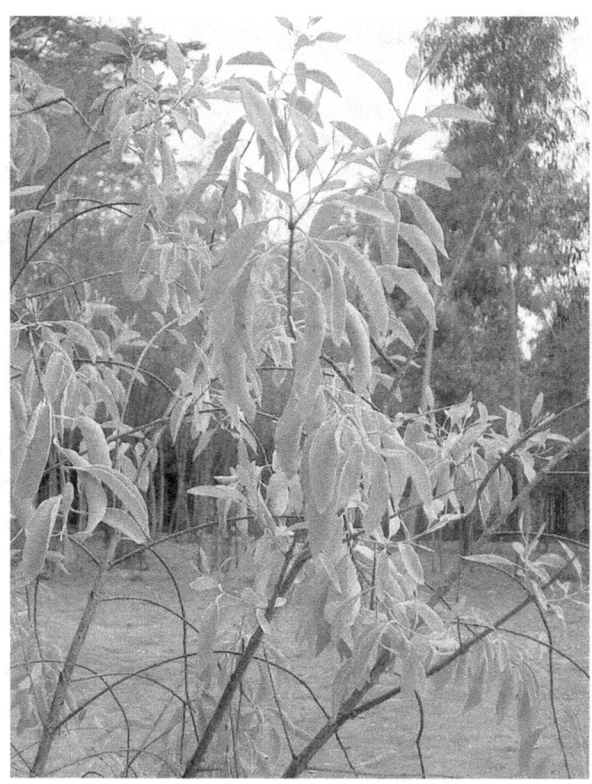

Young sapling

2.52.5 Conservation

The species is threatened by over-exploitation and degradation to habitat through altered land use; fire, agriculture and land-clearing are the factors of most concern. To preserve this vulnerable resource from over-exploitation, legislation protects the species, and cultivation is researched and developed.[5][6][7]

The Indian government has placed a ban on the export of the timber.[1]

2.52.6 Uses

S. album has been the primary source of sandalwood and the derived oil. These often hold an important place within the societies of its naturalised distribution range. The high value of the plant has led to attempts at cultivation, this has increased the distribution range of the plant. The ISO Standard for the accepted characteristics of this essential oil is ISO 3518:2002.[8] HPTLC and GC,[9] GC-MS based methods are used for qualitative and quantitative analyses of the volatile [10] essential oil constituents. The long maturation period and difficulty in cultivation have been restrictive to extensive planting within the range. Harvest of the tree involves several curing and processing stages, also adding to the commercial value. These wood and oil have high demand and are an important trade item in the regions of:

India The use of *S. album* in India is noted in literature for over two thousand years. It has use as wood and oil in religious practices. It also features as a construction material in temples and elsewhere. The Indian government has banned the export of the species to reduce the threat by over-harvesting. In the southern Indian state of Karnataka, all trees of greater than a specified girth are the property of the state. Cutting of trees, even on private property, is regulated by the Forest Department.[11] The infamous forest bandit Veerappan was involved in the illegal felling of sandalwood trees from forests.

Sri Lanka The harvesting of sandalwood is preferred to be of trees that are advanced in age. Saleable wood can, however, be of trees as young as seven years. The entire plant is removed rather than cut to the base, as in coppiced species. The extensive removal of *S. album* over the past century led to increased vulnerability to extinction.[1]

Australia Utilisation of native Australian *Santalum* species in has been extensive; *Santalum spicatum* was extensively harvested and exported from Western Australia during colonisation, this was used as a less expensive alternative to this species. There are two commercial Indian sandalwood plantations in full operation based in Kununurra, Western Australia.[12] [13]

Ethnopharmacological Uses

Sandalwood oil has been widely used in folk medicine for treatment of common colds, bronchitis, skin disorders, heart ailments, general weakness, fever, infection of the urinary tract, inflammation of the mouth and pharynx, liver and gallbladder complaints and other maladies.[14] Recently, the *in vivo* anti-hyperglycemic and antioxidant potentials[15] of α-santalol and sandalwood oil were demonstrated in Swiss Albino mice. Additionally, different *in vitro* and *in vivo* parts of the plant have been shown to possess antimicrobial[16] and antioxidant[16] properties, possibly attributed to sesquiterpenoids,[17] shikimic acid,[18] etc.

2.52.7 See also

- Sandal spike phytoplasma - disease of *S. album*

2.52.8 References

[1] Asian Regional Workshop (1998). *Santalum album*. 2006. *IUCN Red List of Threatened Species*. IUCN 2006. www.iucnredlist.org. Retrieved on 2007-02-08.

[2] http://www.etymonline.com/index.php?term=sandalwood

[3] *Santalum* (IPNI)

[4] "*Santalum ovatum*". *Australian Plant Name Index (APNI), IBIS database*. Centre for Plant Biodiversity Research, Australian Government. George, A.S. & Hewson, H.J. in George, A.S. (Ed) (1984), *Flora of Australia* 22: 61, 63, Fig. 18D, Map 71

[5] http://www.newcrops.uq.edu.au/newslett/ncnl2-54.htm University of Queensland site's detail

[6] Australian Arid Lands Botanic Garden - Plants: Sandalwood, Santalum spicatum

[7] http://www.fpc.wa.gov.au/pdfs/sandalwood_detail.pdf WA Gov site's detail

[8] ISO 3518:2002

[9] Misra, B. B.; Dey, S. "Quantitative and qualitative evaluation of esquiterpenoids from essential oil and in vitro somatic embryos of east Indian Sandalwood (Santalum album) tree by HPTLC and GC.". *Journal of Medicinal and Aromatic Plants* 4 (1): 1–9.

[10] Misra, Biswapriya B.; Das, Shibendu S.; Dey, Satyahari. "Volatile profiling from heartwood of East Indian sandalwood tree". *Journal of Pharmacy Research* 7 (4): 299–303. doi:10.1016/j.jopr.2013.04.030.

[11] Karnataka Forest Department Rules

[12] Indian Sandalwood Plantations in Australia. Tropical Forest Services (TFS) Ltd.

[13] Indian Sandalwood in Western Australia. Santanol

[14] Misra, BB; Dey, S (2013). "Biological Activities of East Indian Sandalwood Tree, Santalum album". *PeerJ PrePrints* 1: e96. doi:10.7287/peerj.preprints.96v1.

[15] Misra, Biswapriya B.; Dey, Satyahari (2013). "Evaluation of in vivo anti-hyperglycemic and antioxidant potentials of α-santalol and sandalwood oil". *Phytomedicine* 20 (5): 409–16. doi:10.1016/j.phymed.2012.12.017. PMID 23369343.

[16] Misra, B.B.; Dey, S. (2012). "Comparative phytochemical analysis and antibacterial efficacy of in vitro and in vivo extracts from East Indian sandalwood tree (Santalum album L.)". *Letters in Applied Microbiology*: n/a. doi:10.1111/lam.12005. PMID 23020220.

[17] Misra, Biswapriya B.; Dey, Satyahari (2012). "Differential Extraction and GC-MS based Quantification of Sesquiterpenoids from Immature Heartwood of East Indian Sandalwood Tree". *Journal of Natural Sciences Research* 2 (6): 29–33.

[18] Misra, Biswapriya B.; Dey, Satyahari (2013). "Shikimic Acid (Tamiflu Precursor) Production in Suspension Cultures of East Indian Sandalwood (Santalum album) in Airlift Bioreactor". *Journal of Postdoctoral Research* 1 (1): 1–9.

2.52.9 External links

- Tennakoon, Kushan U.; Cameron, Duncan D. (2006). "The anatomy of *Santalum album* (Sandalwood) haustoria". *Canadian Journal of Botany* 84 (10): 1608–16. doi:10.1139/b06-118.

- Media related to Santalum album at Wikimedia Commons

- Data related to Santalum album at Wikispecies

- Scoop. It ! On Indian Sandalwood Tree, India, highlighting all major 'recent' research activities and achievements involving Sandalwood

- Homepage of Professor Satyahari Dey, at Department of Biotechnology, IIT Kharagpur, India: Working on Indian Sandalwood since 20 years

- Caldecott, Todd (2006). *Ayurveda: The Divine Science of Life*. Elsevier/Mosby. ISBN 0-7234-3410-7. Contains a detailed monograph on *Santalum album* (Chandana) as well as a discussion of health benefits and usage in clinical practice. Available online at http://www.toddcaldecott.com/index.php/herbs/learning-herbs/379-chandana

2.53 Santalum spicatum

Santalum spicatum, **Australian sandalwood**, is a tree native to semiarid[1] areas at the edge of Southwest Australia. It is traded as sandalwood, and its valuable oil has been used as an aromatic, a medicine, and a food source. *S. spicatum* is one of four high-value *Santalum* species occurring in Australia.

2.53.1 Description

It is one of four species of the family Santalaceae to occur in Western Australia. It has a similar distribution to quandong (*Santalum acuminatum*) and is a hemiparasite requiring macronutrients from the roots of hosts. It has a shrubby to small tree habit, but can grow to 6 metres and is tolerant of drought and salt. The foliage is grey-green in colour. The fruit of *S. spicatum* is spherical, about 3 cm in diameter and is orange. An edible kernel with a hard shell forms the bulk of the fruit; the shell is smoother than *S. acuminatum's* deeply pitted surface. Germination occurs during warm and moist conditions. The impact of overcultivation and land clearing for agriculture, since the 1880s, has greatly reduced the range of the species. The oils produced by the tree contain a greater complexity of chemicals, many of which have antimicrobial qualities.[2]

2.53.2 Commercial use

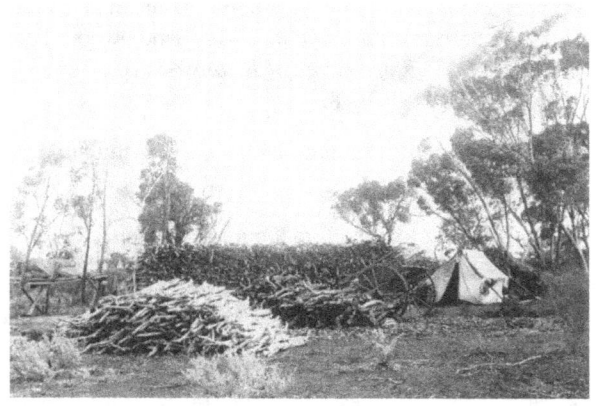

A sandalwood cutters camp in the Wheatbelt of Western Australia

The harvest and export of *S. spicatum* has been an important part of the Western Australian economy, at one time forming more than half of the state's revenue. Settlement of the Wheatbelt area was accelerated by the funds generated by sandalwood found there. Distribution and population of the endemic stands were significantly affected during periods of rural development and economic downturn.

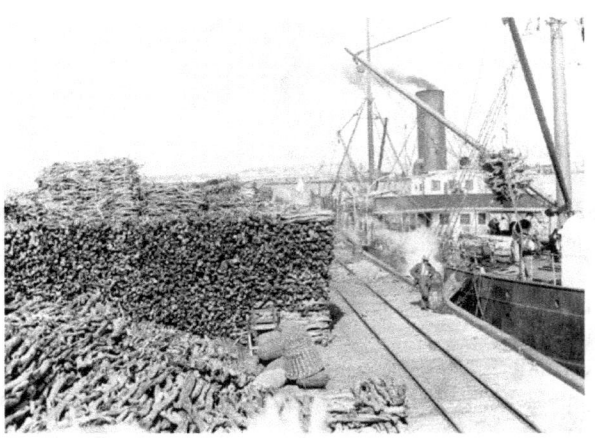

Exported from Fremantle Harbour, 1905

Research by the Forestry Products Commission (Western Australia), state universities and private industry is being undertaken into the cultivation of the tree and the properties of its wood and nuts.[3][4] Replanting has occurred at some properties as a land restoration strategy, a food crop and in the long term for harvest. Oil valued at $1 000(AUD) per kilogram is produced at Mount Romance in Albany, Western Australia.[5] The area of commercial plantations has risen from seven to 70 km^2 between 2000 and 2006. The export of 2 000 tonnes of sandalwood a year is primarily sourced from wild stands of the remote rangelands and Goldfields Region of Western Australia. The harvest of naturally occurring trees is reduced when compared to the industry of the 19th century. Exports of over 50 000 tonnes in the last decade were related to agricultural expansion by increased access and harvesters.[6]

Cultivation

Germination is difficult, and may depend on the El Niño cycle. Success has been reported by placing the kernels in moist vermiculite in sealed plastic bags at room temperature. Once germinated, seeds should be planted next to a (preferably Australian native) seedling, and watered adequately.

Host species

The main host species is *Acacia acuminata*, which is used in plantations, which sustains a 15- to 30-year long-term host species in loamy sands over clay duplex soils. Rock sheaok *Allocasuarina huegeliana*, wodjil *Acacia resinimarginea* and mulga *Acacia aneura* are also used.[7]

2.53.3 References

[1] Sandalwood(Santalum Spicatum) Guide for Farmers - Tree Facts pamphlet- Forest Products Commission - April 2007 specifically states Wheatbelt and areas with minimum 400 mm annual rainfall

[2] *"Santalum"*. *Florabase*. Department of Environment and conservation. August 2002. Retrieved 2007-04-29. /browse/flora?f=092&level=g&id=523 et al.

[3] University of Queensland site's detail

[4] Australian Arid Lands Botanic Garden - Plants: Sandalwood, Santalum spicatum

[5] Murphy, Sean (reporter) (2007-04-27). "High hopes for native sandalwood". *Landline (transcript)*. ABC. Retrieved 2007-05-01. Most of WA's native sandalwood harvest ends up at the Mt Romance essential oil factory in Albany, on the south coast of WA. It is converted into a liquid fetching as much as $1,000 a kilogram.

[6] WA Gov site's detail

[7] Sandalwood Guide for Farmers states 'being a root hemi-parasitic tree.. it is planted with a nitrogen-fixing host species such as jam *Acacia acuminata*"

2.54 Sfumatura

The *sfumatura* or **slow-folding** process is a traditional technique for manually extracting the essential oils from citrus peel using sponges. Dating back to 18th-century Italy, the process is still carried out in Sicily today, although it is increasingly rare.[1] Despite the modern array of sophisticated machines for extracting citrus oil, even the best machinery does not approach the quality of *sfumatura*-produced oil.[2]

Using a *rastrello*, a special spoon-shaped knife, the fresh peel is de-pulped. It is then thoroughly washed with limewater and drip-dried on woven mats or special baskets for 3 to 24 hours, depending on the ripeness of the fruit, the temperature, and the humidity. These steps harden the peel, causing the oil to spurt from the oil glands more easily, and the lime helps neutralize the acidity of the peel.[3]

A series of natural sponges is fixed upon a terracotta basin or *concolina* and held in place with a wooden bar laid across the rim. The dried peel is folded and pressed against the sponges several times in a circular motion, causing a mixture of essential oil and peel liquids to pass into the *concolina*. After finishing with the peel, the sponges are squeezed to recover additional oil and liquids. Finally, the oil is decanted away from the heavier watery phase, which contains detritus from breaking the peel.[3]

2.54.1 References

[1] Di Giacomo p.63-64

[2] Di Giacomo and Di Giacomo p.124

[3] Di Giacomo p.64, Di Giacomo and Di Giacomo pp.125-126

- Giovanni Dugo and Angelo Di Giacomo, eds., ed. (2002). *Citrus*. London: Taylor & Francis. ISBN 0-415-28491-0.

- Angela Di Giacomo. "Development of the citrus industry: historical note". pp. 63–70.

- Angela Di Giacomo and Giovanni Di Giacomo. "Essential oil production". pp. 114–147

2.55 Spearmint

For other uses, see Spearmint (disambiguation).

Spearmint or **spear mint** (***Mentha spicata***) is a species of mint native to much of Europe and Asia (Middle East, Himalayas, China etc.), and naturalized in parts of northern and western Africa, North and South America, as well as various oceanic islands.[2][3][4][5]

Subspecies[2]

1. *Mentha spicata* subsp. *condensata* (Briq.) Greuter & Burdet - Mediterranean region; naturalized in New Zealand

2. *Mentha spicata* subsp. *spicata* - most of species range

2.55.1 Description

It is a herbaceous, rhizomatous, perennial plant growing 30–100 cm tall, with variably hairless to hairy stems and foliage, and a wide-spreading fleshy underground rhizome. The leaves are 5–9 cm long and 1.5–3 cm broad, with a serrated margin. The stem is square-shaped, a trademark of the mint family of herbs. Spearmint produces flowers in slender spikes, each flower pink or white, 2.5–3 mm long, and broad.[3][6]

Hybrids involving spearmint include *Mentha* × *piperita* (peppermint; hybrid with *Mentha aquatica*), *Mentha* × *gracilis* (ginger mint, syn. *M. cardiaca*; hybrid with *Mentha arvensis*), and *Mentha* × *villosa* (large apple mint, hybrid with *Mentha suaveolens*).

The name 'spear' mint derives from the pointed leaf tips.[7]

2.55.2 Cultivation and uses

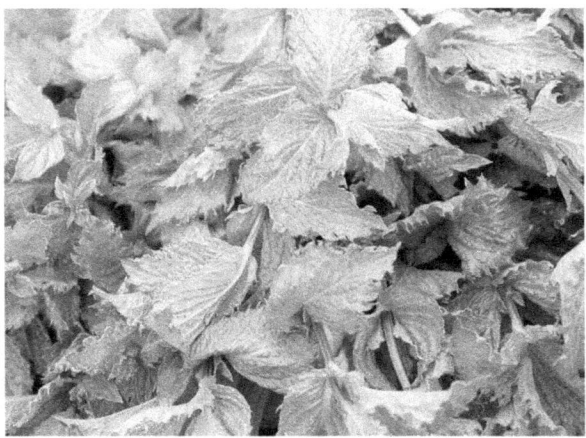

Fresh spearmint offered for sale at a market

Spearmint grows well in nearly all temperate climates. Gardeners often grow it in pots or planters due to its invasive, spreading rhizomes. The plant prefers partial shade, but can flourish in full sun to mostly shade. Spearmint is best suited to loamy soils with abundant organic material.

Spearmint leaves can be used fresh, dried, or frozen. They can also be preserved in salt, sugar, sugar syrup, alcohol, or oil. The leaves lose their aromatic appeal after the plant flowers. It can be dried by cutting just before, or right (at peak) as the flowers open, about one-half to three-quarters the way down the stalk (leaving smaller shoots room to grow). Some dispute exists as to what drying method works best; some prefer different materials (such as plastic or cloth) and different lighting conditions (such as darkness or sunlight).

Spearmint is often cultivated for its aromatic and carminative oil, referred to as **oil of spearmint**. The most abundant compound in spearmint oil is R-(−)-carvone, which gives spearmint its distinctive smell. Spearmint oil also contains significant amounts of limonene, dihydrocarvone, and 1,8-cineol.[8] Unlike peppermint oil, oil of spearmint contains minimal amounts of menthol and menthone.[9] It is used as a flavoring for toothpaste and confectionery, and is sometimes added to shampoos and soaps.

2.55.3 Tea

The cultivar *Mentha spicata* 'Nana', the nana mint of Morocco, possesses a clear, pungent, but mild aroma, and is an essential ingredient of Touareg tea.

Spearmint is an ingredient in several mixed drinks, such as the mojito and mint julep. Sweet tea, iced and flavored with spearmint, is a summer tradition in the Southern United States. As a medicinal plant, spearmint is steeped as tea for the treatment of stomach ache.

2.55.4 Health effects

Spearmint has been studied for antifungal activity; its essential oil was found to have some antifungal activity, although less than oregano.[10] Its essential oil did not show any evidence of mutagenicity in the Ames test.[10] It can have a calming effect when used for insomnia or massages.

2.55.5 References

[1] *"Mentha L.". Germplasm Resources Information Network*. United States Department of Agriculture. 2004-09-10. Retrieved 2010-01-30.

[2] "World Checklist of Selected Plant Families: Royal Botanic Gardens, Kew". *kew.org*.

[3] Flora of China Vol. 17 Page 238 ⬚⬚⬚ liu lan xiang *Mentha spicata* Linnaeus, Sp. Pl. 2: 576. 1753.

[4] Altervista Flora Italiana, Menta romana, *Mentha spicata* L. includes photos + distribution maps for Europe + North America

[5] Biota of North America Program, 2013 county distribution map

[6] Huxley, A., ed. (1992). *New RHS Dictionary of Gardening*. Macmillan ISBN 0-333-47494-5.

[7] Turner, W. (1568). *Herbal*. Cited in the *Oxford English Dictionary*.

[8] Hussain, Abdullah I; Anwar, Farooq; Nigam, Poonam S; Ashraf, Muhammad; Gilani, Anwarul H (2010). "Seasonal variation in content, chemical composition and antimicrobial and cytotoxic activities of essential oils from four *Mentha* species". *Journal of the Science of Food and Agriculture* **90** (11): 1827–36. doi:10.1002/jsfa.4021. PMID 20602517.

[9] , Chemical composition of essential oils from several species of mint (*Mentha*).

[10] Adam, Konstantia; Sivropoulou, Afroditi; Kokkini, Stella; Lanaras, Thomas; Arsenakis, Minas (1998). "Antifungal Activities of *Origanum vulgare* subsp. *hirtum*, *Mentha spicata*, *Lavandula angustifolia*, and *Salvia fruticosa* Essential Oils against Human Pathogenic Fungi". *Journal of Agricultural and Food Chemistry* **46** (5): 1739–45. doi:10.1021/jf9708296.

2.55.6 Gallery

- Plant in flower
- flowers
- 1887 illustration
- Grown in Malaysia

2.56 Styrax balsam

For the Storax tree, see Styrax.

Styrax (storax) balsam is a recent natural resin isolated from the wounded bark of Liquidambar orientalis Mill. (Asia Minor) and Liquidambar styraciflua L. (Central America) (Hamamelidaceae).[1] It is often called benzoic resin, a similar resin obtained from the Styracaceae plant family.

2.56.1 Composition

Purified storax contains circa 33 to 50 % storesin, an alcoholic resin, both free and as cinnamic esters. Contains 5 to 15 % cinnamic acid, 5 to 15 % cinnamyl cinnamate, circa 10 % phenylpropyl cinnamate; small amounts of ethyl cinnamate, benzyl cinnamate, and styrene, Some may contain traces of vanillin. Some sources report a resin containing triterpenic acids (oleanolic and 3-epioleanolic acids).[2]

2.56.2 Uses

Styrax has a pleasant, sweet, balsamic, slightly spicy odor. Storax and its derivatives (resinoid, essential oil, absolute) are used as flavors, fragrances, and in pharmaceuticals (Friar's Balsam).[1][3][4]

American styrax resin (Liquidambar styraciflua) is chewed like gum to freshen breath and clean teeth.[5]

2.56.3 History

Mnesimachus, Aristoteles, Theophrastus (*Historia Plantarum*), Herodotus, and Strabo are the first ones to mention the styrax tree and its balsam. In ancient Greece, styrax also denoted the spike at the lower end of a spearshaft.[6]

Pliny (*Historia Naturalis* 12.98, 15.26; 24.24) notes the use of styrax as a perfume, while Scribonius Largus drank wine flavored with styrax.[7] Ciris mentions storax as a fragrant hair dye.[8] Dioscorides (*De materia medica* 1.79) reports its

use as incense, similar to frankincense, having expectorant and soothing properties.[9]

The 10th century Arab historian al-Masudi listed storax gum (*may'a*) as a spice in his book *Murūḍi al-dhahab* (*Meadows of Gold*).[10]

Chao Ju-Kuan, a 13th century trade commissioner in Fukien province, described liquid storax gum as a product of the Somali (*Po-pa-li*) coast.[11]

Linnaeus, who determined the scientific names of plants, thought that storax was extracted from the tree called in modern Hebrew *livneh refu'i* which he termed Styrax officinalis. However in the light of tests made in Israel it is very doubtful if a sap with medicinal or aromatic qualities can be extracted from this tree. The storax of the ancients was probably extracted from a different tree, seemingly from the Liquidambar orientalis which grows wild in northern Syria and may even have been grown in Israel; from it is extracted an aromatic sap with healing qualities called *storax liquidis*. This may possibly be the biblical balm, though other sources conclude that the biblical balm is Balsam (opobalsamum).[12]

Styrax officinalis is a more humid Asian species, reported from India, Cambodia, Laos, Myanmar, Thailand, Vietnam, Java, Sumatra, and Malaysia. Thus, this species historically would have needed to be imported from outside Israel.[5]

In the nineteenth century, styrene was isolated by distillation of storax balsam.[13]

In North Africa, for mystical purposes, women burn benzoin and styrax in potsherds.[14]

2.56.4 Safety

Storax resin is "generally regarded as safe" (GRAS), but at low levels, for example, circa 15 ppm in candy and 25 ppm in baked goods.[2]

2.56.5 See also

- Opopanax

2.56.6 References

[1] Karl-Georg Fahlbusch; et al. (2007), "Flavors and Fragrances", *Ullmann's Encyclopedia of Industrial Chemistry* (7th ed.), Wiley, p. 115

[2] James A. Duke (2008), "Storax (Liquidambar orientalis Mill. and L., Styraciflua L.)", *Duke's Handbook of Medicinal Plants of the Bible*, Taylor & Francis, pp. 258–259

[3] George A. Burdock (2010), "Styrax", *Fenaroli's Handbook of Flavor Ingredients* (6th ed.), Taylor & Francis, pp. 1853–1854

[4] "Compound Benzoin Tincture", *British Pharmacopoeia* **3**, 2009

[5] James A. Duke (2008), "Benzoin (Styrax benzoin Dryander.)", *Duke's Handbook of Medicinal Plants of the Bible*, Taylor & Francis, p. 445

[6] Henry George Liddell; Robert Scott, eds. (1897), "στύραξ", *Greek-English Lexicon* (8th ed.), Harper & Brothers, p. 1442

[7] "styrax", *Oxford Latin Dictionary*, Oxford University Press, 1968, p. 1832

[8] "storax", *Oxford Latin Dictionary*, Oxford University Press, 1968, p. 1825

[9] Dioscorides (1902), "Styrax", in Julius Berendes, *De materia medica* (PDF), PharmaWiki.ch, p. 89

[10] A. Dietrich (2004), "AFĀWĪH", *The Encyclopaedia of Islam*, 12 (supplement) (2nd ed.), Brill, pp. 42–43

[11] E. Cerulli; M. Orwin; G. S. P. Freeman-Greenville (1997), "SOMALI", *The Encyclopaedia of Islam* **9** (2nd ed.), Brill, pp. 713–727

[12] Jehuda Feliks (2007), "Storax", *Encyclopaedia Judaica* **19** (2nd ed.), Thomson Gale, p. 238

[13] Denis H. James; William M. Castor (2007), "Styrene", *Ullmann's Encyclopedia of Industrial Chemistry* (7th ed.), Wiley, p. 1

[14] D. S. Margoliouth (1997), "ḴĀDIRIYYA", *The Encyclopaedia of Islam* **4** (2nd ed.), Brill, pp. 380–383

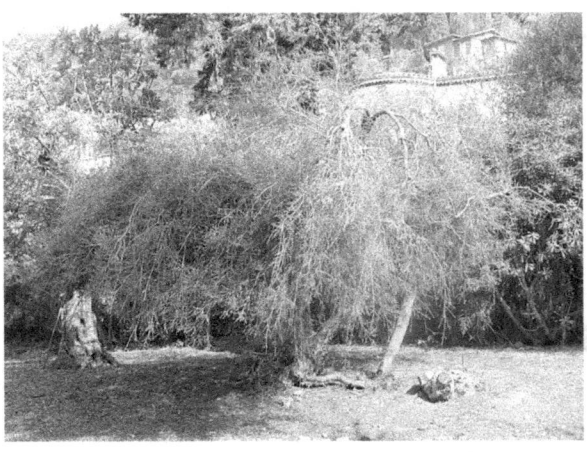

Origin of this essential oil, the tea tree, Melaleuca alternifolia.

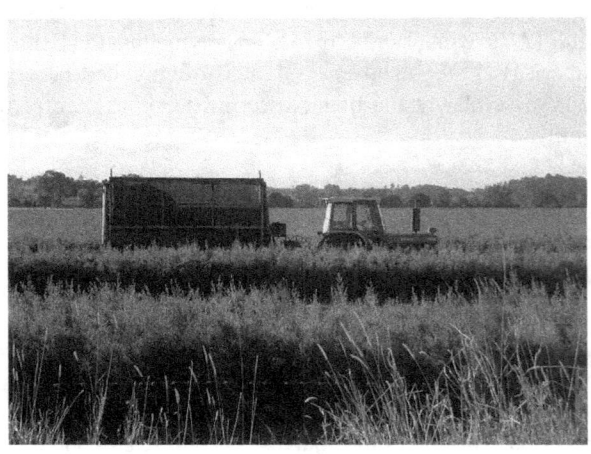

Tea tree plantation, Coraki.

2.57   Tea tree oil

This article is about essential oil isolated form the leaves of the tea tree, *Melaleuca alternifolia*. For the sweet seasoning oil pressed from *Camellia* seeds, *C. sinensis* or *C. oleifera*, see tea seed oil.

Tea tree oil (TTO), or **melaleuca oil**, is an essential oil with a fresh camphoraceous odor and a color that ranges from pale yellow to nearly colorless and clear.[2] It is taken from the leaves of the *Melaleuca alternifolia*, which is native to Southeast Queensland and the Northeast coast of New South Wales, Australia.

Tea tree oil is toxic when taken by mouth,[3][4] but is widely used in low concentrations in cosmetics and skin washes.[1] Tea tree oil has been claimed to be useful for treating a wide variety of medical conditions. It shows some promise as an antimicrobial. Tea tree oil may be effective in a variety of dermatologic conditions including dandruff, acne, lice, herpes, and other skin infections.[5]

2.57.1   History and extraction

The name tea tree is used for several plants, mostly from Australia and New Zealand, from the family Myrtaceae, related to the myrtle. The use of the name probably originated from Captain Cook's description of one of these shrubs, that he used to make an infusion, to drink in place of tea.

The commercial tea tree oil industry originated in the 1920s when Arthur Penfold, an Australian, investigated the business potential of a number of native extracted oils; he reported that tea tree oil had promise as it exhibited powerful antiseptic properties.[6]

Tea tree oil was first extracted from *Melaleuca alternifolia* in Australia, and this species remains the most important commercially. Several other species are cultivated for their extracted oil: *Melaleuca armillaris* and *Melaleuca styphelioides* in Tunisia and Egypt; *Melaleuca leucadendron* in Egypt, Malaysia and Vietnam; *Melaleuca acuminata* in Tunisia; *Melaleuca ericifolia* in Egypt; and *Melaleuca quin-*

quenervia in the United States. Similar oils can also be produced by water distillation from *Melaleuca linariifolia* and *Melaleuca dissitiflora*.[7]

2.57.2 Composition and characteristics

Tea tree oil is defined by the International Standard ISO 4730 ("Oil of *Melaleuca*, Terpinen-4-ol type"), which specifies levels of 15 components which are needed to define the oil as "tea tree oil." The oil has been described as having a fresh, camphor-like smell.[8]

Tea tree oils have six types, oils with different chemical compositions. These include a terpinen-4-ol type, a terpinolene type, and four 1,8-cineole types. These various oil types contain over 98 compounds, with terpinen-4-ol the major component responsible for antimicrobial and anti-inflammatory properties.[9] A second component 1,8-cineole, is likely responsible for most allergies in TTO products. Adverse reactions to TTO diminish with minimization of 1,8-cineole content. In commercial production, TTO is prepared as a terpinen-4-ol type.[5]

2.57.3 Medical use

In vitro studies have shown that tea tree oil kills methicillin-resistant Staphylococcus aureus (MRSA),[10] in nasal or extra-nasal (topical) colonisation studies possibly comparable to treatment with mupirocin,[11] but as of 2005 there appeared to be insufficient evidence to recommend it for clinical use.[10] A 2008 article from the American Cancer Society says that studies have found some promise of a possible role for the topical application of tea tree oil as an antiseptic,[3] but that "despite years of use, available clinical evidence does not support the effectiveness of tea tree oil for treating skin problems and infections in humans".[3] A 2012 review by the NIH rates tea tree oil as "possibly effective" for three applications, saying that "a 5% tea tree oil gel appears to be as effective as 5% benzoyl peroxide" for treating mild to moderate acne, that "topical application of 100% tea tree oil solution, twice daily for six months, can cure fungal toenail infection in about 18% of people who try it," and that "a 10% tea tree oil cream works about as well as tolnaftate 1% cream" in treating symptoms of athlete's foot, although being less effective than clotrimazole or terbinafine.[12]

A 2006 review of the toxicity of tea tree oil concludes that it may be used externally in its diluted form by the majority of individuals without adverse effect (provided oxidization is avoided).[13] Tea tree oil is poisonous when taken internally.[3] Tea tree oil may be effective in a variety of dermatologic conditions including dandruff, acne, lice, herpes, and other skin infections.[5] A 2012 review of head lice

treatment recommended against the use of tea tree oil on children because it could cause skin irritation or allergic reactions, because of contraindications, and because of a lack of knowledge about the oil's safety and effectiveness.[14]

2.57.4 Safety

Tea tree oil is a commercially refined composition of several naturally occurring chemical compounds and is hazardous if misused. Available literature suggests that tea tree oil can be used topically in diluted form by the majority of individuals without adverse effects. Topical application of tea tree oil can cause adverse reactions at high concentration. Adverse effects including skin irritation, allergic contact dermatitis, systemic contact dermatitis, linear immunoglobulin A disease, erythema multiforme like reactions, and systemic hypersensitivity reactions.[5][15]

Tea tree oil is toxic when swallowed.[15] According to the American Cancer Society, ingesting tea tree oil has been reported to cause drowsiness, confusion, hallucinations, coma, unsteadiness, weakness, vomiting, diarrhea, stomach upset, blood cell abnormalities, and severe rashes. It should be kept away from pets and children.[3] Tea tree oil should not be used in or around the mouth.[4] There is at least one case of poisoning reported in medical literature.[16]

Exposure of tea tree oil to air and light results in oxidation of some of its components. Oxidized tea tree oil should not be used.[17] Some people experience allergic contact dermatitis as a reaction to dermal contact with tea tree oil. Allergic reactions may be due to the various oxidation products that are formed by exposure of the oil to light and/or air.[15][18]

In vitro testing of tea tree oil shows that it contains chemicals which are weakly estrogenic, causing particular concern for use with children. However, in tests, the chemicals which show this effect failed to show absorption into the skin, and evidence of a hormonal effect is therefore considered implausible by an EU scientific committee.[1]

In dogs and cats, death[19][20] or transient signs of toxicity (lasting 2 to 3 days), such as depression, weakness, incoordination and muscle tremors, have been reported after external application at high doses.[21] In rats the LD50 is 1.9–2.4 ml/kg.[22]

Undiluted tea tree oil can cause some hearing loss when used in the ears of non-human animals; however, a 2% concentration has not been shown to have any lasting effect. It is not known whether the same is true for humans.[23]

2.57.5 See also

- Cajeput oil – derived from *Melaleuca leucadendra*

2.57.6   References

[1] SCCP/1155/08 Scientific Committee on Consumer Products SCCP OPINION ON Tea tree oil – European Union Commission Health and Consumer Union protection director general – adopted 18th plenary of 16 December 2008

[2] "Directory of Essential Oils for Aromatherapy: Tea-Tree Oil (Melaleuca alternifolia)". Holistics Online.

[3] "Tea Tree Oil". American Cancer Society. November 2008. Retrieved September 2013.

[4] "Tea Tree Oil". National Capital Poison Center. Retrieved 4 December 2013.

[5] Pazyar, N; Yaghoobi, R; Bagherani, N; Kazerouni, A (July 2013). "A review of applications of tea tree oil in dermatology". *International Journal of Dermatology* **52** (7): 784–90. doi:10.1111/j.1365-4632.2012.05654.x. PMID 22998411.

[6] Carson, C. F.; Hammer, K. A.; Riley, T. V. (2006). "Melaleuca alternifolia (Tea Tree) Oil: A Review of Antimicrobial and Other Medicinal Properties". *Clinical Microbiology Reviews* **19** (1): 50–62. doi:10.1128/CMR.19.1.50-62.2006. PMC 1360273. PMID 16418522.

[7] Sávia Perina Portilho Falci (2015-07). "Antimicrobial activity of Melaleuca sp. oil against clinical isolates of antibiotics resistant Staphylococcus aureus". *Acta Cirurgica Brasileira* **30** (7). Check date values in: |date= (help)

[8] Billee Sharp (18 September 2013). *Lemons and Lavender: The Eco Guide to Better Homekeeping*. Cleis Press. pp. 43–. ISBN 978-1-936740-11-6.

[9] Hart, P.H.; Brand, C.; Carson, C.F.; Riley, T.V.; Prager, R.H.; Finlay-Jones, J.J. (2000). "Terpinen-4-ol, the main component of the essential oil of Melaleuca alternifolia (tea tree oil), suppresses inflammatory mediator production by activated human monocytes.". *Inflammation Research* **49** (11): 619–26. doi:10.1007/s000110050639. PMID 11131302.

[10] Flaxman, D.; Griffiths, P. (2005). "Is tea tree oil effective at eradicating MRSA colonization? A review". *Br. J. Community Nurs.* **10** (3, March): 123–126. PMID 15824699.

[11] Bradley, Suzanne F (January 2011). "MRSA colonisation (eradicating colonisation in people without active/invasive infection)". *Clinical Evidence* **2011**. PMID 21477403.

[12] "Tea tree oil". U.S. National Library of Medicine. Retrieved 15 December 2014.

[13] Hammer, KA; Carson, CF; Riley, TV; Nielsen, JB (May 2006). "A review of the toxicity of Melaleuca alternifolia (tea tree) oil.". *Food and chemical toxicology : an international journal published for the British Industrial Biological Research Association* **44** (5): 616–25. doi:10.1016/j.fct.2005.09.001. PMID 16243420.

[14] Eisenhower, Christine; Farrington, Elizabeth Anne (2012). "Advancements in the Treatment of Head Lice in Pediatrics". *Journal of Pediatric Health Care* **26** (6): 451–61; quiz 462–4. doi:10.1016/j.pedhc.2012.05.004. PMID 23099312.

[15] Hammer, K; Carson, C; Riley, T; Nielsen, J (2006). "A review of the toxicity of Melaleuca alternifolia (tea tree) oil". *Food and Chemical Toxicology* **44** (5): 616–25. doi:10.1016/j.fct.2005.09.001. PMID 16243420.

[16] "Ingestion of tea tree oil (Melaleucaoil) by a 4-year-old boy".

[17] "THE EFFECTIVENESS AND SAFETY OF AUSTRALIAN TEA TREE OIL". Australian Government - Rural Industries and Development Corporation. Retrieved 26 February 2014.

[18] Aberer, W (January 2008). "Contact allergy and medicinal herbs". *Journal der Deutschen Dermatologischen Gesellschaft = Journal of the German Society of Dermatology : JDDG* **6** (1): 15–24. doi:10.1111/j.1610-0387.2007.06425.x. PMID 17919303.

[19] "Tea Tree Oil and Dogs, Tea Tree Oil and Cats". Petpoisonhelpline.com. Retrieved December 13, 2012.

[20] "Tea Tree Oil Toxicity". Veterinarywatch. Retrieved December 13, 2012.

[21] Villar, D; Knight, MJ; Hansen, SR; Buck, WB (April 1994). "Toxicity of melaleuca oil and related essential oils applied topically on dogs and cats". *Veterinary and human toxicology* **36** (2): 139–42. PMID 8197716.

[22] Clinical Microbiological Reviews: Melaleuca alternifolia (Tea Tree) Oil: a Review of Antimicrobial and Other Medicinal Properties-C. F. Carson,1 K. A. Hammer,1 and T. V. Riley

[23] "Tea tree oil". Medline Plus, a service of the U.S. National Library of Medicine from the National Institutes of Health. 27 July 2012.

2.57.7   External links

- "The Marshall Centre: Tea Tree Oil"., research group at the University of Western Australia

- "Tea Tree Oil". at the American Cancer Society

- "Australian Tea Tree Oil database"., a searchable abstract database containing 1200+ journal articles on Tea Tree Oil.

2.58 Volatility (chemistry)

In chemistry and physics, **volatility** is the tendency of a substance to vaporize. Volatility is directly related to a substance's vapor pressure. At a given temperature, a substance with higher vapor pressure vaporizes more readily than a substance with a lower vapor pressure.[1][2][3][4]

The term is primarily written to be applied to liquids; however, it may be used to describe the process of sublimation which is associated with solid substances, such as dry ice (solid carbon dioxide) and ammonium chloride, which can change directly from the solid state to a vapor without becoming liquid.

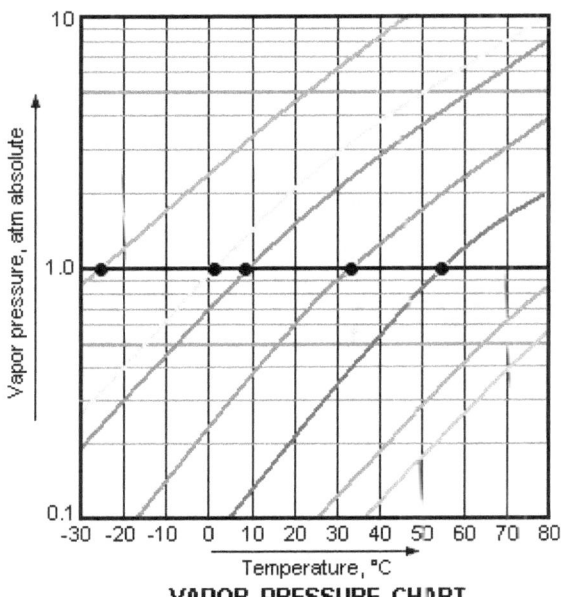

VAPOR PRESSURE CHART

Color code:
— Methyl chloride   — Methyl acetate
   Butane   — Fluorobenzene
— neo-Pentane   — 2-Heptene
— Diethyl ether   ● Normal boiling point

A typical vapor pressure chart for various liquids

2.58.1 Relations between vapor pressure, temperature, and boiling point

Main article: Vapor pressure

The vapor pressure of a substance is the pressure at which its gas phase is in equilibrium with its condensed phases (liquid or solid). It is a measure of the tendency of molecules and atoms to escape from a liquid or a solid. A liquid's atmospheric pressure boiling point corresponds to the temperature at which its vapor pressure is equal to the surrounding atmospheric pressure and it is often called the *normal boiling point*.

The higher the vapor pressure of a liquid at a given temperature, the higher the volatility and the lower the normal boiling point of the liquid. The vapor pressure chart (right hand side) displays the vapor pressures dependency for a variety of liquids as a function of temperature.[5]

For example, at any given temperature, methyl chloride has the highest vapor pressure of any of the liquids in the chart. It also has the lowest normal boiling point (−24.2 °C), which is where the vapor pressure curve of methyl chloride (the blue line) intersects the horizontal pressure line of one atmosphere (atm) of absolute vapor pressure.

2.58.2 See also

- Clausius–Clapeyron relation
- Distillation
- Fractional distillation
- Partial pressure
- Raoult's law
- Relative volatility
- Vapor–liquid equilibrium
- Volatile organic compound

2.58.3 References

[1] Gases and Vapor (University of Kentucky website)

[2] Definition of Terms (University of Victoria website)

[3] James G. Speight (2006). *The Chemistry and Technology of Petroleum* (4th Edition ed.). CRC Press. ISBN 978-0-8493-9067-8.

[4] Kister, Henry Z. (1992-02-01). *Distillation Design* (1st Edition ed.). McGraw-hill. ISBN 978-0-07-034909-4.

[5] Perry, R.H. and Green, D.W. (Editors); Don W. Green; James O. Maloney (1997). *Perry's Chemical Engineers Handbook* (7th Edition ed.). McGraw-Hill. ISBN 978-0-07-049841-9.

2.58.4 External links

- Volatility from ilpi.com
- Definition of volatile from Wiktionary

2.59 Wintergreen

This article is about the plants of the genus *Gaultheria* that are commonly known as wintergreen. For other uses, see Wintergreen (disambiguation).

Wintergreen is a group of aromatic plants. The

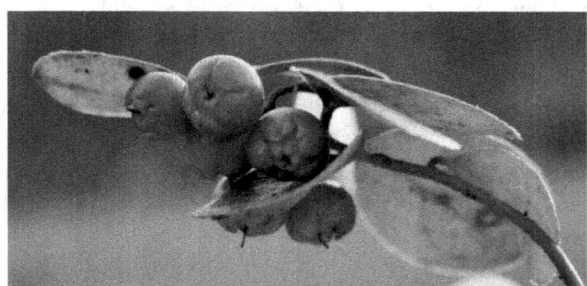

Gaultheria *from Fountain Springs, Pennsylvania*

term "wintergreen" once commonly referred to plants that remain green (continue photosynthesis) throughout the winter. The term "evergreen" is now more commonly used for this characteristic.

Most species of the shrub genus *Gaultheria* demonstrate this characteristic and are called wintergreens in North America, the most common generally being the American wintergreen (*Gaultheria procumbens*). Wintergreens in the genus *Gaultheria* contain an aromatic compound, methyl salicylate, and are used as a mintlike flavoring.

2.59.1 Uses

Wintergreen berries, from *Gaultheria procumbens*, are used medicinally. Native Americans brewed a tea from the leaves to alleviate rheumatic symptoms, headache, fever, sore throat, and various aches and pains. These therapeutic effects likely arose because the primary metabolite of methyl salicylate is salicylic acid, a proven NSAID that is also the metabolite of acetylsalicylic acid, commonly known as aspirin. During the American Revolution, wintergreen leaves were used as a substitute for tea, which was scarce.[1]

Wintergreen is a common flavoring in American products ranging from chewing gum, mints, and candies to smokeless tobacco such as dipping tobacco (American "dip" snuff) and snus. It is also a common flavoring for dental hygiene products such as mouthwash and toothpaste.

Wintergreen oil can also be used in fine art printing applications to transfer a color photocopy image or color laser print to a high-rag-content art paper, such as a hot-press watercolor paper. The transfer method involves coating the source image with the wintergreen oil then placing it face-

down on the target paper and pressing the pieces of paper together under pressure using a standard etching press.

Artificial wintergreen oil, which is pure methyl salicylate, is used in microscopy because of its high refractive index.[2]

2.59.2 Oil of wintergreen

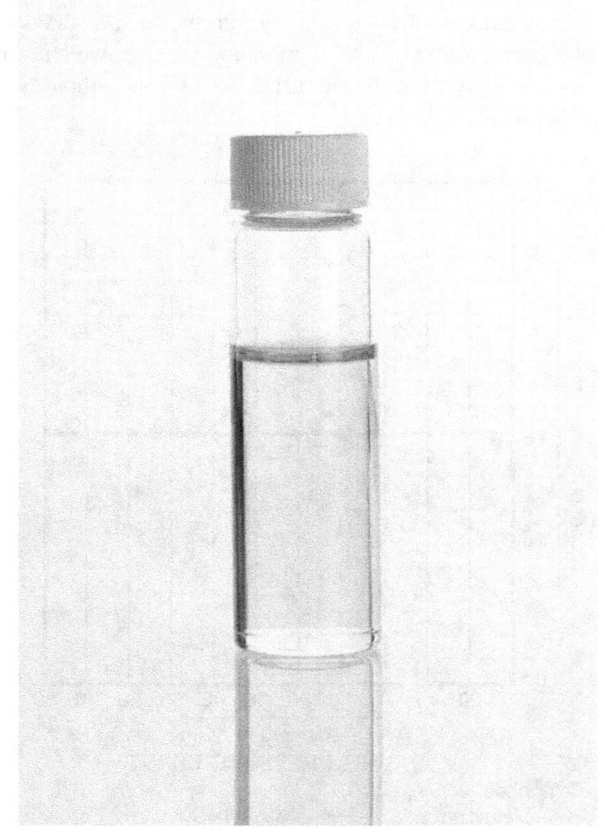

Wintergreen (Gaultheria procumbens) *essential oil*

The *Gaultheria* species share the common characteristic of producing oil of wintergreen. Wintergreen oil is a pale yellow or pinkish fluid liquid that is strongly aromatic with a sweet, woody odor (components: methyl salicylate (about 98%), a-pinene, myrcene, delta-3-carene, limonene, 3,7-guaiadiene, and delta-cadinene)[3] that gives such plants a distinctive "medicinal" smell whenever bruised. Salicylate sensitivity is a common adverse reaction to the methyl salicylate in oil of wintergreen; it can produce allergy-like symptoms or asthma.

Wintergreen essential oil is usually obtained by steam distillation of the leaves of the plant following maceration in warm water. Methyl salicylate is not present in the plant until formed by enzymatic action from a glycoside within the leaves as they are macerated in warm water.[4] Oil of wintergreen is also manufactured from some species of birch, but these deciduous trees are not called wintergreens. *Spiraea* plants also contain methyl salicylate in large amounts and are used similarly to wintergreen. Wintergreen has a strong "minty" odor and flavor, the *Gaultheria*-genus plants are not true mints, which belong to the genus *Mentha*.

Wintergreen oil is used topically (diluted) or aromatheraputically as a folk remedy for muscle and joint discomfort, arthritis, cellulite, obesity, edema, poor circulation, headache, heart disease, hypertension, rheumatism, tendinitis, cramps, inflammation, eczema, hair care, psoriasis, gout, ulcers, and broken or bruised bones. The liquid salicylate dissolves into tissue and also into capillaries, so overuse is as risky as overuse of aspirin. Wintergreen also is used in some perfumery applications and as a flavoring agent for toothpaste, chewing gum, soft drinks,[3] confectionery, Listerine, and mint flavorings. One application is rust removal and degreasing of machinery. Wintergreen is particularly effective for breaking through sea water corrosion.

2.59.3 Toxicity of wintergreen oil

Further information: Methyl salicylate § Safety and toxicity

Thirty ml (about 1 fl oz) of oil of wintergreen is equivalent to 55.7 g of aspirin, or about 171 adult aspirin tablets (US). This conversion illustrates the potency and potential toxicity of oil of wintergreen even in small quantities.[5]

Illiteracy may be a common factor in accidental overdoses and ingestions in adults. Treatment is identical to the other salicylates. Early use of hemodialysis in conjunction with maximal supportive measures is encouraged in any significant ingestion of methyl salicylate.[6]

Strong warning labels are recommended for household salicylate-containing compounds such as oil of wintergreen.

2.59.4 See also

- *Gaultheria humifusa* - alpine wintergreen

- *Gaultheria ovatifolia* - western teaberry or Oregon spicy wintergreen

- *Chimaphila maculata* - striped wintergreen

2.59.5 References

[1] Prescription for Herbal Healing By Phyllis A. Balch, Robert Rister

[2] Cecilia W. Lo, 2000. *Developmental biology protocols*, Volume 1, Springer in google books

[3] Khilendra Gurung 2007. *Analysis of wintergreen oil*, Ecology Agriculture and Rural Development Society, Dolakha, Nepal

[4] Essential Oil Profile of Wintergreen by Ingrid Krein

[5] Johnson PN: Methyl salicylate/aspirin equivalence: Vet Hum Toxicol 1985; 26:317-318

[6] Howrie DL, Moriaty R, Breit R: Candy flavoring as a source of salicylate poisoning. Pediatrics 1985; 75:869-871

- Beck TR, Beck JB 1963. *Elements of Medical Jurisprudence, ed 11*. Philadelphia, JB Lippincott, 1963

- Stevenson CA 1937 Oil of wintergreen poisoning. *Med Sci* 193:772-788

- McGuigan MA 1987 A two-year review of salicylate deaths in Ontario. *Arch Intern Med* 147:510-512

2.60 Yarrow oil

Yarrow essential oil is a volatile oil including a chemical called proazulenes.

The dark blue essential oil, extracted by steam distillation of the flowers, is generally used as an anti-inflammatory[1] or in chest rubs for colds and influenza.

2.60.1 See also

- Yarrow

- Essential oil

2.60.2 References

[1] http://www.aromaweb.com/essential-oils/yarrow-oil.asp

2.61 List of essential oils

Essential oils are volatile and liquid aroma compounds from natural sources, usually plants. Essential oils are not oils in a strict sense, but often share with oils a poor solubility in water. Essential oils often have an odor and are therefore used in food flavoring and perfumery. Essential oils are usually prepared by fragrance extraction techniques (such as distillation, pressing, or maceration). Essential oils are distinguished from aroma oils (essential oils and aroma compounds in an oily solvent), infusions in a vegetable oil,

Essential oil of Eucalyptus

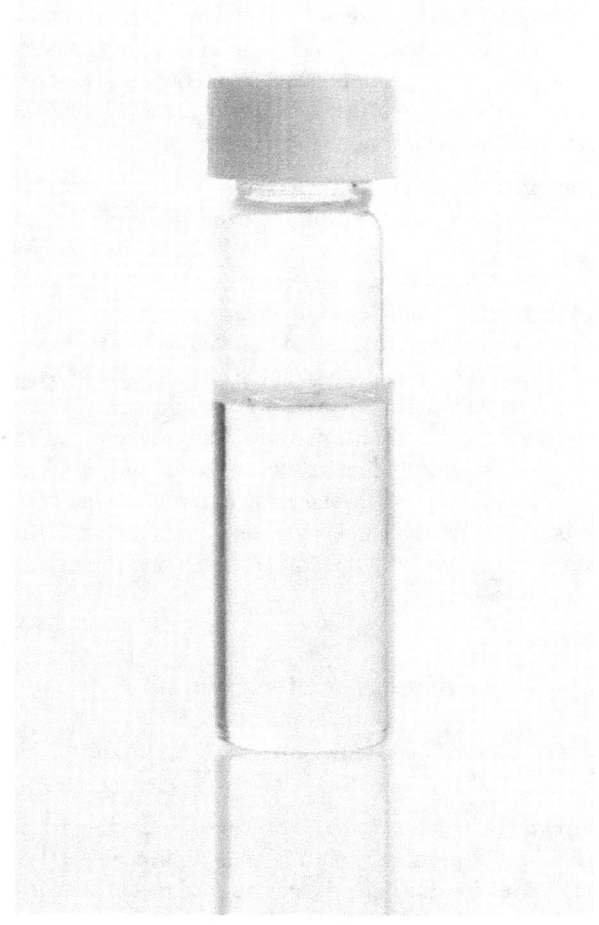

A glass vial containing sandalwood oil

absolutes, and concretes. Typically, essential oils are highly complex mixtures of often hundreds of individual aroma compounds.

- Agar oil or oodh, distilled from Agarwood (*Aquilaria malaccensis*). Highly prized for its fragrance.[1]

- Ajwain oil, distilled from the leaves of Bishop's weed (*Carum copticum*). Oil contains 35–65% thymol.

- Angelica root oil, distilled from the *Angelica archangelica*.

- Anise oil, from the *Pimpinella anisum*, rich odor of licorice, used medicinally.

- Asafoetida, used medicinally and to flavor food.

- Balsam of Peru, from the *Myroxylon*, used in food and drink for flavoring, in perfumes and toiletries for fragrance, and in medicine and pharmaceutical items for healing properties.

- Basil oil is used in making perfumes, as well as in aromatherapy

- Bay oil is used in perfumery; Aromatherapeutic for sprains, colds, flu, insomnia, rheumatism.

- Bergamot oil, used in aromatherapy and in perfumes.

- Black Pepper essential oil is distilled from the berries of *Piper nigrum*. The warm, soothing effect makes it ideal for treating muscle aches, pains and strains and promoting healthy digestion.

- Buchu oil, made from the buchu shrub. Considered toxic and no longer widely used. Formerly used medicinally.

- Birch is aromatheapeutic for gout, Rheumatism, Eczema, Ulcers.

- Camphor is used for cold, cough, fever, rheumatism, and arthritis

- Cannabis flower essential oil, used as a flavoring in foods, primarily candy and beverages. Also used as a scent in perfumes, cosmetics, soaps, and candles.[2]

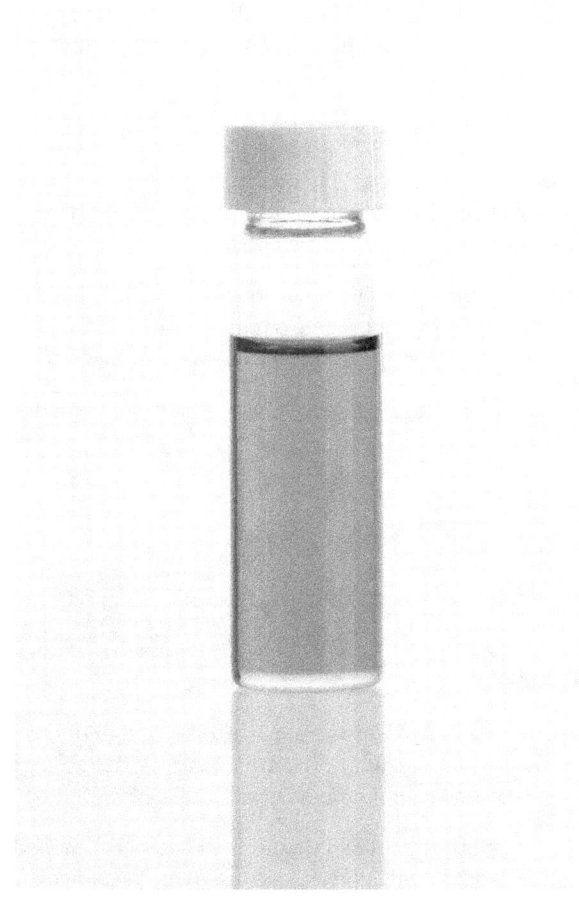

Davana essential oil

- Caraway oil, used a flavoring in foods. Also used in mouthwashes, toothpastes, etc. as a flavoring agent.[3]

- Cardamom seed oil, used in aromatherapy and other medicinal applications. Extracted from seeds of sub-species of Zingiberaceae (ginger). Also used as a fragrance in soaps, perfumes, etc.

- Carrot seed oil (essential oil), used in aromatherapy.

- Cedarwood oil, primarily used in perfumes and fragrances.

- Chamomile oil, There are many varieties of chamomile but only two are used in aromatherapy-Roman and German. Both have similar healing properties but German chamomile contains a higher level of azulin (an anti-inflammatory agent).

- Calamus Root, used medicinally

- Cinnamon oil, used for flavoring and medicinally.

- *Cistus* species

- Citron

- Citronella oil, from a plant related to lemon grass is used as an insect repellent, as well as medicinally.

- Clary Sage

- Clove oil, used as a topical anesthetic to relieve dental pain.

- Coffee, used to flavor food.

- Coriander

- Costmary oil (bible leaf oil), from the *Tanacetum balsamita*

- Costus Root, used medicinally

- Cranberry seed oil, equally high in omega-3 omega-6 fatty acids. primarily used in the cosmetic industry.

- Cubeb, used medicinally and to flavor foods.

- Cumin oil/Black seed oil, used as a flavor, particularly in meat products. Also used in veterinary medicine.

- Cypress

- Cypriol

- Curry leaf, used medicinally and to flavor food.

- Davana oil, from the *Artemisia pallens*, used as a perfume ingredient and as a germicide.

- Dill oil, chemically almost identical to caraway seed oil. High carvone content.

- Elecampane. used medicinally.

- Eucalyptus oil, historically used as a germicide. Commonly used in cough medicine, among other medicinal uses.[4]

- Fennel seed oil, used medicinally, particularly for treating colic in infants.

- Fenugreek oil, used medicinally and for cosmetics from ancient times.

- Fir

- Frankincense oil, used for aromatherapy and in perfumes.

- Galangal, used medicinally and to flavor food.

- Galbanum

- Geranium oil, used medicinally, particularly in aromatherapy, used for hormonal imbalance, for this reason geranium is often considered to be "female" oil.

- Ginger oil, used medicinally in many cultures.

- Goldenrod

- Grapefruit oil, extracted from the peel of the fruit. Used in aromatherapy. Contains 90% limonene.

- Henna oil, used medicinally.

- Helichrysum

- Hickory nut oil

- Horseradish oil

- Hyssop

- Idaho Tansy

- Jasmine oil, used for its flowery fragrance.

- Juniper berry oil, used as a flavor. Also used medicinally, including traditional medicine.

- *Laurus nobilis*

- Lavender oil, used primarily as a fragrance. Also used medicinally.

- *Ledum*

- Lemon oil, similar in fragrance to the fruit. Unlike other essential oils, lemon oil is usually cold pressed. Used medicinally, as an antiseptic, and in cosmetics.

- Lemongrass. Lemongrass is a highy fragrant grass from India. In India, it is used to help treat fevers and infections. The oil is very useful for insect repellent.

- Lime, anti septic, anti viral, astringent, aperitif, bactericidal, disinfectant, febrifuge, haemostatic, restorative and tonic.

- *Litsea cubeba* oil, lemon-like scent, often used in perfumes and aromatherapy.

- Linaloe

- Mandarin

- Marjoram

- Melaleuca See Tea tree oil

- Melissa oil (Lemon balm), sweet smelling oil used primarily medicinally, particularly in aromatherapy.

- Mentha arvensis *oil/Mint oil, used in flavoring toothpastes, mouthwashes and pharmaceuticals, as well as in aromatherapy and other medicinal applications.*

- Moringa oil, can be used directly on the skin and hair. It can also be used in soap and as a base for other cosmetics.

- Mountain Savory

- Mugwort oil, used in ancient times for medicinal and magical purposes. Currently considered to be a neurotoxin.

- Mustard oil (essential oil), containing a high percentage of allyl isothiocyanate or other isothiocyanates, depending on the species of mustard

- Myrrh oil, warm, slightly musty smell. Used medicinally.

- Myrtle

- Neem oil or Neem Tree Oil

- Neroli is produced from the blossom of the bitter orange tree.

- Nutmeg

- Orange oil, like lemon oil, cold pressed rather than distilled. Consists of 90% d-Limonene. Used as a fragrance, in cleaning products and in flavoring foods.

- Oregano oil, contains thymol and carvacrol, making it a useful fungicide. Also used to treat digestive problems.[5]

- Orris oil is extracted from the roots of the Florentine iris (*Iris florentina*), *Iris germanica'* and Iris pallida. *It is used as a flavouring agent, in perfume, and medicinally.*[6]

- Palo Santo

- Parsley oil, used in soaps, detergents, colognes, cosmetics and perfumes, especially men's fragrances.

- Patchouli oil, very common ingredient in perfumes.

- Perilla essential oil, extracted from the leaves of the perilla plant. Contains about 50–60% perillaldehyde.

- Pennyroyal oil, highly toxic. It is abortifacient and can even in small quantities cause acute liver and lung damage.

- Peppermint oil, used in a wide variety of medicinal applications.

- Petitgrain

- Pine oil, used as a disinfectant, and in aromatherapy.

- Ravensara

- Red Cedar

- Roman Chamomile

- Rose oil, distilled from rose petals, Used primarily as a fragrance.

- Rosehip oil, distilled from the seeds of the *Rosa rubiginosa* or *Rosa mosqueta*. Used medicinally.

- Rosemary oil, distilled from the flowers of *Rosmarinus officinalis*. Used in aromatherapy, topically to sooth muscles, and medicinal for its antibacterial and antifungal properties.[7]

- Rosewood oil, used primarily for skin care applications. Also used medicinally.

- Sage oil, used medicinally.

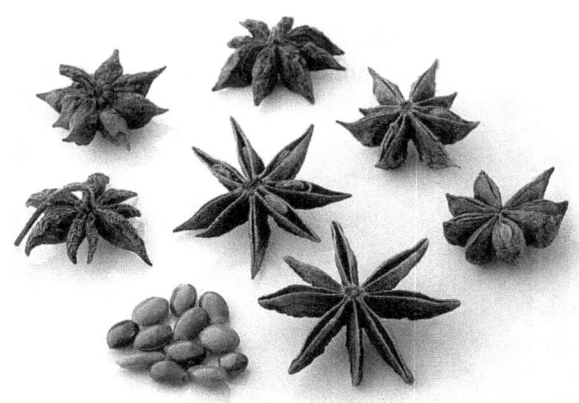

The spice star anise is distilled to make star anise oil

- Sandalwood oil, used primarily as a fragrance. for its pleasant, woody fragrance.[8]

- Sassafras oil, from sassafras root bark. Used in aromatherapy, soap-making, perfumes, and the like. Formerly used as a spice, and as the primary flavoring of root beer, *inter alia*.

- Savory oil, from Satureja species. Used in aromatherapy, cosmetic and soap-making applications.

- Schisandra oil, from *Schisandra chinensis*, used medicinally.

- Spearmint oil, often used in flavoring mouthwash and chewing gum, among other applications.

- Spikenard, used medicinally.

- Spruce has calming and elevating properties. It can be used as a topical application for muscular aches and pains, poor circulation, and rheumatism. Spruce Oil has also been used to improve breathing conditions of asthma, bronchitis, coughs, and general weakness.

- Star anise oil, highly fragrant oil using in cooking. Also used in perfumery and soaps, has been used in toothpastes, mouthwashes, and skin creams.[9] 90% of the world's star anise crop is used in the manufacture of Tamiflu, a drug used to treat influenza, and is hoped to be useful for avian flu

- Tangerine

- Tarragon oil, distilled from Artemisia dracunculus, used medicinally.

- Tea tree oil, extracted from Melaleuca alternifolia; promoted for medicinal use, but with limited evidence of effectiveness.

- Thyme oil, used medicinally.

- Tsuga belongs to the pine tree family. It is used as analgesic, antirheumatic, blood cleanser, and stimulant. It treats cough, respiratory conditions, kidney ailments, urinary infections.

- Turmeric, used medicinally and to flavor food

- Valerian is used for insomnia, migraines, nervous dyspepsia, and dandruff.

- Vetiver oil (khus oil) a thick, amber oil, primarily from India. Used as a fixative in perfumery, and in aromatherapy

- Western red cedar

- Wintergreen can be used as an analgesic, anodyne, anti rheumatic & anti arthritic, anti spasmodic. anti septic, aromatic, astringent, carminative, diuretic, emenagogue and stimulant

- Yarrow oil is used medicinally, to relieve joint pain.

- Ylang-ylang is used for calming, antiseptic, and aphrodisiac purposes, as well as hypertension and skin diseases.

- Zedoary, used medicinally and to flavor food.

2.61.1 See also

- Eau de Cologne and perfume

2.61.2   Books

- Julia Lawless, *The Illustrated Encyclopedia of Essential Oils: The Complete Guide to the Use of Oils in Aromatherapy and Herbalism* (ISBN 1852307218) 1995

- *The Complete Book of Essential Oils & Aromatherapy*

2.61.3   References

[1] "Agar". Nagaon. Archived from the original on 2006-09-20. Retrieved 2006-11-17.

[2] Hemp: A New Crop with New Uses for North America, from the Purdue University NewCROP Web site.

[3] Caraway oil, from the Victoria, Australia Department of Primary Industries Web site.

[4] Eucalyptus oil

[5] Oregano oil

[6] "Orris oil". Encyclopaedia Britannica. Retrieved 2006-11-20.

[7] Rosemary

[8] FAO. "Sandalwood oil". *Flavours and fragances of plant origin*. Retrieved 2006-07-25.

[9] J.E. Simon, A.F. Chadwick and L.E. Craker (1984). "Anise". *Herbs: An Indexed Bibliography.*, cited on the Purdue Center for New Crops Web site

2.62   List of vegetable oils

Vegetable oils are triglycerides extracted from plants. Such oils have been part of human culture for millennia.[1] Edible vegetable oils are used in food, both in cooking and as supplements. Many oils, edible and otherwise, are burned as fuel, such as in oil lamps and as a substitute for petroleum-based fuels. Some of the many other uses include wood finishing, oil painting, and skin care.

There are several types of plant oils, distinguished by the method used to extract the oil from the plant. The relevant part of the plant may be placed under pressure to extract the oil, giving an expressed (or pressed) oil. The oils included in this list are of this type. Oils may also be extracted from plants by dissolving parts of plants in water or another solvent. The solution may be separated from the plant material and concentrated, giving an extracted or leached oil. The mixture may also be separated by distilling the oil away from the plant material. Oils extracted by this latter method are called essential oils. Essential oils often have different properties and uses than pressed or leached vegetable oils.

Finally, macerated oils are made by infusing parts of plants in a base oil, a process called liquid-liquid extraction.

The term "vegetable oil" can be narrowly defined as referring only to substances that are liquid at room temperature,[2] or broadly defined without regard to a substance's state of matter at a given temperature.[3] While a large majority of the entries in this list fit the narrower of these definitions, some do not qualify as vegetable oils according to all understandings of the term.

Although most plants contain some oil, only the oil from certain major oil crops[4] complemented by a few dozen minor oil crops[5] is widely used and traded.

Vegetable oils can be classified in several ways, for example:

- By source: most, but not all vegetable oils are extracted from the fruits or seeds of plants, and the oils may be classified by grouping oils from similar plants, such as "nut oils".

- By use: as described above, oils from plants are used in cooking, for fuel, for cosmetics, for medical purposes, and for other industrial purposes.

The vegetable oils are grouped below in common classes of use.

2.62.1   Edible oils

See also: Cooking oil

Major oils

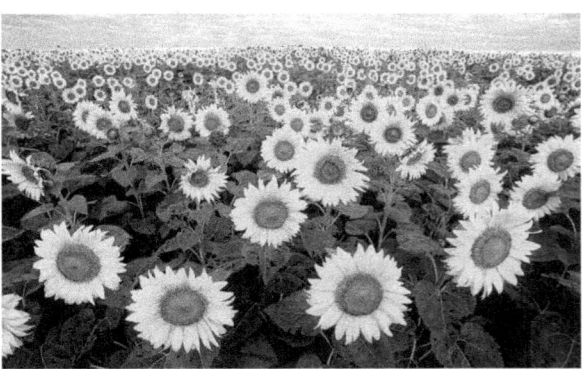

Sunflowers, the seeds of which are the source of sunflower oil.

These oils make up a significant fraction of worldwide edible oil production. All are also used as fuel oils.

- Coconut oil, a cooking oil, with medical and industrial applications as well. Extracted from the kernel or meat of the fruit of the coconut palm. Common in the tropics, and unusual in composition, with medium chain fatty acids dominant.[6]

- Corn oil, one of the principal oils sold as salad and cooking oil.[7]

- Cottonseed oil, used as a salad and cooking oil, both domestically and industrially.[8]

- Olive oil, used in cooking, cosmetics, soaps, and as a fuel for traditional oil lamps.[9]

- Palm oil, the most widely produced tropical oil.[10] Popular in West African and Brazilian cuisine.[11] Also used to make biofuel.[12]

- Peanut oil (Ground nut oil), a clear oil with some applications as a salad dressing, and, due to its high smoke point, especially used for frying.[13]

- Rapeseed oil, including Canola oil, one of the most widely used cooking oils.[14]

- Safflower oil, until the 1960s used in the paint industry, now mostly as a cooking oil.[15]

- Sesame oil, cold pressed as light cooking oil, hot pressed for a darker and stronger flavor.[16]

- Soybean oil, produced as a byproduct of processing soy meal.[17]

- Sunflower oil, a common cooking oil, also used to make biodiesel.[18]

Nut oils

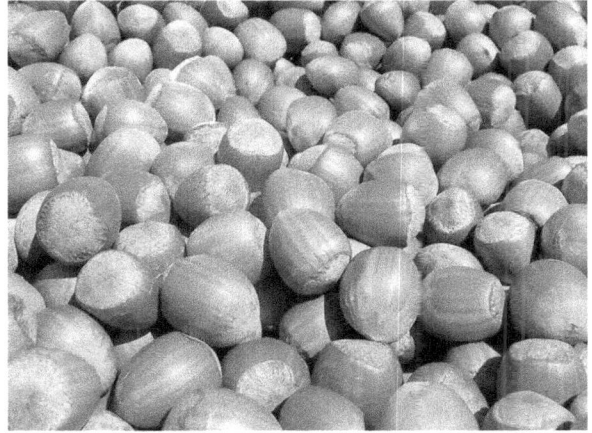

Hazelnuts from the Common Hazel, used to make Hazelnut oil.

Nut oils are generally used in cooking, for their flavor Most are quite costly, because of the difficulty of extracting the oil.

- Almond oil, used as an edible oil, but primarily in the manufacture of cosmetics.[19]

- Beech nut oil, from *Fagus sylvatica* nuts, is a well-regarded edible oil in Europe, used for salads and cooking.[20]

- Brazil nut oil contains 75% unsaturated fatty acids composed mainly of oleic and linolenic acids, as well as the phytosterol, beta-sitosterol,[21] and fat-soluble vitamin E.[22] Extra virgin oil can be obtained during the first pressing of the nuts, possibly for use as a substitute for olive oil due to its mild, pleasant flavor.

- Cashew oil, somewhat comparable to olive oil. May have value for fighting dental cavities.[23]

- Hazelnut oil, mainly used for its flavor. Also used in skin care, because of its slight astringent nature.[24]

- Macadamia oil, with a mild nutty flavor and a high smoke point.[25]

- Mongongo nut oil (or *manketti oil*), from the seeds of the *Schinziophyton rautanenii*, a tree which grows in South Africa. High in vitamin E. Also used in skin care.[26]

- Pecan oil, valued as a food oil, but requiring fresh pecans for good quality oil.[27]

- Pine nut oil, sold as a gourmet cooking oil,[28][29] and of potential medicinal interest as an appetite suppressant.[30]

- Pistachio oil, a strongly flavored oil with a distinctive green color.[25]

- Walnut oil, used for its flavor,[25] also used by Renaissance painters in oil paints.[31][32]

Citrus oils

A number of citrus plants yield pressed oils. Some, such as lemon and orange oil, are used as essential oils, which is uncommon for pressed oils.[note 1][33] The seeds of many if not most members of the citrus family yield usable oils.[33][34][35][36]

- Grapefruit seed oil, extracted from the seeds of grapefruit (*Citrus × paradisi*). Grapefruit seed oil was extracted experimentally in 1930 and was shown to be suitable for making soap.[37]

- Lemon oil, similar in fragrance to the fruit. One of a small number of cold pressed essential oils.[38] Used as a flavoring agent[39] and in aromatherapy.[40]

- Orange oil, like lemon oil, cold pressed rather than distilled.[41] Consists of 90% d-Limonene. Used as a fragrance, in cleaning products and in flavoring foods.[42]

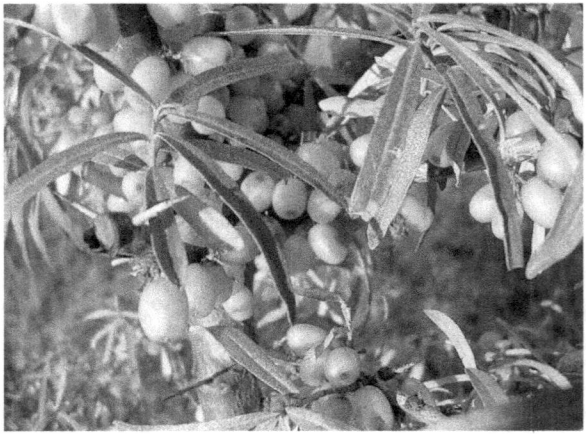

The fruit of the sea-buckthorn

Oils from melon and gourd seeds

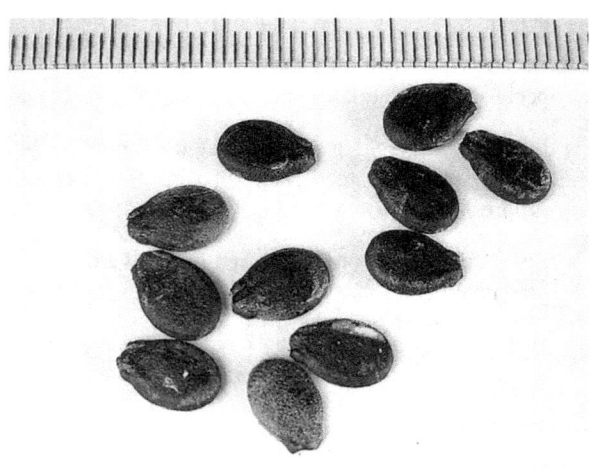

Watermelon seed oil, extracted from the seeds of Citrullus vulgaris, *is used in cooking in West Africa.*

Members of the Cucurbitaceae include gourds, melons, pumpkins, and squashes. Seeds from these plants are noted for their oil content, but little information is available on methods of extracting the oil. In most cases, the plants are grown as food, with dietary use of the oils as a byproduct of using the seeds as food.[43]

- Bitter gourd oil, from the seeds of *Momordica charantia*. High in α-Eleostearic acid. Of current research interest for its potential anti-carcinogenic properties.[44]

- Bottle gourd oil, extracted from the seeds of the *Lagenaria siceraria*, widely grown in tropical regions. Used as an edible oil.[45]

- Buffalo gourd oil, from the seeds of the *Cucurbita foetidissima*, a vine with a rank odor, native to southwest North America.[46]

- Butternut squash seed oil, from the seeds of *Cucurbita moschata*, has a nutty flavor that is used for salad dressings, marinades, and sautéeing.[47]

- Egusi[note 2] seed oil, from the seeds of *Cucumeropsis mannii naudin*, is particularly rich in linoleic acid.[48]

- Pumpkin seed oil, a specialty cooking oil, produced in Austria, Slovenia and Croatia. Used mostly in salad dressings.[49]

- Watermelon seed oil, pressed from the seeds of *Citrullus vulgaris*. Traditionally used in cooking in West Africa.[50][51]

Food supplements

A number of oils are used as food supplements (or "nutraceuticals"), for their nutrient content or purported medicinal effect. Borage seed oil, blackcurrant seed oil, and evening primrose oil all have a significant amount of gamma-Linolenic acid (GLA) (about 23%, 15–20% and 7–10%, respectively), and it is this that has drawn the interest of researchers.

- Açaí oil, from the fruit of several species of the Açaí palm (*Euterpe*) grown in the Amazon region.[52][53]

- Black seed oil, pressed from *Nigella sativa* seeds, has a long history of medicinal use, including in ancient Greek, Asian, and Islamic medicine, as well as being a topic of current medical research.[54][55][56]

- Blackcurrant seed oil, from the seeds of *Ribes nigrum*, used as a food supplement. High in gamma-Linolenic, omega-3 and omega-6 fatty acids.[57]

- Borage seed oil, from the seeds of *Borago officinalis*.[57]

- Evening primrose oil, from the seeds of *Oenothera biennis*,[58] the most important plant source of gamma-Linolenic acid, particularly because it does not contain alpha-Linolenic acid.[57][59]

- Flaxseed oil (called linseed oil when used as a drying oil), from the seeds of *Linum usitatissimum*. High in omega-3 and lignans, which can be used medicinally. A good dietary equivalent to fish oil.[60] Easily turns rancid.[61]

Other edible oils

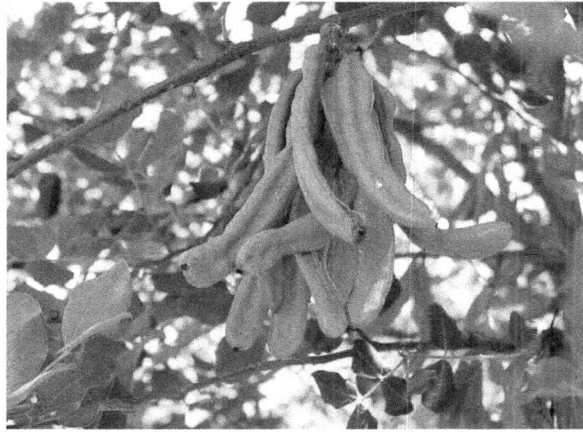

Carob seed pods, used to make carob pod oil.

- Amaranth oil, from the seeds of grain amaranth species, including *Amaranthus cruentus* and *Amaranthus hypochondriacus*, high in squalene and unsaturated fatty acids.[62]

- Apricot oil, similar to almond oil, which it resembles. Used in cosmetics.[63]

- Apple seed oil, high in linoleic acid.[64]

- Argan oil, from the seeds of the *Argania spinosa*, is a food oil from Morocco[65] developed through a women's cooperative founded in the 1990s,[note 3] that has also attracted recent attention in Europe.

- Avocado oil, an edible oil[66] used primarily in the cosmetics and pharmaceutical industries.[67][68] Unusually high smoke point of 510 °F.[69]

- Babassu oil, from the seeds of the *Attalea speciosa*, is similar to, and used as a substitute for, coconut oil.[70]

- Ben oil, extracted from the seeds of the *Moringa oleifera*. High in behenic acid. Extremely stable edible oil. Also suitable for biofuel.[71]

- Borneo tallow nut oil, extracted from the fruit of species of genus *Shorea*. Used as a substitute for cocoa butter, and to make soap, candles, cosmetics and medicines in places where the tree is common.[72]

- Cape chestnut oil, also called yangu oil, is a popular oil in Africa for skin care.[73]

- Carob pod oil (Algaroba oil), from carob, with an exceptionally high essential fatty acid content.[74][75]

- Cocoa butter, from the cacao plant, is used in the manufacture of chocolate, as well as in some ointments and cosmetics; sometimes known as theobroma oil [76]

- Cocklebur oil, from species of genus *Xanthium*, with similar properties to poppyseed oil, similar in taste and smell to sunflower oil.[77][78]

- Cohune oil, from the *Attalea cohune* (cohune palm) used as a lubricant, for cooking, soapmaking and as a lamp oil.[79]

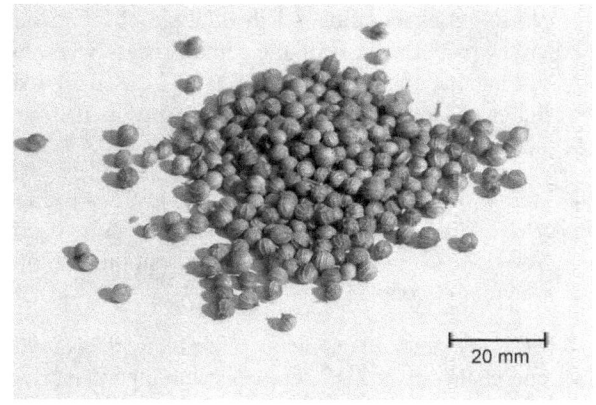

Coriander seeds are the source of an edible pressed oil, Coriander seed oil.

- Coriander seed oil, from coriander seeds, used in a wide variety of flavoring applications, including gin and seasoning blends.[80] Recent research has shown promise for use in killing food-borne bacteria, such as *E. coli*.[81]

- Date seed oil, extracted from date pits.[82] Its low extraction rate and lack of other distinguishing characteristics make it an unlikely candidate for major use.[83]

- Dika oil, from *Irvingia gabonensis* seeds, native to West Africa. Used to make margarine, soap and pharmaceuticals, where is it being examined as a tablet lubricant. Largely underdeveloped.[84][85]

- False flax oil made of the seeds of *Camelina sativa*. One of the earliest oil crops, dating back to the 6th millennium B.C.[86] Produced in modern times in Central and Eastern Europe; fell out of production in the 1940s.[87] Considered promising as a food or fuel oil.[88]

- Grape seed oil, a cooking and salad oil, also sprayed on raisins to help them retain their flavor.[89]

- Hemp oil, a high quality food oil[90] also used to make paints, varnishes, resins and soft soaps.[91]

- Kapok seed oil, from the seeds of *Ceiba pentandra*, used as an edible oil, and in soap production.[92]

- Kenaf seed oil, from the seeds of *Hibiscus cannabinus*. An edible oil similar to cottonseed oil, with a long history of use.[93][94]

- Lallemantia oil, from the seeds of *Lallemantia iberica*, discovered at archaeological sites in northern Greece.[95]

- Mafura oil, extracted from the seeds of *Trichilia emetica*. Used as an edible oil in Ethiopia. Mafura butter, extracted as part of the same process when extracting the oil, is not edible, and is used in soap and candle making, as a body ointment, as fuel, and medicinally.[96]

- Marula oil, extracted from the kernel of *Sclerocarya birrea*. Used as an edible oil with a light, nutty flavor. Also used in soaps. Fatty acid composition is similar to that of olive oil.[97][98]

- Meadowfoam seed oil, highly stable oil, with over 98% long-chain fatty acids. Competes with rapeseed oil for industrial applications.[99]

- Mustard oil (pressed), used in India as a cooking oil. Also used as a massage oil.[100]

- Niger seed oil is obtained from the edible seeds of the Niger plant, which belongs to the Asteraceae family and of the Guizotia genus. The botanical name of the plant is *Guizotia abyssinica*. Cultivation for the plant originated in the Ethiopian highlands, and has since spread from Malawi to India.[101]

- Nutmeg butter, extracted by expression from the fruit of cogeners of genus *Myristica*. Nutmeg butter has a large amount of trimyristin. Nutmeg oil, by contrast, is an essential oil, extracted by steam distillation.[102]

- Okra seed oil, from *Abelmoschus esculentus*. Composed predominantly of oleic and linoleic acids.[103] The greenish yellow edible oil has a pleasant taste and odor.[104]

- Papaya seed oil, high in omega-3 and omega-6, similar in composition to olive oil.[105] Not to be confused with papaya oil produced by maceration.[106]

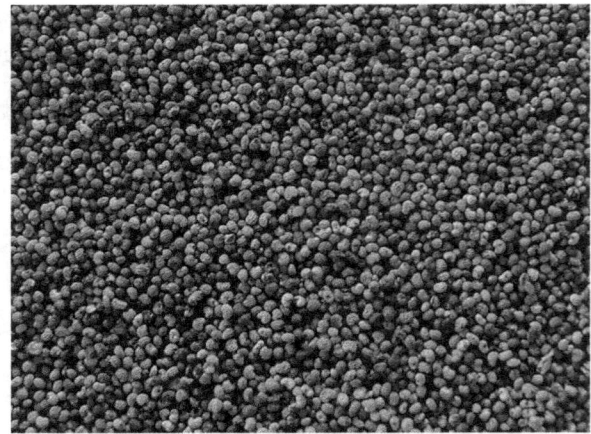

Poppy seeds, used to make poppyseed oil

- Perilla seed oil, high in omega-3 fatty acids. Used as an edible oil, for medicinal purposes in Asian herbal medicine, in skin care products and as a drying oil.[107][108]

- Persimmon seed oil, extracted from the seeds of *Diospyros virginiana*. Dark, reddish brown color, similar in taste to olive oil. Nearly equal content of oleic and linoleic acids.[109]

- Pequi oil, extracted from the seeds of *Caryocar brasiliense*. Used in Brazil as a highly prized cooking oil.[110]

- Pili nut oil, extracted from the seeds of *Canarium ovatum*. Used in the Philippines as an edible oil, as well as for a lamp oil.[111]

- Pomegranate seed oil, from *Punica granatum* seeds, is very high in punicic acid (which takes its name from pomegranates). A topic of current medical research for treating and preventing cancer.[112][113]

- Poppyseed oil, long used for cooking, in paints, varnishes, and soaps.[114][115][116][117]

- Pracaxi oil, extracted from the seeds of Pentaclethra macroloba. Similar to peanut oil, but has a high concentration of behenic acid (19%).[118]

- Prune kernel oil, marketed as a gourmet cooking oil[119][120] Similar in composition to peach kernel oil.[121]

- Quinoa oil, similar in composition and use to corn oil.[122]

- Ramtil oil, pressed from the seeds of the one of several species of genus *Guizotia abyssinica* (Niger pea) in India and Ethiopia.[123][124]

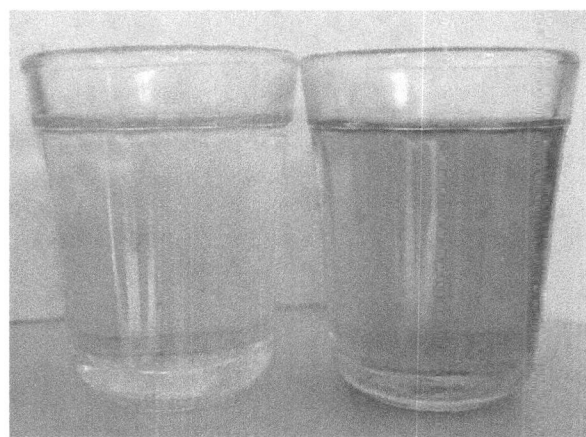

Virgin pracaxi oil

- Rice bran oil is a highly stable cooking and salad oil, suitable for high-temperature cooking.[69][125] It also has potential as a biofuel.[126]

- Royle oil, pressed from the seeds of *Prinsepia utilis*, a wild, edible oil shrub that grows in the higher Himalayas. Used medicinally in Nepal.[127]

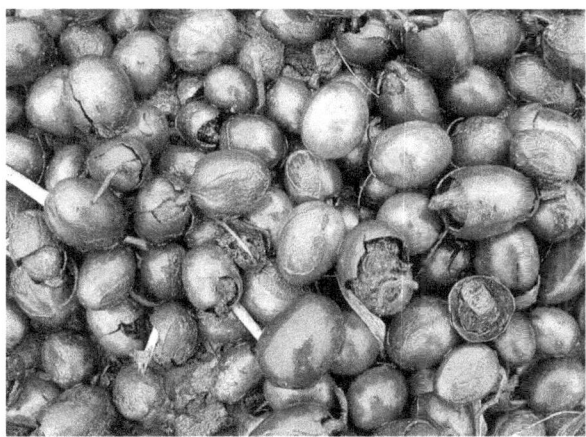

Shea nuts, from which shea butter is pressed

- Sacha inchi oil, from the Peruvian Amazon. High in behenic, omega-3 and omega-6 fatty acids.[128][129]

- Sapote oil, used as a cooking oil in Guatemala.[130]

- Seje oil, from the seeds of *Jessenia bataua*. Used in South America as an edible oil, similar to olive oil, as well as for soaps and in the cosmetics industry.[131]

- Shea butter, much of which is produced by poor, African women. Used primarily in skin care products and as a substitute for cocoa butter in confections and cosmetics.[132][133]

- Taramira oil, from the seeds of the arugula (*Eruca sativa*), grown in West Asia and Northern India. Used as a (pungent) edible oil after aging to remove acridity.[134][135]

- Tea seed oil (Camellia oil), widely used in southern China as a cooking oil. Also used in making soaps, hair oils and a variety of other products.[136][137]

- Thistle oil, pressed from the seeds of *Silybum marianum*.[138] A good potential source of special fatty acids, carotenoids, tocopherols, phenol compounds and natural anti-oxidants,[139] as well as for generally improving the nutritional value of foods.[140]

- Tigernut oil (or nut-sedge oil) is pressed from the tuber of *Cyperus esculentus*. It has properties similar to soybean, sunflower and rapeseed oils.[141] It is used in cooking and making soap[142] and has potential as a biodiesel fuel.[141]

- Tobacco seed oil, from the seeds of *Nicotiana tabacum* and other *Nicotiana* species. Edible if purified.[143]

- Tomato seed oil is a potentially valuable by-product, as a cooking oil, from the waste seeds generated from processing tomatoes.[144]

- Wheat germ oil, used nutritionally and in cosmetic preparations, high in vitamin E and octacosanol.[145]

2.62.2 Oils used for biofuel

See also: Vegetable oil used as fuel

A number of oils are used for biofuel (biodiesel and Straight Vegetable Oil) in addition to having other uses. Other oils are used only as biofuel.[note 4][146]

Although diesel engines were invented, in part, with vegetable oil in mind,[147] diesel fuel is almost exclusively petroleum-based. Vegetable oils are evaluated for use as a biofuel based on:

1. Suitability as a fuel, based on flash point, energy content, viscosity, combustion products and other factors

2. Cost, based in part on yield, effort required to grow and harvest, and post-harvest processing cost

Multipurpose oils also used as biofuel

The oils listed immediately below are all (primarily) used for other purposes – all but tung oil are edible – but have been considered for use as biofuel.

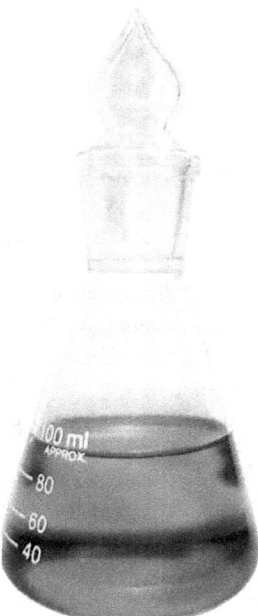

A flask of biodiesel

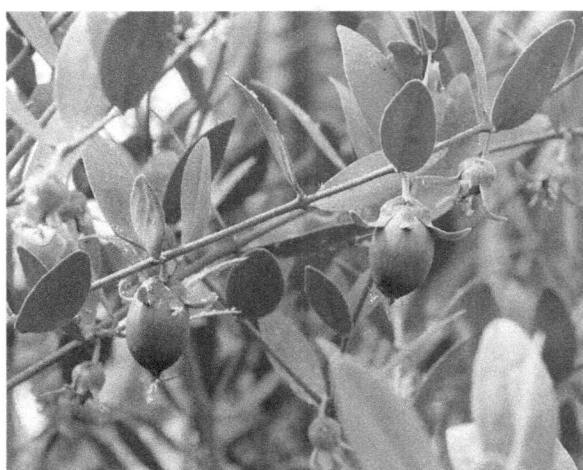

Jojoba fruit

- Corn oil, appealing because of the abundance of maize as a crop.

- Cottonseed oil, the subject of study for cost-effectiveness as a biodiesel feedstock.[151][152]

- False flax oil, from *Camelina sativa*, used in Europe in oil lamps until the 18th century.[88]

- Hemp oil, relatively low in emissions. Production is problematic in some countries because of its association with marijuana.[153][154]

- Mustard oil, shown to be comparable to Canola oil as a biofuel.[155]

- Palm oil, very popular for biofuel, but the environmental impact from growing large quantities of oil palms has recently called the use of palm oil into question.[156]

- Peanut oil, used in one of the first demonstrations of the Diesel engine in 1900.[147]

- Radish oil. Wild radish contains up to 48% oil, making it appealing as a fuel.[157]

- Rapeseed oil, the most common base oil used in Europe in biodiesel production.[146]

- Ramtil oil, used for lighting in India.[158]

- Rice bran oil, appealing because of lower cost than many other vegetable oils. Widely grown in Asia.[159]

- Safflower oil, explored recently as a biofuel in Montana.[160]

- Salicornia oil, from the seeds of *Salicornia bigelovii*, a halophyte (salt-loving plant) native to Mexico.[161]

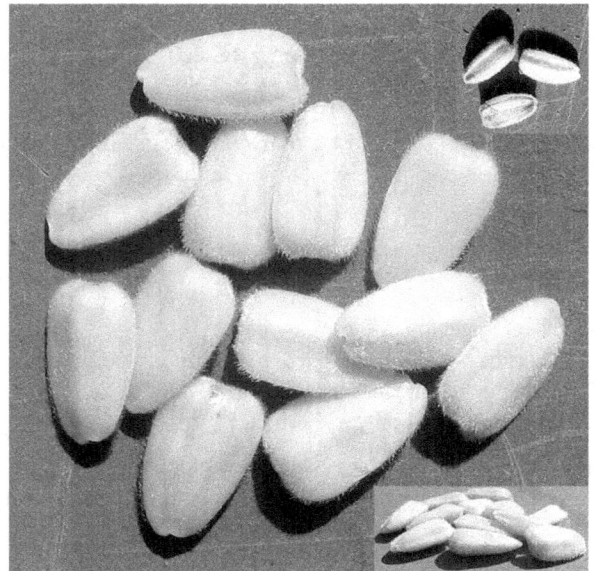

Sunflower kernels

- Castor oil, lower cost than many candidates. Kinematic viscosity may be an issue.[148]

- Coconut oil (copra oil), promising for local use in places that produce coconuts.[149]

- Colza oil, from *Brassica rapa, var. oleifera* (turnip) is closely related to rapeseed (or canola) oil. It is a major source of biodiesel in Germany.[150]

- Soybean oil, not economical as a fuel crop, but appealing as a byproduct of soybean crops for other uses.[146]

- Sunflower oil, suitable as a fuel, but not necessarily cost effective.[162]

- Tigernut oil has been described by researchers in China as having "great potential as a biodiesel fuel."[141]

- Tung oil, referenced in several lists of vegetable oils that are suitable for biodiesel.[163] Several factories in China produce biodiesel from tung oil.[164]

Inedible oils used only or primarily as biofuel

See also: Algae fuel

These oils are extracted from plants that are cultivated solely for producing oil-based biofuel.[note 5] These, plus the major oils described above, have received much more attention as fuel oils than other plant oils.

- Copaiba, an oleoresin tapped from species of genus *Copaifera*. Used in Brazil as a cosmetic product and a major source of biodiesel.[165]

- Jatropha oil, widely used in India as a fuel oil. Has attracted strong proponents for use as a biofuel.[166][167]

- Jojoba oil, from the *Simmondsia chinensis*, a desert shrub.[168]

- Milk bush, popularized by chemist Melvin Calvin in the 1950s. Researched in the 1980s by Petrobras, the Brazilian national petroleum company.[169]

- Nahor oil, pressed from the kernels of *Mesua ferrea*, is used in India as a lamp oil.[170]

- Paradise oil, from the seeds of *Simarouba glauca*, has received interest in India as a feed stock for biodiesel.[171]

- Petroleum nut oil, from the Petroleum nut (*Pittosporum resiniferum*) native to the Philippines. The Philippine government once explored the use of the petroleum nut as a biofuel.[172]

- Pongamia oil (also known as Honge oil), extracted from *Millettia pinnata* and pioneered as a biofuel by Udipi Shrinivasa in Bangalore, India.[173][174]

2.62.3 Drying oils

See also: Drying oil

Drying oils are vegetable oils that dry to a hard finish at normal room temperature. Such oils are used as the basis of oil paints, and in other paint and wood finishing applications. In addition to the oils listed here, walnut, sunflower and safflower oil are also considered to be drying oils.[175]

- Dammar oil, from the *Canarium strictum*, used in paint as an oil drying agent.[176] Can also be used as a lamp oil.[177]

- Linseed oil's properties as a polymer make it highly suitable for wood finishing, for use in oil paints, as a plasticizer and hardener in putty and in making linoleum.[178] When used in food or medicinally linseed oil is called flaxseed oil.

- Poppyseed oil, similar in usage to linseed oil but with better color stability.[175]

- Stillingia oil (also called *Chinese vegetable tallow oil*), obtained by solvent from the seeds of *Sapium sebiferum*. Used as a drying agent in paints and varnishes.[179][180]

- Tung oil, used as an industrial lubricant and highly effective drying agent. Also used as a substitute for linseed oil.[181]

- Vernonia oil is produced from the seeds of the *Vernonia galamensis*. It is composed of 73–80% vernolic acid, which can be used to make epoxies for manufacturing adhesives, varnishes and paints, and industrial coatings.[182]

2.62.4 Other oils

A number of pressed vegetable oils are either not edible, or not used as an edible oil.

- Amur cork tree fruit oil, pressed from the fruit of the *Phellodendron amurense*. It has been studied for insecticidal use.[183][184]

- Artichoke oil, extracted from the seeds of the artichoke fruit, is an unsaturated semi-drying oil with potential applications in making soap, shampoo, alkyd resin and shoe polish.[185]

- Astrocaryum murumuru butter is employed in lotions, creams, soaps hair conditioners, facial masks, shampoo, oils and emulsions, skin moisturizer, products for

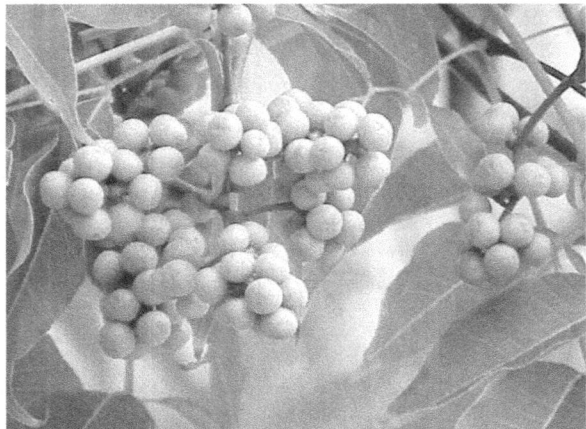

The fruit of the amur cork tree

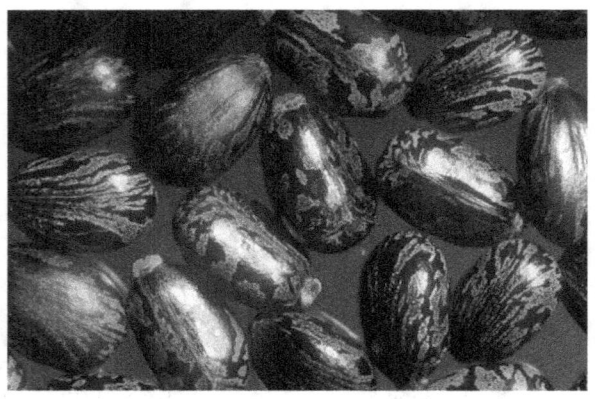

Castor beans are the source of castor oil

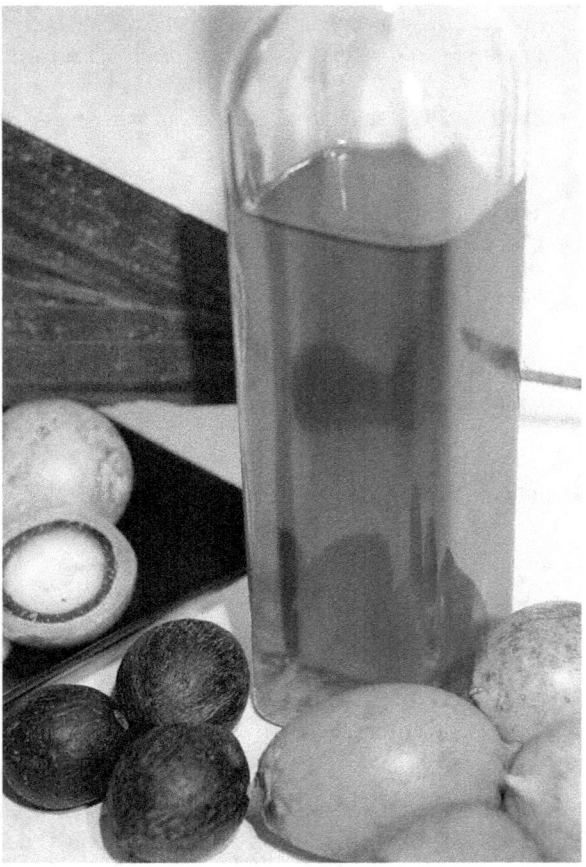

Astrocaryum vulgare (Tucumã) oil

the nutrition of the hair and restore damaged hair, depilatory waxes.[186]

- Balanos oil, pressed from the seeds of *Balanites aegyptiaca*, was used in ancient Egypt as the base for perfumes.[71]

- Bladderpod oil, pressed from the seeds of *Physaria fendleri*, native to North America. Rich in lesquerolic acid, which is chemically similar to the ricinoleic acid found in castor oil. Many industrial uses. Possible substitute for castor oil as it requires much less moisture than castor beans.[187]

- Brucea javanica oil, extracted from the seeds of the *Brucea javanica*. The oil has been shown to be effective in treating certain cancers.[188][189]

- Burdock oil (Bur oil) extracted from the root of the burdock. Used as an herbal remedy for scalp conditions.[190]

- Buriti oil, extracted from the Mauritia flexuosa fruit, is high in carotenoids and monounsaturated fatty acids, and of consequent nutritional interest. It is also used in the cosmetics industry.[191]

- Candlenut oil (Kukui nut oil), produced in Hawai'i, used primarily for skin care products.[192]

- Carrot seed oil (pressed), from carrot seeds, used in skin care products.[note 6][193]

- Castor oil, with many industrial and medicinal uses. Castor beans are also a source of the toxin ricin.[146]

- Chaulmoogra oil, from the seeds of *Hydnocarpus wightiana*, used for many centuries, internally and externally, to treat leprosy.[194] Also used to treat secondary syphilis, rheumatism, scrofula, and in phthisis.[195][196]

- Crambe oil, extracted from the seeds of the *Crambe abyssinica*. High in erucic acid, used as an industrial lubricant, a corrosion inhibitor, and as an ingredient in the manufacture of synthetic rubber.[197][198]

- Croton oil (tiglium oil) is pressed from the seeds of *Croton tiglium*. Highly toxic, it was formerly used as a drastic purgative.[199]

- Cuphea oil, from a number of species of genre *Cuphea*. Of interest as sources of medium chain triglycerides.[200]

- Cupuaçu butter is closely analogous to cocoa, and is used to make white chocolate.[201]

- Honesty oil, from the seeds of *Lunaria annua*, which contain 30–40% oil. The oil is particularly rich in long chain fatty acids, including erucic and nervonic acid, making it suitable for certain industrial purposes.[51][202]

- Illipe butter, from the nuts of the *Shorea stenoptera*. Similar to cocoa butter, but with a higher melting point. Used in cosmetics.[203][204]

- Jojoba oil, used in cosmetics as an alternative to whale oil spermaceti.[205]

- Mango oil, pressed from the stones of the mango fruit, is high in stearic acid, and can be used for making soap.[206]

- Mowrah butter, from the seeds of the *Madhuca latifolia* and *Madhuca longifolia*, both native to India. Crude Mowrah butter is used as a fat for spinning wool, for making candles and soap. The refined fat is used as an edible fat and vegetable ghee in India.[46]

- Neem oil, from *Azadirachta indica*, a brownish-green oil with a high sulfur content, used in cosmetics, for medicinal purposes, and as an insecticide.[207]

- Ojon oil extracted from the nut of the American palm (*Elaeis oleifera*). Oil extracted from both the nut and husk is also used as an edible oil in Central and South America. Commercialized by a Canadian businessman in the 1990s.[208][209]

- Passiflora edulis Passion fruit oil is extracted from the seeds and composed mainly of linoleic acid (62%) with smaller amounts of oleic acid (20%) and palmitic acid (7%). It has varied applications in cosmetics manufacturing and for uses as a human or animal food.[210]

- Rose hip seed oil, used primarily in skin care products, particularly for aging or damaged skin.[211]

- Rubber seed oil, pressed from the seeds of the Rubber tree (*Hevea brasiliensis*), has received attention as a potential use of what otherwise would be a waste product from making rubber. It has been explored as a drying oil in Nigeria,[212] as a diesel fuel in India[213] and as food for livestock in Cambodia and Vietnam.[214]

- Sea buckthorn oil, derived from *Hippophae rhamnoides*, produced in northern China, used primarily medicinally.[215]

- Sea rocket seed oil, from the halophyte *Cakile maritima*, native to north Africa, is high in erucic acid, and therefore has potential industrial applications.[216]

- Snowball seed oil (Viburnum oil), from *Viburnum opulus* seeds. High in tocopherol, carotenoides and unsaturated fatty acids. Used medicinally.[217]

- Tall oil, produced as a byproduct of wood pulp manufacture. A further byproduct called *tall oil fatty acid* (TOFA) is a cheap source of oleic acid.[218]

- Tamanu or foraha oil[219] from the *Calophyllum tacamahaca*, is important in Polynesian culture, and, although very expensive,[219] is used for skin care.[220]

- Tonka bean oil (Cumaru oil), popular ingredient in cologne, used medicinally in Brazil.[221]

- Tucumã butter is extracted from the both the pulp and seed of the fruit of Astrocaryum vulgare, a South American oil palm.[222] The pulp oil is used as a skin conditioner. The seed oil is sold for use as a cooking oil and for making soap due to its high lauric acid content.[223]

- Ucuhuba seed oil, extracted from the seeds of *Virola surinamensis*, is unusually high in myristic acid.[220]

2.62.5 See also

- Carrier oil discusses the use of (pressed) vegetable oils, mixed with essential oils

- Fatty acid discusses the components of most vegetable fats and oils

- International Nomenclature of Cosmetic Ingredients explains naming conventions for oils used in cosmetics and soaps

- List of essential oils

2.62.6 Notes

[1] Lime oil, for example, is distilled, not pressed. See Jackson, p. 131

[2] Note that "egusi" is the common name of several species of melons, including *Citrullus vulgaris* cultivars and *Lagenaria sicerari*.

[3] The Targanine cooperative was founded by Prof. Zoubida Charrouf in the 1990s to help local poor, widowed and divorced women derive an income from producing and exporting high-quality argan oil. See Rainer Höfer, ed. (2009). *Sustainable Solutions for Modern Economies*. Royal Society of Chemistry (Great Britain). p. 401. ISBN 1847559050.

[4] Ethanol and, to a lesser degree, methanol and butanol are the other major types of biofuel.

[5] There are some plants that yield a commercial vegetable oil, that are also used to make other sorts of biofuel. Eucalyptus, for example, has been explored as a means of biomass for producing ethanol. These plants are not listed here.

[6] Carrot seeds are also used to obtain an essential oil with quite different properties than carrot seed pressed oil.

2.62.7 References

[1] "4,000-year-old 'kitchen' unearthed in Indiana". Archaeo News. January 26, 2006. Retrieved 2011-12-30.

[2] Parwez Saroj. *The Pearson Guide to the B.Sc. (Nursing) Entrance Examination*. Pearson Education India. p. 109. ISBN 81-317-1338-5.

[3] Robin Dand (1999). *The International Cocoa Trade*. Woodhead Publishing. p. 169. ISBN 1-85573-434-6.

[4] Economic Research Service (1995–2011). *Oil Crops Outlook*. United States Department of Agriculture. Retrieved 2011-11-19. This publication is available via email subscription.

[5] Axtell, B.L. from research by R.M. Fairman (1992). *Minor oil crops*. FAO. Retrieved 2011-10-24.

[6] Gursche, Siegfried (2008). *Coconut Oil: Discover the Key to Vibrant Health*. Book Publishing Company. p. 12. ISBN 1-55312-043-4. Retrieved 2012-01-21.

[7] *Food Fats and Oils* (PDF) (9 ed.). Institute of Shortening and Edible Oils. 2006. p. 27. Retrieved 2011-11-19.

[8] "Twenty Facts about Cottonseed Oil". National Cottonseed Producers Association. Retrieved 2011-10-17.

[9] "Difference Between Olive oil and Extra Virgin Olive oil". Difference Between.net. Retrieved 2011-10-19.

[10] "Palm Oil Facts". Soyatech. Retrieved 2011-10-19.

[11] "Palm oil". *Food dictionary*. Epicurious. Retrieved 2011-10-19.

[12] "Corporate power: The palm-oil-biodiesel nexus". *Seedling* (GRAIN). July 2007.

[13] Dean, Lisa L.; Davis, Jack P.; Sanders, Timothy H. (2011). "Groundnut (Peanut) Oil". In Frank Gunstone. *Vegetable Oils in Food Technology: Composition, Properties and Uses*. John Wiley & Sons. p. 225. ISBN 1-4443-3268-6. Retrieved 2014-10-05.

[14] "Canola Oil - The Myths Debunked". Canola Council of Canada. Retrieved 2014-10-05.

[15] Boland, Michael (January 2011). "Safflower". Agriculture Marketing Resource Center. Retrieved 2011-10-17.

[16] Hansen, Ray (August 2011). "Sesame profile". Agriculture Marketing Resource Center. Retrieved 2011-11-19.

[17] Bennett, David (February 5, 2003). "World soybean consumption quickens". Southeast Farm Press. Retrieved 2014-10-05.

[18] Boland, Michael; Stroade, Jeri (August 2011). "Sunflower profile". Agricultural Marketing Resource Center. Retrieved 2011-10-17.

[19] Axtell, "I. Individual monographs".

[20] Janick, Jules; Paull, Robert E. (2008). *The encyclopedia of fruit & nuts*. Cabi Publishing. p. 405. ISBN 0-85199-638-8. Retrieved 2011-11-21.

[21] Kornsteiner-Krenn M, Wagner KH, Elmadfa I (2013). "Phytosterol content and fatty acid pattern of ten different nut types". *Int J Vitam Nutr Res* **83** (5): 263–70. doi:10.1024/0300-9831/a000168. PMID 25305221.

[22] Ryan E, Galvin K, O'Connor TP, Maguire AR, O'Brien NM (2006). "Fatty acid profile, tocopherol, squalene and phytosterol content of brazil, pecan, pine, pistachio and cashew nuts". *Int J Food Sci Nutr* **57** (3-4): 219–28. PMID 17127473.

[23] Himejima, Masaki; Kubo, Isao (1991). "Antibacterial agents from the cashew Anacardium occidentale (Anacardiaceae) nut shell oil". *Journal of Agricultural and Food Chemistry* **39** (2): 418–21. doi:10.1021/jf00002a039. Lay summary – *Science News* (March 23, 1991).

[24] Madhaven, N (2001). "Final Report on the Safety Assessment of Corylus Avellana (Hazel) Seed Oil, Corylus Americana (Hazel) Seed Oil, Corylus Avellana (Hazel) Seed Extract, Corylus Americana (Hazel) Seed Extract, Corylus Rostrata (Hazel) Seed Extract, Corylus Avellana (Hazel) Leaf Extract, Corylus Americana (Hazel) Leaf Extract, and Corylus Rostrata (Hazel) Leaf Extract". *International Journal of Toxicology* **20** (1 Suppl): 15–20. doi:10.1080/109158101750300928. PMID 11358108.

[25] Simmons, Marie (2008). *Things Cooks Love*. Andrews McMeel Publishing. p. 295. ISBN 0-7407-6976-6. Retrieved 2014-10-05.

[26] Bafana, Busani (July 2009). "Mongongo–a tough nut worth cracking". New Agriculturist. Retrieved 2011-04-28.

[27] Storey, J. Benton. "Pecans as a health food". Texas AgriLIFE Extension Service. Retrieved 2013-12-03.

[28] John Shi, Chi-Tang Ho, Fereidoon Shahidi eds., ed. (May 15, 2010). "Antioxidant Functional Factors in Nuts". *Functional Foods of the East*. p. 353. ISBN 1-4200-7192-0.

[29] Daley, Regan (2001). *In the Sweet Kitchen: The Definitive Baker's Companion*. Artisan Books. p. 159. ISBN 1-57965-208-5. Retrieved 2014-10-05.

[30] Yu Liangli; Slavin, Margaret (2008). "Nutraceutical Potential of Pine Nut". In Cesarettin Alasalvar, Fereidoon Shahidi. *Tree nuts: composition, phytochemicals, and health effects*. CRC Press. p. 289. ISBN 0-8493-3735-5. Retrieved 2014-10-05.

[31] Powell, William F. (1990). *Oil Painting Materials*. Walter Foster. p. 43. ISBN 1-56010-056-7.

[32] Gottsegen, Mark. *Painter's Handbook*. p. 77. ISBN 0-8230-3496-8. Retrieved 2014-10-05.

[33] Jackson, John F.; Linskens, H.F. (2002). *Analysis of Taste and Aroma* **21**. Springer. p. 131. ISBN 3540417532.

[34] Ajewole, Kola; Adeyeye, A. (1993). "Characterisation of Nigerian citrus seed oils". *Food Chemistry* **47** (1): 77–8. doi:10.1016/0308-8146(93)90306-Z.

[35] Habib, M. A.; Hammam, M. A.; Sakr, A. A.; Ashoush, Y. A. (1986). "Chemical evaluation of egyptian citrus seeds as potential sources of vegetable oils". *Journal of the American Oil Chemists' Society* **63** (9): 1192–6. doi:10.1007/BF02663951.

[36] Filsoof, M.; Mehran, M. (1976). "Fatty acid composition of Iranian citrus seed oils". *Journal of the American Oil Chemists' Society* **53** (10): 654–5. doi:10.1007/BF02586282.

[37] Jamieson, G. S.; Baughman, W. F.; Gertler, S. I. (1930). "Grape fruit seed oil". *Oil & Fat Industries* **7** (5): 181–3. doi:10.1007/BF02564074.

[38] S. R. J. Robbins, ed. (1983). "The Citrus Oils: An Introductory Review". *Selected markets for the essential oils of lime, lemon and orange*. p. 17.

[39] Fenaroli, Giovanni (1975). *Handbook of flavor ingredients*. Taylor & Francis US. p. 577. ISBN 0-87819-533-5.

[40] Rose, Jeanne; Hulburd, John (1993). *The aromatherapy book: applications & inhalations*. North Atlantic Books. p. 110. ISBN 1-55643-073-6.

[41] Wong, Dominic W. S. (1989). *Mechanism and theory in food chemistry*. Springer. p. 253. ISBN 0-442-20753-0. Retrieved 2014-10-05.

[42] Ashurst, Philip R. (994). *Production and Packaging of Non-Carbonated Fruit Juices and Fruit Beverages*. Springer. p. 81. ISBN 0-8342-1289-7. Retrieved 2014-10-05.

[43] Axtell, "Cucurbitaceae

[44] Kohno, Hiroyuki; Yasui, Yumiko; Suzuki, Rikako; Hosokawa, Masashi; Miyashita, Kazuo; Tanaka, Takuji (2004). "Dietary seed oil rich in conjugated linoleic acid from bitter melon inhibits azoxymethane-induced rat colon carcinogenesis through elevation of colonic PPARγ expression and alteration of lipid composition". *International Journal of Cancer* **110** (6): 896–901. doi:10.1002/ijc.20179. PMID 15170673.

[45] Axtell, "Bottle gourd"

[46] Meitzner, Laura S.; Price, Martin L. (1996). "Oil Crops". *Amaranth to Zai Holes*. ECHO. Retrieved 2014-10-06.

[47] Ogrodnick, Joe (Spring 2009). "Butternut Squash Seed Oil Goes to Market". CALS News. Retrieved 2011-01-14.

[48] Kapseu, C.; Kamga, R.; Tchatchueng, J.B. (1993). "Triacylglycerols and fatty acids composition of egusi seed oil (*Cucumeropsis Marnii Naudin')*". Grasas y Aceites **44** (6): 354. doi:10.3989/gya.1993.v44.i6.1062. *External link in |work= (help)*

[49] Bavec, F.; Grobelnik Mlakar, S.; Rozman, Č.; Bavec, M. (2007). J. Janick and A. Whipkey, ed. "Oil Pumpkins: Niche for Organic Producers" (PDF). *Issues in new crops and new uses* (ASHS Press, Alexandria, VA.).

[50] G. J. H. Grubben (ed.). "Citrullus". *Plant resources of tropical Africa: Vegetables*. Plant Resources of Tropical Africa. p. 185. ISBN 90-5782-147-8.

[51] Salunkhe, D. K. (1992). *World oilseeds: chemistry, technology, and utilization*. Springer. p. 460. ISBN 0-442-00112-6. Retrieved 2014-10-05.

[52] Schauss, Alexander G.; Jensen, Gitte S.; Wu, Xianli. "Açai (Euterpe oleracea)". *Flavor and Health Benefits of Small Fruits*. pp. 213–223. doi:10.1021/bk-2010-1035.ch013.

[53] Pacheco-Palencia, LA; Mertens-Talcott S; Talcott ST (Jun 2008). "Chemical composition, antioxidant properties, and thermal stability of a phytochemical enriched oil from Acai (Euterpe oleracea Mart.)". *J Agric Food Chem* **56** (12): 4631–6. doi:10.1021/jf800161u. PMID 18522407

[54] Jacobson, Hilary (2004). *Mother Food for Breastfeeding Mothers*. PageFree Publishing, Inc. p. 364. ISBN 1-58961-229-9. Retrieved 2014-10-05.

[55] Worku, Mulumabet; Gerald, Carresse (2007). "*C. elegans* Chemotaxis and Reproduction Following Environmental Exposure". *Proceedings of the 2007 National Conference on Environmental Science and Technology*. Springer. ISBN 0-387-88482-3. Retrieved 2014-10-05.

[56] al-Jawzīyah, Muḥammad ibn Abī Bakr Ibn Qayyim; Al Jauziyah, Imam Ibn Qayyim; Abdullah, Abdul Rahman (2003). second, ed. *Healing with the Medicine of the Prophet*. Darussalam. p. 261. ISBN 9960-892-91-3. Retrieved 2014-10-05.

[57] Shahidi, Fereidoon (2006). *Nutraceutical and specialty lipids and their co-products*. CRC Press. pp. 13–14. ISBN 1-57444-499-9. Retrieved 2014-10-05.

[58] Shahidi, Fereidoon; Miraliakbari, Homan (2005). "Evening primrose (Oenothera biennis)". In Paul M. Coates. *Encyclopedia of dietary supplements*. CRC Press. p. 197. ISBN 0-8247-5504-9. Retrieved 2014-10-05.

[59] "Evening Primrose Oil". Drugs.com. Retrieved 2011-10-25.

[60] Cousens, Gabriel (2009). *Conscious Eating* (2 ed.). North Atlantic Books. pp. 459–460. ISBN 1-55643-858-3. Retrieved 2014-10-05.

[61] Oomah, B. David; Mazza, G. (2000). "Bioactive Components of Flaxseed: Occurrence and Health Benefits". In Fereidoon Shahidi, Chi-Tang Ho. *Phytochemicals and phytopharmaceuticals*. The American Oil Chemists Society. pp. 106–116. ISBN 1-893997-05-7. Retrieved 2014-10-05.

[62] Pina-Rodriguez, AM; Akoh, CC (June 10, 2009). "Enrichment of amaranth oil with ethyl palmitate at the sn-2 position by chemical and enzymatic synthesis". *J Agric Food Chem* **57** (11): 4657–62. doi:10.1021/jf900242g. PMID 19413361.

[63] Grieve, Margaret (1931). "Apricot". *A Modern Herbal*. Dover Publications. ISBN 0-486-22798-7. Retrieved 2014-10-05. Originally published in 1931, and republished regularly since.

[64] Yu Xiuzhu; van de Voort, Frederick R.; Li Zhixi; Yue Tianli (October 25, 2007). "Proximate Composition of the Apple Seed and Characterization of Its Oil". *International Journal of Food Engineering* **3** (5). doi:10.2202/1556-3758.1283. Retrieved 2011-10-24.

[65] Jacobs, Daniel (2010). *The Rough Guide to Morocco*. Penguin. p. 498. ISBN 1-84836-977-8. Retrieved 2014-10-05.

[66] Whiley, Antony William; Schaffer, Bruce; Wolstenholme, B. Nigel (2002). *The avocado: botany, production, and uses*. CABI. p. 390. ISBN 0-85199-357-5. Retrieved 2014-10-05.

[67] Magness, J.R.; Markle, G.M.; Compton, C.C. (1971). *Food and feed crops of the United States. Interregional Research Project IR-4, IR Bul. 1 (Bul. 828 New Jersey Agr. Expt. Sta.)*. Retrieved 2014-10-05., quoted in "Purdue New Crops: Avocado oil".

[68] Ash, Irene (2004). *Handbook of green chemicals*. Synapse Info Resources. p. 531. ISBN 1-890595-79-9. Retrieved 2014-10-05.

[69] Chu, Michael. "Smoke Points of Various Fats". Cooking for Engineers. Retrieved 2011-10-20.

[70] "Codex standard for named vegetable oils" (PDF). *Codex Alimentarius* **8**. Codex Alimentarius Commission. 2001. Retrieved 2014-10-05.

[71] "Beauty Secrets of the Ancient Egyptians". Tour Egypt online magazine. Retrieved 2011-10-24.

[72] Axtell, "Borneo tallow nut

[73] D. Louppe, A.A. Oteng-Amoako, M. Brink, ed. (2008). *Plant resources of tropical Africa* **7**. PROTA. p. 110. ISBN 90-5782-209-1.

[74] Orhan, I.; Sener, B. (2002). "Fatty acid content of selected seed oils". *J Herb Pharmacother* **2** (3): 29–33. doi:10.1080/J157v02n03_03. PMID 15277087.

[75] Dakia, Patrick Aubin; Wathelet, Bernard; Paquot, Michel (2007). "Isolation and chemical evaluation of carob (Ceratonia siliqua L.) seed germ". *Food Chemistry* **102** (4): 1368–1374. doi:10.1016/j.foodchem.2006.05.059.

[76] "Cocoa butter – Britannica Online Encyclopedia". *Britannica Encyclopedia article*. July 1998. Retrieved 2007-09-10.

[77] Maximov, N. (1963). "Physico-Chemical Investigation of Cocklebur Oil". *Comptes Rendus* (Akademiia nauk SSSR): 381ff.

[78] McHargue, J. S. (April 1921). "Some Points of Interest Concerning the Cocklebur and Its Seeds". *Ecology* **2** (2): 110–119. doi:10.2307/1928923. JSTOR 1928923.

[79] McLendon, Chuck (July 28, 2000). "Attalea cohune". Floridata. Retrieved 2011-10-21.

[80] Ashurst, P. R. (1999). *Food Flavorings*. Springer. pp. 17–18. ISBN 0-8342-1621-3. Retrieved 2014-10-05.

[81] Bhanoo, Sindya N. (August 20, 2011). "A Bacteria-Busting Oil Behind a Popular Spice". *New York Times*.

[82] Besbes, S; Bleckerb, C; Deroanneb, C; Drirac, NE and Attiaa, H (March 2004). "Date seeds: chemical composition and characteristic profiles of the lipid fraction". *Food Chemistry* **84** (4): 577–584. doi:10.1016/S0308-8146(03)00281-4.

[83] Barreveld, W.H. (1993). "By-products of Date Packing and Processing". *Date Palm Products*. FAO. Retrieved 2011-11-19.

[84] United States National Research Council (2006). "Dika". *Lost Crops of Africa: Volume II: Vegetables*. National Academies Press. ISBN 0-309-10333-9. Retrieved 2014-10-05.

[85] Udeala, OK; Onyechi, JO; Agu, SI (January 1980). "Preliminary evaluation of dika fat, a new tablet lubricant". *J Pharm Pharmacol* **32** (1): 6–9. doi:10.1111/j.2042-7158.1980.tb12834.x. PMID 6102130.

[86] Mascia, Peter N. (2010). *Plant Biotechnology for Sustainable Production of Energy and Co-Products*. Springer. p. 231. ISBN 3-642-13439-4. Retrieved 2014-10-05.

[87] Zohary, Daniel; Hopf, María (2000). *Domestication of plants in the old world: the origin and spread of cultivated plants in West Asia, Europe, and the Nile Valley*. Oxford University Press. p. 138. ISBN 0-19-850356-3. Retrieved 2014-10-05.

[88] El Bassam, Nasir (2010). *Handbook of bioenergy crops: a complete reference to species, development and applications*. Earthscan. p. 18. ISBN 1-84407-854-X. Retrieved 2014-10-05.

[89] Bewley, J. Derek; Black, Michael; Halmer, Peter (2006). *The encyclopedia of seeds: science, technology and uses.* CABI. ISBN 0-85199-723-6. Retrieved 2014-10-05.

[90] France, Louise (November 7, 2004). "Hemp oil: A true superfood?". *The Guardian* (London). Retrieved 2011-10-24.

[91] Harborne, p. 100

[92] "Kapok seed oil". German Transport Information Service. Retrieved 2011-10-24.

[93] Lewy, Mario (1946). "Kenaf seed oil". *Journal of the American Oil Chemists' Society* **24** (1): 3–5. doi:10.1007/BF02645761.

[94] Bledsoe, Venita (1999). *Kenaf: alternative fiber : the Bledsoe experience.* Countryside Pub.

[95] Jones, Glynis; Valamoti, Soultana M. (2005). "Lallemantia, an imported or introduced oil plant in Bronze Age northern Greece". *Vegetation History and Archaeobotany* **14** (4): 571–7. doi:10.1007/s00334-005-0004-z.

[96] van der Vossen, H.A.M.; Mkamilo, G.S. (2007). "Vegetable oils". *Plant Resources of Tropical Africa* **14**. Plant Resources of Tropical Africa. p. 172. ISBN 90-5782-191-5.

[97] Shackleton, Sheona E.; Shackleton, Charlie M.; Cunningham, Tony; Lombard, Cyril; Sullivan, Caroline A.; Netshiluvhi, Thiambi R. (2002). "Knowledge on *Sclerocarya birrea* subsp. *caffra* with emphasis on its importance as a non-timber forest product in South and southern Africa: A Summary: Part 1: Taxonomy, ecology and role in rural livelihoods". *The Southern African Forestry Journal* **194** (1): 27–41. doi:10.1080/20702620.2002.10434589.

[98] United States National Research Council Board on Science and Technology for International Development (2008). "Marula". *Lost Crops of Africa: Fruits* **III**. National Academies Press. p. 23. ISBN 9780309164436. Retrieved 2013-10-25.

[99] Burden, Dan. "Meadowfoam". Agricultural Marketing Resource Center. Retrieved 2011-10-24.

[100] "Mustard oil". German Transport Information System. Retrieved 2011-10-22.

[101] Quinn, J.; Myers, R.L. (2002). "Trends in new crops and new uses". *Nigerseed: Specialty grain opportunity for Midwestern US.* ASHS Press. pp. 174–82. Retrieved 2013-10-15.

[102] "Nutmeg butter". Encyclopædia Britannica. Retrieved 2011-10-24.

[103] Holser, R.; Bost, G. (May 2004). "Hibiscus seed oil compositions". *Journal of the American Oil Chemists' Society* **95**.

[104] Martin, Franklin W. (1982). "Okra, Potential Multiple-Purpose Crop for the Temperate Zones and Tropics". *Economic Botany* **36** (3): 340–345. doi:10.1007/BF02858558.

[105] Raina Niskanen, ed. (2003). *Crop Management and Postharvest Handling of Horticultural Products: Crop Fertilization, Nutrition and Growth* **3**. Science Publishers. p. 178. ISBN 1-57808-140-8.

[106] Somonsohn, Barbara (2002). *Healing Power of Papaya.* Lotus Press. p. 153. ISBN 81-7769-066-3. Retrieved 2014-10-05.

[107] Brenner, David M. (1993). "Perilla: Botany, Uses and Genetic Resources". Retrieved 2011-10-24.

[108] Harborne, p. 102

[109] Cloughly, Cecil P.; Burlage, Henry M. (August 1959). "An examination of the oil of the seeds of persimmon (Diospyros Virginiana L., Fam. Ebenaceae)". *Journal of the American Pharmaceutical Association* **48** (8): 449–451. doi:10.1002/jps.3030480807. PMID 13672839.

[110] Axtell, "Caryocar spp.

[111] Axtell, "Pili nut"

[112] Stoner, Gary D. (2010). *Berries and Cancer Prevention.* Springer. p. 218. ISBN 1-4419-7553-5. Retrieved 2014-10-05.

[113] Watson, Ronald Ross; Preedy, Victor R. (2010-11-11). *Bioactive Foods and Extracts: Cancer Treatment and Prevention.* Taylor & Francis US, 2010. p. 60. ISBN 1-4398-1619-0.

[114] Lewkowitsch, Julius (1914). George H. Warburton ed., ed. *Chemical technology and analysis of oils, fats and waxes* **2** (5 ed.). Macmillan. p. 119.

[115] *Modern Technology Of Oils, Fats & Its Derivatives.* National Institute of Industrial Research. 2002. p. 105. ISBN 81-7833-085-7. Retrieved 2014-10-05.

[116] Creevy, Bill (1999). *The Oil Painting Book: Materials and Techniques for Today's Artist.* Watson-Guptill. ISBN 0-8230-3274-4.

[117] Gonsalves, John (2010). *Economic botany and ethnobotany.* Mittal Publications. p. 102. ISBN 81-8293-067-7. Retrieved 2014-10-05.

[118] Pesce, Celestino (1941). *Oleaginosas da Amazonia.* Composto e impresso Nas.

[119] "ACNFP Meeting minutes 14 March 2001". Advisory Committee on Novel Foods and Processes. March 14, 2001. Retrieved 2011-10-22.

[120] "Virgin Plum Oil cold pressed from d'Agen prune seeds". Vidalou Farm. Retrieved 2011-10-22.

[121] *Modern Technology Of Oils, Fats & Its Derivatives.* National Institute of Industrial Research. 2002. p. 108. ISBN 81-7833-085-7. Retrieved 2014-10-05.

[122] Koziol, Michael J. (1993). "Quinoa: A Potential New Oil Crop". *New crops* **2**.

[123] Siegbert Uhlig, ed. (2007). "Nug oil". *Encyclopaedia Aethiopica: He-N*. Otto Harrassowitz Verlag. p. 1202. ISBN 3-447-05607-X. Retrieved 2014-10-05.

[124] Getinet, A.; Sharma, S. M. (1996). *Niger, Guizotia abyssinica (L.f.) Cass*. Bioversity International. p. 35. ISBN 92-9043-292-6. Retrieved 2014-10-05.

[125] Gunstone, Frank (2009). *The Chemistry of Oils and Fats: Sources, Composition, Properties and Uses*. John Wiley & Sons. p. 8. ISBN 1-4051-5002-5. Retrieved 2014-10-05.

[126] Ju Yi-Hsu; Rayat, C.M.E. (2009). "Biodiesel from Rice Bran Oil". In Ashok Pandey. *Handbook of plant-based biofuels*. CRC Press. pp. 241–253. ISBN 1-56022-175-5. Retrieved 2014-10-05.

[127] Kunwar, Ripu M.; Adhikari, Nirmal (July 2005). "Ethnomedicine of Dolpa district, Nepal: the plants, their vernacular names and uses". *Lyonia*. ISSN 0888-9619. Retrieved 2011-10-24.

[128] "Sacha Inchi: Oil from the Amazon Takes Gold in Paris". Peru Food. September 22, 2006. Retrieved 2011-10-24.

[129] Krivankova, Blanka; Polesny, Zbynek; Lojka, Bohdan; Lojkova, Jana; Banout, Jan; Preininger, Daniel (October 2007). Eric Tielkes (ed.), ed. *Sacha Inchi (Plukenetia volubilis, Euphorbiaceae): A Promising Oilseed Crop from Peruvian Amazon*. Tropentag. Cuvillier Verlag Göttingen. Retrieved 2011-10-24.

[130] Jamieson, G. S.; McKinney, R. S. (1931). "Sapote (mammy apple) seed and oil". *Journal of the American Oil Chemists' Society* **8** (7): 255–256. doi:10.1007/BF02574575.

[131] Axtell, "Seje"

[132] Harsch, Ernest (2001). "Shea butter:making trade work for poor women". *Africa Recovery* **15** (4).

[133] Moranz, Steve; Masters, Eliot (2005). "What's in your chocolate?". In R. Selvarajah-Jaffery, B. Wagner, E. Sulzberger. *World Agroforestry Centre annual report 2005: Agroforestry science to support the millennium development goals*. World Agroforestry Centre. p. 19. ISBN 92-9059-199-4. Retrieved 2014-10-05.

[134] Kanya, T.C. Sindhu; Urs, M. Kantaraj (January 1989). "Studies on taramira (eruca sativa) seed oil and meal". *Journal of the American Oil Chemists' Society* **66** (1): 139. doi:10.1007/BF02661804.

[135] Grubben, G.J.H.; Denton, O.A., ed. (2004). "Vegetables". *Plant Resources of Tropical Africa* **2**. p. 295. ISBN 90-5782-147-8.

[136] Ruter, John M. (1993). "Nursery Production of Tea Oil Camellia Under Different Light Levels". *Trends in new crops and new uses*. Retrieved 2014-10-05.

[137] Axtell, "Teased" [*sic*]

[138] Parry Jr., John Wynne (2006). *Value-adding factors in cold-pressed edible seed oils and flours*. ProQuest. ISBN 978-0-542-96237-0. Retrieved 2014-10-05., p. 22

[139] Parry, p. 89

[140] Parry, p. 112

[141] He Yuan Zhanga; Hannab, Milford A.; Alib, Yusuf; Lu Nana (September 1996). "Yellow nut-sedge (Cyperus esculentus L.) tuber oil as a fuel". *Industrial Crops and Products* **5** (3): 177–181. doi:10.1016/0926-6690(96)89446-5.

[142] "Cyperus esculentus". Plants for a Future. Retrieved 2011-10-21.

[143] Harborne, p. 104

[144] Eller, F.J.; Moser, J.K.; Kenar, J.A.; Taylor, S.L. (2010). "Extraction and Analysis of Tomato Seed Oil". *Journal of the American Oil Chemists' Society* **87** (7): 755–762. doi:10.1007/s11746-010-1563-4.

[145] Mrak, E. Emil Marcel; Chichester, C. O.; Stewart, George Franklin, eds. (1977). *Advances in Food Research* **23**. Academic Press. ISBN 0080567681. Retrieved 2014-10-05.

[146] "Bio fuels". Castoroil.in. Retrieved 2011-11-19.

[147] Lee, Sunggyu; Shah, Y.T. (2012). *Biofuels and Bioenergy: Processes and Technologies*. CRC Press. p. 41. ISBN 1420089552. Retrieved 2014-10-05.

[148] "Castor Oil as Biodiesel & Biofuel". CastorOil.in. Retrieved 2011-10-24.

[149] Cloin, Jan. "Coconut Oil as a Biofuel in Pacific Islands–Challenges & Opportunities" (PDF). South Pacific Applied Geoscience Commission. Retrieved 2011-11-19.

[150] Kraminska, N.; Teleto, O. "The as the way to energy safety of the economy of the Ukraine" (PDF). Sumy State University, Sumy, Ukraine. Retrieved 2011-11-19.

[151] Morgan, Ben. "Economic Analysis and Feasibility of Cottonseed Oil as a Biodiesel Feedstock" (PDF). Texas Tech University, Industrial Engineering Department. Retrieved 2011-11-19.

[152] Laws, Forrest (August 29, 2007). "Can cottonseed join biodiesel race?". Southeast Farm Press. Retrieved 2011-11-19.

[153] Deitch, Robert (2003). *Hemp: American history revisited: the plant with a divided history*. Algora Publishing. p. 223. ISBN 0-87586-205-5. Retrieved 2014-10-05.

[154] Benhaim, Paul (2003). "Hemp as a Biofuel". *H.E.M.P.: Healthy Eating Made Possible*. Raw With Life. pp. 76–77. ISBN 1-901250-64-4. Retrieved 2014-10-05.

[155] Peterson, C.L.; Thompson, J.; Jones, S.. Hollenbeck, D. (November 2001). "Biodiesel from Yellow Mustard Oil". U.S. Department of Transportation. Retrieved 2013-10-25. Office of University Research and Education

[156] Jackson, Wes (Fall 1999). "Clearcutting the Last Wilderness". *The Land Report* (The Land Institute) (65).

[157] Hobbs, Steve. "Bio-diesel, farming for the future". Australian Agronomy Society. Retrieved 2011-10-22.

[158] Axtell, "Noog abyssinia"

[159] Rachmaniah, Orchidea; Ju Yi-Hsu; Vali, Shaik Ramjan; Tjondronegoro, Ismojowati; and Musfil, A.S. (2004). "A Study on Acid-Catalyzed Transesterification of Crude Rice Bran Oil for Biodiesel Production" (PDF). *World Energy Congress* (19). Retrieved 2011-11-19.

[160] Chef Boy Ari (January 5, 2006). "Safflower Oil in your Tank". *The Durango Telegraph*. Retrieved 2011-10-22.

[161] Dickenson, Marty (July 10, 2008). "The old man who farms with the sea". *Los Angeles Times*. Retrieved 2011-10-24.

[162] Peterson, Charles L.; Auld, Dick L. (1991). "Technical Overview of Vegetable Oil as a Transportation Fuel". *FACT: Solid Fuel Conversion for the Transportation Sector* (ASME) **12**.

[163] "Journey to Forever: Bio-diesel Yield". Retrieved 2011-10-24.

[164] Farago, Robert (July 15, 2008). "China Builds Tung Tree Oil Biodiesel Plants". The Truth about Cars. Retrieved 2011-11-19.

[165] Duke Handbook, "Copaifera langsdorfii Desf."

[166] Kanter, James (2011-12-30). "Air New Zealand Flies on Engine With Jatropha Biofuel Blend". *The New York Times*.

[167] Pramanik, K. (February 2003). "Properties and use of jatropha curcas oil and diesel fuel blends in compression ignition engine". *Renewable Energy* **28** (2): 239–248. doi:10.1016/S0960-1481(02)00027-7.

[168] Duke Handbook, "Simmondsia chinensis'

[169] Duke Handbook, "Euphorbia tirucalli

[170] Salunkhe, p 522

[171] "Lakshmi Taru tree answer to climate change problems: experts". oneIndia News. April 15, 2007. Retrieved 2011-11-05.

[172] Duke Handbook, "Pittosporum resiniferum

[173] Chandraju, S.; Prathima, B. K. (2003). "Ethyl ester of pongamia (Honge) oil: ecologically safe fuel". *Chemical & Environmental Research* **12** (3 & 4). ISSN 0971-2151. Retrieved 2013-10-08.

[174] Ramoo, S.K. (April 6, 2001). "A case for Honge oil as substitute for diesel". *The Hindu*. Retrieved 2011-06-19.

[175] "The Encyclopedia of Painting Materials: Drying oils" Retrieved 2011-10-24.

[176] Smyth, Herbert Warington (1906). *Mast & Sail in Europe & Asia*. p. 416. Retrieved 2011-10-19. (Mentions the use of dammar oil in marine paints)

[177] Database of Oil Yielding Plants

[178] Postell, Jim; Gesimondo, Nancy (2011). *Materiality and Interior Construction*. John Wiley and Sons. p. 137 ISBN 1-118-01969-5 Retrieved 2012-01-21.

[179] "Vegetable and Animal Oils and Fats". *Definition and Classification of Commodities*. FAO. 1992. Retrieved 2011-10-24.

[180] Axtell, "Chinese vegetable tallow

[181] Commodity Research Bureau (2007). *The CRB Commodity Yearbook 2007*. John Wiley and Sons. p. 288. ISBN 0-470-08015-9. Retrieved 2011-10-24.

[182] Teynor, T.M. (1992). "Vernonia". *Alternative Field Crops Manual*. Retrieved 2011-10-24.

[183] Schery, Robert W. (1972). *Plants for man*. Prentice-Hall. p. 325. ISBN 0-13-681254-6.

[184] Schechter, M.S.; Haller, H.L. (1943). "The insecticidal principle in the fruit of Amur corktree (Phellodendron amurense)". *Journal of Organic Chemistry* **8** (2): 194–197. doi:10.1021/jo01190a012.

[185] Miceli, A.; De Leo, P. (September 1996). "Extraction, characterization and utilization of artichoke-seed oil". *Bioresource Technology* **57** (3): 301–302. doi:10.1016/S0960-8524(96)00075-2.

[186] PLANTAS DA AMAZÔNIA PARA PRODUÇÃO COSMÉTICA: uma abordagem química - 60 espécies do extrativismo florestal não-madeireiro da Amazônia / Floriano Pastore Jr. (coord.); Vanessa Fernandes de Araújo [et. al.];– Brasília, 2005. 244 p.

[187] Kleiman, R. (1990). J. Janick and J.E. Simon (eds.), ed. "Chemistry of new industrial oilseed crops". *Advances in new crops* (Timber Press, Portland, OR): 196–203. Retrieved 2011-10-24.

[188] Zhang, Hong; Yang, Jing Yu; Zhou, Fan; Wang, Li Hui; Zhang, Wen; Sha, Sha; Wu, Chun Fu (2011). "Seed Oil of *Brucea javanica* Induces Apoptotic Death of Acute Myeloid Leukemia Cells via Both the Death Receptors and the Mitochondrial-Related Pathways". *Evidence-Based Complementary and Alternative Medicine* **2011**:

1.   doi:10.1155/2011/965016.   PMC 3132896.   PMID 21760826.

[189]   Lou, Guo-Guang; Yao, Hang-Ping; Xie, Li-Ping (2010). "*Brucea javanica* Oil Induces Apoptosis in T24 Bladder Cancer Cells via Upregulation of Caspase-3, Caspase-9, and Inhibition of NF-κB and COX-2 Expressions". *The American Journal of Chinese Medicine* **38** (3): 613–24. doi:10.1142/S0192415X10008093. PMID 20503476.

[190]   Duke, James A. (1997). *The green pharmacy: new discoveries in herbal remedies for common diseases and conditions from the world's foremost authority on healing herbs.* Rodale. ISBN 0-87596-316-1. Retrieved 2014-10-05.

[191]   Rostagno, Mauricio A.; Prado, Juliana M. (2013). *Natural Product Extraction: Principles and Applications.* Royal Society of Chemistry. p. 35. ISBN 1849736065. Retrieved 2015-02-27.

[192]   Elevitch, Craig R.; Manner, Harley I. (2006). *Traditional trees of Pacific Islands: their culture, environment, and use.* PAR. p. 53. ISBN 0-9702544-5-8. Retrieved 2014-10-05.

[193]   Yu, Lucy Liangli; Zhou, Kevin Kequan; Parry, John (2005). "Antioxidant properties of cold-pressed black caraway, carrot, cranberry, and hemp seed oils". *Food chemistry* **91** (4): 723–729. doi:10.1016/j.foodchem.2004.06.044. ISSN 0308-8146. INIST:16541373.

[194]   Axtell, "Chaulmoogra"

[195]   Felter, Harvey Wickes; Lloyd, John Uri (1898). "Gynocardia—Chaulmoogra". *King's American Dispensatory.* Retrieved 2011-10-24.

[196]   Cottle, Wyndham (28 June 1879). "Chaulmoogra Oil in Leprosy". *The British Medical Journal* **1** (965): 968–969. doi:10.1136/bmj.1.965.968. JSTOR 25251370.

[197]   Oplinger, E.S. (1991). "Crambe". *Alternative Field Crops Manual.* Retrieved 2011-10-24.

[198]   Salunkhe, p. 488

[199]   Harborne, Jeffrey B.; Baxter, Herbert (2001). *Chemical dictionary of economic plants.* John Wiley and Sons. p. 99. ISBN 0-471-49226-4. Retrieved 2014-10-05.

[200]   Kleiman, Robert (1990). "Chemistry of New Industrial Oilseed Crops". *Advances in new crops*: 196–203. Retrieved 2011-10-24.

[201]   *Food and Fruit-bearing Forest Species: Examples from Latin America.* FAO. 1986. p. 298. ISBN 9251023727.

[202]   Martin, R. J.; Porter, N. G.; Deo, B. (2005). "Initial studies on seed oil composition of Calendula and Lunaria" (PDF). *Agronomy N.Z.* **35**.

[203]   Goreja, W.G. (2004). "Comparison of Shea Butter to Other Oils and Emollients". *Shea Butter: The Nourishing Properties of Africa's Best-Kept Natural Beauty Secret.* TNC International Inc. p. 20. ISBN 0-9742962-5-2. Retrieved 2014-10-05.

[204]   Kochhar, S. Prakash (2011). "Minor and Specialty Oils". In Frank Gunstone. *Vegetable Oils in Food Technology: Composition, Properties and Uses.* John Wiley & Sons. p. 323. ISBN 1-4443-3268-6. Retrieved 2014-10-05.

[205]   Black, Michael; Bewle, J. Derek, eds. (2000). *Seed Technology and Its Biological Basis.* CRC Press. p. 149. ISBN 0849397499. Retrieved 2014-10-05.

[206]   Morton, Julia F. "Mango". *Fruits of Warm Climates.* ISBN 0-9610184-1-0. Retrieved 2014-10-05.

[207]   Puri, Harbans Singh (1999). *Neem: the divine tree : Azadirachta indica.* CRC Press. p. 74ff. ISBN 90-5702-348-2. Retrieved 2011-11-15.

[208]   See "Ojon.com Web site". Ojon.com. Retrieved 2011-11-19.

[209]   Munguia, Osvaldo; Collins, Judith (December 5, 2005). "Ojon Oil". *Footsteps* (Tear Fund International) **65**.

[210]   Pruthi, J. (1963). "Physiology, Chemistry and Technology of Passion Fruit". *Advances in Food Research* **12**: 268.

[211]   Scott, Timothy Lee; Buhner, Stephen Harrod (2010). *Invasive Plant Medicine: The Ecological Benefits and Healing Abilities of Invasives.* Inner Traditions / Bear & Co. ISBN 1-59477-305-X. Retrieved 2014-10-05.

[212]   "Rubber Seed Oil : Finding Uses for a Waste Product (Nigeria)". International Development Research Centre. May 29, 2000. Retrieved 2011-10-24.

[213]   Ramadha, A.S.; Jayaraj, S.; Muraleedharan, C. (April 2003). "Characterization and effect of using rubber seed oil as fuel in the compression ignition engines". *Renewable Energy* **20** (5): 795–803. doi:10.1016/j.renene.2004.07.002.

[214]   Bùi Huy Như Phúc (March 25–28, 2003). Reg Preston and Brian Ogle, ed. *Ileal digestibility of coconut oil meal and rubber seed oil meal in growing pigs.* Proceedings of Final National Seminar-Workshop on Sustainable Livestock Production on Local Feed Resources. Retrieved 2011-10-24.

[215]   Dharmananda, Subhuti. "Sea buckthorn". Institute for Traditional Medicine. Retrieved 2011-10-24.

[216]   Zarouk, M.; El Almi, H.; Ben Youssef, N.; Sleimi, N.; Smaoui, A.; Bin Miled, D.; Abdelly, C. (2003). "Lipid Composition of Seeds of Local Halophytes: *Cakile maritima, Zygophyllum album* and *Crithmum maritimum*". In Helmut Lieth, Marina Mochtchenko (eds.). *Cash crop halophytes: recent studies : 10 years after the Al Ain meeting. Tasks for vegetation science* (Springer). p. 124. ISBN 1-4020-1202-0. Retrieved 2013-10-25.

[217]   Grebneva, E.V.; Nesterova, O.V. (July 25, 2006). "Berry Marc Oils as Untraditional Resourse for Functional Food and Fitopreparation". In Danik M. Martirosyan. *Functional Foods for Chronic Diseases.* p. 152. ISBN 0-9767535-2-9.

[218] Panda, Himadri (2002). "Tall Oil and its Derivatives". *The Complete Technology Book On Natural Products (Forest Based)*. Asia Pacific Business Press. pp. 361–376. ISBN 81-7833-072-5. Retrieved 2014-10-05.

[219] D. Louppe; A.A. Oteng-Amoako; M. Brink, ed. (2008). *Plant resources of tropical Africa* 7. PROTA. ISBN 90-5782-209-1.

[220] Gunstone, F. D.; Harwood, John L.; Dijkstra, Albert J. (2007). *The lipid handbook with CD-ROM*. CRC Press. p. 86. ISBN 0-8493-9688-3. Retrieved 2014-10-05.

[221] Duke, James A.; DuCellier, Judith L. (1993). *CRC handbook of alternative cash crops*. CRC Press. p. 238. ISBN 0-8493-3620-1.

[222] Pesce, Celestino (2009). *Oleaginosas da Amazônia*. Belém: Museu Paraense Emilio Goeldi. p. 334. ISBN 978-85-61377-06-9.

[223] Smith, Nigel (2014). *Palms and People in the Amazon*. p. 81. ISBN 3319055097.

2.62.8 Further reading

- "Fats and Cholesterol: Out with the Bad, In with the Good". *The Nutrition Source*. Harvard School of Public Health. Retrieved 2011-10-22.

- "Bulk Oil Trading". Archived from the original on 2006-07-18. Retrieved 2006-07-25. An older version of this site was very helpful in making this list more comprehensive.

- "Vegetable Oil Yields and Characteristics". Retrieved 2011-10-24. Compiles useful information on vegetable oils from a number of sources.

- "Castor Oil". Retrieved 2006-07-25. The site contains a large set of resources on castor oil and many other oils, particularly those used to make biodiesel.

- Botanical Garden of Indian Republic (BGIR) (April 5, 2004). "Database of Oil Yielding Plants" (PDF). *Botanical Survey of India*. Archived from the original (PDF) on 2011-07-21. Retrieved 2010-10-19. List of about 300 plants that grow in India, and that yield oil. Also includes common names in languages spoken in India.

- Macmillan, H.F. "Oils and Vegetable Fats". *Handbook of Tropical Plants*. Herbdata New Zealand. ISBN 81-7041-177-7. Archived from the original on 2011-07-21. Old reference with basic information on an unusually large variety of plant oils.

- Ashurst, P. R. (1999). *Food Flavorings*. Springer. ISBN 0-8342-1621-3. Retrieved 2014-10-05. Comprehensive information on cooking oils that are used for flavoring foods.

- Duke, James A. (1982). *Handbook of Energy Crops*. Purdue University Center for New Crops. Retrieved 2011-11-19.

Chapter 3

Text and image sources, contributors, and licenses

3.1 Text

- **Essential oil** *Source:* https://en.wikipedia.org/wiki/Essential_oil?oldid=686853942 *Contributors:* AxelBoldt, The Anome, Tarquin, PierreAbbat, Tedernst, Edward, Brainsik, Sannse, Mkweise, Ahoerstemeier, Ronz, Ootachi, Imc, Tempshill, Wetman, Pollinator, Shantavira, Robbot, Texture, Dbroadwell, Giftlite, Mintleaf~enwiki, Wolfkeeper, Kabulykos, Dmmaus, Ryanaxp, Wmahan, Utcursch, Quarl, Mrtrey99, Jklamo, Thorwald, Kmccoy, Wfaulk, Rich Farmbrough, Cacycle, Eskrima, Vsmith, Smyth, Dour High Arch, Bender235, ESkog, Mwanner, Bobo192, Che090572, Davidruben, Duk, Mtruch, Viriditas, Cmdrjameson, Dungodung, Cayte, Alastairgbrown, Wendell, Keenan Pepper, Sjschen, Walkerma, Alisonsage, Shoefly, Versageek, Gene Nygaard, Tainter, Ceyockey, Stuartyeates, Feezo, Woohookitty, LostAccount, StradivariusTV, MrWhipple, MGTom, Futhark, BD2412, FreplySpang, Rjwilmsi, Loniceas, Ricardo Carneiro Pires, FlaBot, Mister Matt, CarolGray, Marsve, Akhenaten0, Physchim62, Chobot, Rewster, WriterHound, YurikBot, Wavelength, Waitak, Huw Powell, Kymacpherson, Liastnir, Dforest, Nick, Malcolma, Mgcsinc, Tsalman, Mysid, Kirper, FF2010, Phgao, 2over0, Pamela J. Leavey, Ninly, Modify, GraemeL, Foolestroupe, Alexandrov, GrinBot~enwiki, Groyolo, Luk, Veinor, SmackBot, Khcbaser, Melchoir, Unyoyega, Delldot, Eskimbot, Gdaypal, Hardyplants, Kintetsubuffalo, Hbackman, Edgar181, Apers0n, Ohnoitsjamie, David.Throop, Chris the speller, Smalltowngirl, RDBrown, Tito4000, Deli nk, DHN-bot~enwiki, Colonies Chris, KojieroSaske, Mike hayes, Zaian, Japeo, Totophe64~enwiki, Cybercobra, BullRangifer, Bejnar, SashatoBot, Six.oh.six, Mbeychok, Beetstra, TastyPoutine, Foolishben, Nehrams2020, Iridescent, JoeBot, Cynthia Blue, Schlagwerk, Daniel5127, Atomobot, Dia^, JForget, Requestion, Shandris, WeggeBot, Mccojr02, Steel, Rifleman 82, Gogo Dodo, Palaeologos, Optimist on the run, Chachilongbow, Barticus88, Typing monkey, Who123, Headbomb, Dalahäst, JustAGal, Aroma-guide, Gregalton, Zorgkang, John Moss, Shivaexportsindia, JAnDbot, Herbjunkie, Epeefleche, Jamesfuhrman, Acroterion, Wasell, Mdurante, Dekimasu, Felix Stember, Tejawe, Prestonmcconkie, Indon, Adrian J. Hunter, Vssun, PoliticalJunkie, Hannah-w, Pyritie, Rolfs, PKLpink, R'n'B, DavidSTaylor, Mfbabcock, Discott, Mininanny123, Cindy Jones1, Sbula, Naniwako, Belovedfreak, FJPB, STBotD, Idioma-bot, EODoc, ABF, Minwu, TXiKiBoT, Lottiotta, Theofenton, Room429, Mattchess, Olav 10, Sochlo, SieBot, Wjreece, Riley Clarke, 3diwl9p02, Bentogoa, Wombatcat, Darladeer, Rightleftright, Anchor Link Bot, Essentialdepot, Hard2Win, ClueBot, Lianiwidjaja, Robbiemuffin, The Thing That Should Not Be, Plankwalking, Fionnasmom, TypoBoy, DragonBot, Excirial, LarryMorseDCOhio, Slidinandridin06, Secret, Brylletc, XLinkBot, Jytdog, Ost316, TFOWR, Addbot, DOI bot, Beyoung, Cblack2, Valoriejl, Goodoodh, Jboud, Tassedethe, Tide rolls, DebKM, Zorrobot, Luckas-bot, Yobot, Cinteotl, Declan.kenny, JeanGeilland, Amirobot, Eric-Wester, Honey badger 08, AnomieBOT, The Parting Glass, Eoilco, Materialscientist, Citation bot, Xqbot, Gigemag76, Tabouretamtam, Wperdue, Elvim, Gilo1969, 1bluerhino, Thehelpfulbot, FrescoBot, Biolandes, Maxx.scent, Monirnstu, Louperibot, Citation bot 1, Givrix~enwiki, Lobito09, Sandcat01, Pinethicket, RedBot, Chobiche, Francis Lima, JamesGrimshaw, Bradensam, TobeBot, DixonDBot, Eisolson, Reach Out to the Truth, Mean as custard, TjBot, EmausBot, TheRealKhaled, Dewritech, Hannah9, AvicBot, ZéroBot, LoR. Caarl Robinson, Fred Gandt, Sodabrew, Erianna, JoeSperrazza, L Kensington, Donner60, ChuispastonBot, G-13114, ClueBot NG, Rich Smith, Gareth Griffith-Jones, Birdmeister, Johnwikiupdater, Helpful Pixie Bot, 9tmaxr, Hyptis, BG19bot, Surftheweb, Northamerica1000, Hallows AG, Harizotoh9, MrBill3, Chip123456, Tfbybyhf, Kraftykyle, Sandhillman, Crouchs, Dhopeshwarsales, Total-MAdMaN, Kaidenj, Hangm n, Organics4horses, Kevinba99, Ice9ismine, Epicgenius, Magnolia677, Habibibibalani, Nickknack00, Kfleisc, RhinoMind, Stamptrader, Somunair, Lagoset, Monkbot, Glharris2011, Scarlettail, NodtheProphet, MinnesotaScholar, Spwg, Cr0cc0H, Jonathanarpith, Resistence2000, Iamawdsin, Smartgirltips, Lalalalallalalallalalalala, Sallywithx, GlendaGuzman, MelissaCstyer, Nleeguitar, Wicki, Arkimbald, Dominick16, John t denison, Thesib12, KasparBot, LeiaChester, Ralph2324eqe and Anonymous: 276

- **Anethole** *Source:* https://en.wikipedia.org/wiki/Anethole?oldid=683553552 *Contributors:* Ehn, Dratman, Bobblewik, Quadell, H Padleckas, Cacycle, Jérôme, Benjah-bmm27, Tabletop, DePiep, Rjwilmsi, Vuong Ngan Ha, FlaBot, Chobot, Hede2000, DAJF, SmackBot, Edgar181, Phillipbeynon, Averette, Chris the speller, Bluebot, Nbarth, Smokefoot, Drphilharmonic, Chymicus, DA3N, Beetstra, Van helsing, Cydebot, Rifleman 82, Christian75, Calvero JP, Thijs!bot, Nick Number, Astavats, John Moss, Karol007, ChemNerd, Nono64, Discott, Enix150, IceDragon64, Una Smith, Mike2vil, Chem-awb, Polyamorph, Sensonet, Jytdog, MystBot, Addbot, Chempedia, Epop fr, Vapeur, CheMoBot, Materialscientist, ArthurBot, Jü, البط علي حسن, Almabot, Citation bot 1, Nirmos, Trappist the monk, Radio89, Aoidh, Jynto, Reach Out to the Truth, RjwilmsiBot, DASHBot, Ebe123, ZéroBot, Prayerfortheworld, Kikolock, ChuispastonBot, ClueBot NG, Helpful Pixie Bot, JohnSRoberts99, NotWith, Stoneglasgow, ArmbrustBot, Stamptrader, Monkbot, Renamed user 51g7z61hz5af2azs6k6, P. S. Sena, PishT, Scifrk and Anonymous: 24

- **Aroma lamp** *Source:* https://en.wikipedia.org/wiki/Aroma_lamp?oldid=680212953 *Contributors:* Bearcat, Cydebot, Mean as custard, This lousy T-shirt, BG19bot, Lagoset, Frlgin, Vivek.bekhabar and Anonymous: 2

- **Aromatherapy** *Source:* https://en.wikipedia.org/wiki/Aromatherapy?oldid=685363035 *Contributors:* Tbc~enwiki, 0, The Anome, Koyaanis Qatsi, PierreAbbat, Stevertigo, Brainsik, Tim Starting, Delirium, Tregoweth, Ahoerstemeier, Ronz, Theresa knott, Angela, Andres, Jiang, le-andré du Toit, Markb, Toph99, Imc, Finlay McWalter, Carbuncle, Robbot, Hankwang, TimothyPilgrim, Rholton, Texture, Ojigiri~enwiki, Auric, Mr-Natural-Health, Bkell, Hadal, Wikibot, Michael Snow, Alan Liefting, Fabiform, Wouterhagens, Ceejayoz, Solipsist, Wmrahen, Utcursch, Sonjaaa, Phil Sandifer, Mike Storm, Salimfadhley, HamYoyo, Mahendra, Rich Farmbrough, Cacycle, Nina Gerlach, Mani., Vi-oletriga, Elwzkipedista~enwiki, El C, Mwanner, JackWasey, CDN99, StoatBringer, Arcadian, Cayte, Famousdog, MPere., Nsaa, Sjschen, Ebeaverton, Spangineer, Callimanda, RJFJR, Zawersh, Versageek, Pwqn, John11235813, Stuartyeates, Feezo, Bobrayner, Woohookitty, Mind-matrix, RHaworth, SusanLarson, WadeSimMiser, John Gohde, Graham87, BD2412, Josh Parris, Rjwilmsi, Vary, Loniceas, Cff12345 FaBot, AED, Nihiltres, RexNL, Gurch, KFP, TheMoog, DaGizza, DVdm, WriterHound, YurikBot, Splintercellguy, SkyCaptain~enwiki, Waitak, Chris Capoccia, Chaser, R. L. Bright, CambridgeBayWeather, Boneheadmx, Grafen, Dforest, Tearlach, Nick, Aaron Brenneman, Mikeblas, Syrthiss, Dbfirs, Pamela J. Leavey, Zzuuzz, Ninly, Closedmouth, GraemeL, Wjousts, Cotoco, Alexandrov, DVD R W, NickelShoe, Luk, Sar-danaphalus, Veinor, Crystallina, SmackBot, Herostratus, BenBurch, Jagged 85, Eskimbot, Hardyplants, Paxse, Edgar181, Cazort, Apers0n, Ohnoitsjamie, Smalltowngirl, Deli nk, HerbsNSuch, JREL, Frap, Xiner, Realberserker, Downtown dan seattle, RandomP, BullRangifer, Ee-jnar, Ohconfucius, Will Beback, SashatoBot, T-dot, Bella Swan, Chrisch, Beetstra, George The Dragon, Manov, TastyPoutine, Foolishben, DI2000, Hu12, Judgesurreal777, Filelakeshoe, Atomobot, CRGreathouse, CmdrObot, Jorcoga, Cydebot, Crychan2001, Gogo Dodo, JFree-man, Yinunit, Thijs!bot, Epbr123, OrangePeel, Daniel, Sendbinti, Second Quantization, Dfrg.msc, Nick Number, Escarbot, Aroma-guide, Mentifisto, AntiVandalBot, Milton Stanley, Majorly, TimVickers, Fayenatic london, Nipisiquit, Spencer, Huttarl, Narssarssuaq, YK Times, PhilKnight, SiobhanHansa, VoABot II, Spikeyone, Steven Walling, Froid, Fabrictramp, Indon, Lsern, Naturallythinking, Foregone conclusion, RickSalsman, CliffC, CommonsDelinker, Emeraldlingerie, Fred.e, Adifeldman, Tikiwont, Mike.lifeguard, Mininanny123, Amphora aromatics, Yoongkheong, Cindy Jones1, McSly, Sbula, Bailo26, Namiwako, RoboMaxCyberSem, Belovedfreak, SmilesALot, Stephaniegilmore, Siraj88, Equazcion, Arrisweb, Briandube, Tomcrocker, Idioma-bot, MummyCassie, Al7~enwiki, VolkovBot, Thedjatclubrock, Wizard-Frogs.com p, TXiKiBoT, Java7837, Lottiotta, Nightwatchman, John Carter, Uni.wiki.editor, LeaveSleaves, Webdoc46, BotKung, Penkala, בכ יבול, Cm-bay, Mattchess, Falcon8765, Turgan, GlassFET, Senyor Nuclear, HiDrNick, AlleborgoBot, Burgercat, Ponyo, Wjreece, Nubiatech, Caltas, Jrun, Alexbrr, Darladeer, Wahrmund, Soulja2mv, Loren.wilton, Martarius, ClueBot, Lianiwidjaja, Ferred, MikeVitale, Desoto10, Keryarome, Arakunem, Fionnasmom, Mild Bill Hiccup, Bonnyrigg High School, Auntof6, Delnatura, Valueaddedwater, Aua, Wazupmedia, PixelBot, Slidi-nandridin06, Hollyroseeva, Brylletc, Bhughes916, DumZiBoT, Millpightle, Bev1953, Tam001, Timgaunt, XLinkBot, Jytdog, Mafizah~enwiki, Rror, Pianississimo, Nicolae Coman, Addbot, Orac7, DOI bot, Cblack2, Serrac, Ashanda, Sgt Sharpe, Geratina, Lucian Sunday, LinkFA-Bot, Gail, Zorrobot, Thothbook, Yobot, Kartano, Orac29, Amirobot, Brougham96, A Stop at Willoughby, IW.HG, TestEditBot, Backslash For-wardslash, DiverDave, AnomieBOT, Jim1138, Piano non troppo, Surfcitymama, Citation bot, Tabouretamtam, Kristinamv, 2008forum, Little Flower Eagle, Clayterch, FrescoBot, Aromaqueen, Alarics, Citation bot 1, I dream of horses, Pink Bull, Aromaman2009, Kibi78704, Gambi-ent, Buddy23Lee, Blind cyclist, Mean as custard, Flipflopdoc, DASHBot, Green Minnow, Immunize, Super48paul, Kiliona, L235, Cctreadway, LauraGarride, Cjsunbird, Tama1923, H3llBot, MonoAV, Lauburn, DASHBotAV, ClueBot NG, Frietjes, Rezabot, The Old Trout, Wikiguen, Roses4u2, Jeffshjarback, Benton28031, Daphnenelson, BG19bot, Chris Reed, Mollisha, Allecher, Aromatherapy Council, Nappysgirl, Paulrow-lands76, MrBill3, NotWith, Jacknunn, Kayp22, BattyBot, Marklancs, Aromamonika, Mjsteiner, Dexbot, Xanstar, Munskeptics, I am One of Many, Mys7688, ErnieGeek, cb, Pieking10, Fhanisreal, ممنون حسی‌ها, Kloningan719, Monkbot, Dr. Cory Schultz, Ghas24, Nourelkhatib, KatBerg52, Ccan811, Lalt3617, Simone11pink, Mafroulis, J cab6641, JavieraC123, Julietdeltalima, Stardoman, GlendaGuzman, Ecosumit, KasparBot, Kulbrez2, LeiaChester, Vivek.bekhabar, Merissaluetjen and Anonymous: 349

- **Artemisia pallens** *Source:* https://en.wikipedia.org/wiki/Artemisia_pallens?oldid=680746320 *Contributors:* Jokestress, Hesperian, Stemonitis, Rjwilmsi, FlaBot, DAJF, Asarelah, Sahyadri, Edgar181, Rxitko, Vprajkumar, Cydebot, Hebrides, Headbomb, Sankalpdravid, SchreiberBike, Addbot, Luckas-bot, Ulric1313, Citation bot, Fasiru, Mishae, RjwilmsiBot, EmausBot, ChrisGualtieri, Lagoset, P. S. Sena and Anonymous: 7

- **Backhousia citriodora** *Source:* https://en.wikipedia.org/wiki/Backhousia_citriodora?oldid=681376548 *Contributors:* Dreamyshade, Bogdan-giusca, Cherkash, MPF, Wolfkeeper, Mako098765, DragonflySixtyseven, Bender235, Davidruben, 99of9, Hesperian, Alansohn, Walkerma, Oliphaunt, BD2412, Josh Parris, Rjwilmsi, Joe Decker, Eubot, OpenToppedBus, CJLL Wright, Gdrbot, Badagnani, DAJF, Mugwumpjism, That Guy, From That Show!, Donama, Hmains, JRSP, Melburnian, JGXenite, Eataust, Chefben, Cherikoff, Dchadburn, Storeye, PKT, Beneaththestorm, AntiVandalBot, John Moss, Hotridge, Gypsyware, Acalamari, Berichard, January2007, Jaguarlaser, HelloMojo, ClueBot, Bob1960evens, Unbuttered Parsnip, Mild Bill Hiccup, Alexbot, 02millers, Addbot, DOI bot, Cuaxdon, Flakinho, Lightbot, Luckas-bot, Yobot, Galoubet, LilHelpa, Jmundo, Itineranttrader, Arsenalthefootballchampions, Citation bot 1, Aareo, Look2See1, Racerx11, AvicBot, Re-sprinter123, ClueBot NG, Helpful Pixie Bot, Plantdrew, Shisha-Tom, BattyBot, Dexbot, P. S. Sena and Anonymous: 33

- **Benzoin resin** *Source:* https://en.wikipedia.org/wiki/Benzoin_resin?oldid=653763675 *Contributors:* Stone, Dogface, Francs2000, MPF, Rich Farmbrough, CanisRufus, Longhair, Hooperbloob, Anthony Appleyard, Sjschen, Andrewpmk, SI, Dryman, Allen3, V8rik, Anarchivist, Ws-erd911, SkyCaptain~enwiki, RussBot, Shaddack, Prime Entelechy, El Cazangero, Dysmorodrepanis~enwiki, Trovatore, DAJF, IceCreamAn-tisocial, NielsenGW, The Famous Movie Director, Sei Shonagon~enwiki, Drphilharmonic, Ligulembot, Snowgrouse, SilkTork, Christian75, JAnDbot, Epeefleche, Magioladitis, Maproom, DASonnenfeld, Idioma-bot, Almazi, Wie146, Italtrav, Wikiisawesome, SieBot, Calliope-jen1, LarryMorseDCOhio, Jht4060, Addbot, Mr0t1633, DOI bot, Panfily, SamatBot, Yobot, PMLawrence, Wisg, LilHelpa, Janmeut~enwiki, Dinamik-bot, Gixie, Kamran the Great, EmausBot, WikitanvirBot, Tmrdean, BG19bot, PhnomPencil, Bangalorius, Solar Dynasty Mpiva, Lemnaminor, Arun Skeet, Alluppity, Karish10, P. S. Sena and Anonymous: 23

- **Bergamot essential oil** *Source:* https://en.wikipedia.org/wiki/Bergamot_essential_oil?oldid=653764365 *Contributors:* Rjwilmsi, DAJF, Thnidu, Woodshed, Epeefleche, CommonsDelinker, Dthomsen8, Jht4060, Jacopo Werther, Yobot, FrescoBot, SporkBot, Khazar2, Hmains-bot1, Alp Kunkar, Monkbot, P. S. Sena and Anonymous: 6

- **Black pepper** *Source:* https://en.wikipedia.org/wiki/Black_pepper?oldid=687809743 *Contributors:* Bryan Derksen, William Avery Heron, Montrealais, Edward, PhilipMW, Zocky, Llywrch, Dominus, Menchi, Ixfd64, Shoaler, Gbleem, Mdebets, Mark Foskey, Nikai, Kaysov, Jengod, Tpbradbury, Taxman, Phoebe, Morn, Wetman, David.Monniaux, Francs2000, PuzzletChung, Gentgeen, Hankwang, Rfc1394, Spike, Tex-ture, Bkell, Oobopshark, Ryanrs, MPF, Wolf530, Haeleth, BenFrantzDale, Tom harrison, Lupin, Curps, Jdavidb, Jfdwolff, Revth, Booblewik, Andycjp, Gzuckier, Quadell, Vina, MacGyverMagic, Garymead, Neutrality, Burschik, Oknazevad, Robin klein, Kevyn, Flyhighplato, Kate,

O'Dea, DanielCD, Discospinster, Twinxor, Rich Farmbrough, Cacycle, SpanishJoe, Vsmith, Bishonen, Tsujigiri~enwiki, Kaisershatner, Pjf, Edward Z. Yang, Clk3, Triona, Nrbelex, Guettarda, Fir0002, TheSolomon, Foobaz, Neg, BillyTFried, Hesperian, Idleguy, Krellis, Caeruleancentaur, Ranveig, Alansohn, Eleland, Mo0, Tek022, Eric Kvaalen, Joolz, Hydriotaphia, Wiki-uk, Atlant, Damnreds, Mailer diablo, Ynhockey, Roger2~enwiki, Svartalf, MattWade, Sciurinæ, Coolmallu, Someoneinmyheadbutit'snotme, Gene Nygaard, HenryLi, Kazvorpal, CranialNerves, Stemonitis, Isfisk, Woohookitty, Jacob Haller, Oliphaunt, JeremyA, MONGO, Moormand, Wikiklrsc, SDC, Wayward, Allen3, Kbdank71, Bunchofgrapes, FreplySpang, Pmj, Rjwilmsi, NatusRoma, Jweiss11, Harro5, Mork the delayer, Oblivious, CQJ, Ricardo Carneiro Pires, Brighterorange, Yug, Panterka, Fish and karate, Naraht, Eubot, RobertG, Awotter, Chanting Fox, Meeve, Spudtater, RexNL, Kolbasz, OpenToppedBus, Ronebofh, Le Anh-Huy, Mongreilf, Gdrbot, Bgwhite, NSR, WriterHound, The Rambling Man, YurikBot, Sceptre, SkyCaptain~enwiki, Red Slash, Kvuo, IBook of the Revolution, Stephenb, Mithridates, Gaius Cornelius, Wimt, Curtis Clark, Dysmorodrepanis~enwiki, Nirvana2013, Veledan, Badagnani, Geeksquad, Joelr31, Mccready, Ragesoss, Banes, Coderzombie, Vivaldi, Marknesbitt, Syrthiss, Gadget850, Asarelah, Tachs, 1978~enwiki, Crisco 1492, Leptictidium, Codrinb, Theda, SMcCandlish, Canley, BorgQueen, MrHen, Katieh5584, Kungfuadam, DVD R W, Jaysscholar, A bit iffy, SmackBot, YellowMonkey, Bouette, Erwinrossen, Ma8thew, Gubby, Olorin28, Hydrogen Iodide, Sanjay ach, Blue520, Thunderboltz, Grey Shadow, Eskimbot, Anomaly2002, Stevegallery, TypoDotOrg, Gilliam, Ohnoitsjamie, Cibyd, KaragouniS, Smalltowngirl, CrookedAsterisk, Thumperward, HartzR, Hollow Wilerding, Deli nk, ImpuMozhi, Uthbrian, Octahedron80, Junius49, Royboycrashfan, Scray, Rfwoolf, Flibbert, Andrewin, Yidisheryid, 66664yyiotjwoier, CJ666, Neonow, Jkirish5, Rrburke, Kingdon, TedE, VegaDark, BryanG, Ligulembot, Mu2, Tjrichter, Bejnar, Apalaria, DrJoe, Eliyak, Geach, Teneriff, Kuru, Ian Spackman, Joffeloff, IronGargoyle, A. Parrot, Eternal Equinox, NcSchu, SQGibbon, SandyGeorgia, Ryulong, M855GT, Peyre, OnBeyondZebrax, Tina Brooks, Blehfu, Tawkerbot2, Mschroebel, JForget, KNM, Code E, Ale jrb, Albert.white, IP Address, GargoyleMT, Pgr94, Tomw91, Doctormatt, Cydebot, Webaware, Anthonyhcole, Tawkerbot4, Damianrafferty, Zalgo, Calvero JP, Casliber, SummonerMarc, Epbr123, Devadaskrishnan, Bryanwake, Hammerhorn~enwiki, Dgies, AntiVandalBot, Widefox, CLSwiki, Esesk, Danger, Mutt Lunker, NinaSpeaking, Skarkkai, StrawberryClock, JAnDbot, Tigga, Altairisfar, MER-C, Ericoides, Awien, Colotfox, KaUni, Magioladitis, WolfmanSF, Bongwarrior, VoABot II, JNW, Rivertorch, Trugster, Rimibchatterjee, Jessicapierce, Robotman1974, Rhalden, 28421u2232nfenfcenc, Spellmaster, The cattr, DerHexer, Philg88, Jerem43, MartinBot, Grandia01, R'n'B, CommonsDelinker, Fconaway, Wlodzimierz, J.delanoy, Pharaoh of the Wizards, Thegreenj, Whitebox, Rstevec, Salih, Jigesh, Anonywiki, AntiSpamBot, NewEnglandYankee, Fakewcfrog, Biglovinb, Juliancolton, DorganBot, Treisijs, PurelyNina, Nashville Monkey, DASonnenfeld, Xiahou, Idioma-bot, Redtigerxyz, Valugi, Sniper1rfa, VolkovBot, Saddy Dumpington, GimmeBot, Abtinb, Fcb981, Tusbra, Someguy1221, Naohiro19 revertvandal, Seraphim, BotKung, Pigslookfunny, Spicedoctor, Fotek, Jaguarlaser, Falcon8765, Spinningspark, GoddersUK, SieBot, Ivan Štambuk, Prakash Nadkarni, Dawn Bard, Ghaag, WestCoastMusketeer, Lydiafiedler, Flyer22 Reborn, Jojalozzo, Carnun, Arknascar44, Ftindia, Oxymoron83, Goustien, Lightmouse, Gordonofcartoon, Moletrouser, Afernand74, Dabomb87, Escape Orbit, ClueBot, Ian S. Richards, Abee60, Jmgarg1, The Thing That Should Not Be, Kallidaimaniac, EoGuy, Av99, Mild Bill Hiccup, Niceguyedc, Another Matt, Auntof6, Paulcmnt, Akk7a, Excirial, Yossman97, PixelBot, Vivio Testarossa, NuclearWarfare, Georgiamonet, Lalitstar, SoHome, Slidinandridin06, JasonAQuest, Versus22, MuckFizzou, DumZiBoT, XLinkBot, Drhealthnutty, Vanished 45kd09la13, Wikiuser100, AndreNatas, Senzuri, ZooFari, Airplaneman, HexaChord, Johnny apples, GDibyendu, Addbot, DOI bot, Tcncv, Rav314, Annielogue, Nath1991, CanadianLinuxUser, Bazza1971, Glane23, Bassbonerocks, Chzz, Zanbuist, Ahmad.ghamdi.24, CarTick, Americanfreedom, Kommus, Tide rolls, Lightbot, Luckas-bot, Yobot, TaBOT-zerem, Choosetocount, Legobot II, Sanyi4, KamikazeBot, IW.HG, AnomieBOT, Cicero in utero, Qwertyuiopasdfghjklñ, Piano non troppo, Golb12, Zeisterre, Sz-iwbot, Citation bot, Lightningman26, Quebec99, Capricorn42, Astudent1, ChildofMidnight, Vanished user xlkvmskgm4k, GrouchoBot, Jhbdel, Itineranttrader, Brandon5485, Zefr, Dr.Dunn, Bonerbiter69, Doulos Christos, Grammarfixeruper, Dasaradhawiki, Hamamelis, Dan Wylie-Sears 2, Starwars1791...continued, FrescoBot, XXeggsexXx, Pepper, Racingstripes, Kites11, PiperNigrum, Citation bot 1, Pinethicket, HRoestBot, Abductive, Faerra, Dosinovsky, Wikitza, STEV56, My05hammer, Tyler-willard, Zhonghuo~enwiki, IJBall, Trappist the monk, Xlxfjh, FlamingMoonsOfSaturn, Diannaa, Firebeastm, Tbhotch, Bariapepper, Obsidian Soul, Servbot777, Ripchip Bot, The Stick Man, Sajoshthambi, Binoyjsdk, EmausBot, Acather96, WikitanvirBot, Dewritech, Jkadavoor, Rajkiandris, Slightsmile, Wikipelli, Djembayz, Urbain23, Balisong5, Comesturnruler, ZéroBot, John Cline, Fæ, Schubert80, Traxs7, Access Denied, H3llBot, Wayne Slam, Erianna, Rcsprinter123, Anglais1, Donner60, Phanjuy, Uziel302, Mikhail Ryazanov, ClueBot NG, Mr. Glengarry Glen Ross, Rich Smith, Ishfaq Khan8, Gareth Griffith-Jones, Servbot0303, Jiwa Matahari, Movses-bot, A.D.Balasubramaniyan, Samalambam1, Dr.Cena, Wangond, Diyasp, Widr, Joelcostanzo21, Ante Vranković, Seemerock, Helpful Pixie Bot, Bobby chauhan, ?oygul, Calidum, DBigXray, Plantdrew, Gomada, Blake Burba, Northamerica1000, Cold Season, Jahnavisatyan, OttawaAC, Yowanvista, MsBatfish, YVSREDDY, Vrraybadboy3013, Pratap.sps, Crabapple44, Vanished user lt94ma34le12, Nguyễn Quốc Việt, Sanjaya weerasinghe, ChrisGualtieri, Ancienzus, TylerDurden8823, One-ply, Sumimary, Dexbot, Jesse sidhu, Hmainsbot1, Webclient101, Tommy Pinball, Frosty, Corn cheese, Ihatelettuce, Rocketman2699, Aftabbanoori, The Ajan, Jamie LaDawn, Rockonomics, Ministar Nesigurnosti, JamesMoose, Rybec, Gunny777, Mantedayya, Ugog Nizdast, NottNott, Chindukulkarni, Kind Tennis Fan, Kochay1, Stamptrader, JaconaFrere, Safarigal11, Gbrager, Sanskari, Oiyarbepsy, Einskisson, Julietdeltalima, Aristo Class, Keerthijagannath and Anonymous: 536

- **Cajeput oil** *Source:* https://en.wikipedia.org/wiki/Cajeput_oil?oldid=671393647 *Contributors:* Earth, Salimfadhley, Brian0918, Borgx, Prime Entelechy, DAJF, Pawyilee, SmackBot, Eug, Mairibot, Bluebot, Mike hayes, Geach, Sunjan, A876, Riti~enwiki, AdamRoach, Merbabu, Thomas.W, Chaoborus, Alexbrn, Sphilbrick, Londoner1961, Mattgirling, Mutari, Vigilius, Addbot, Download, AnomieBOT, Itineranttrader, SassoBot, ZéroBot, Cjsunbird, Hugepossum, Manytexts, Mark Marathon, Plantdrew, BG19bot, Northamerica1000, BattyBot, Pravito, Rimba56, P. S. Sena, Teacher was here and Anonymous: 17

- **Calophyllum inophyllum seed oil** *Source:* https://en.wikipedia.org/wiki/Calophyllum_inophyllum_seed_oil?oldid=683897541 *Contributors:* Kolbasz, Malcolma, DAJF, Chris the speller, ChemNerd, Yobot, AnomieBOT, FrescoBot, EmausBot, BG19bot, Hmainsbot1, Palagiri, P. S. Sena and Anonymous: 3

- **Cananga odorata** *Source:* https://en.wikipedia.org/wiki/Cananga_odorata?oldid=687718467 *Contributors:* Magnus Manske, PierreAbbat, Stan Shebs, Jogloran, Grendelkhan, Texture, DanielCD, Cacycle, YUL89YYZ, ESkog, Sten, CanisRufus, Kwamikagami, Ludwigvan beethoven, Rainer Bielefeld~enwiki, Hesperian, Keenan Pepper, Sjschen, Nsswaga, StradivariusTV, Rjwilmsi, Vary, Bensin, Vuong Ngan Ha, Eubot, SiGarb, Gdrbot, WriterHound, YurikBot, Vuvar1, Bobby1011, Dysmorodrepanis~enwiki, DAJF, Asarelah, IceCreamAntisocial, Jacklee, Musashi miyamoto, Alexandrov, The7chakrasintune, SmackBot, EncycloPetey, Alsandro, Eug, Ottawakismet, Smalltowngirl, Deli nk, DHN-bot~enwiki, Chlewbot, Vina-iwbot~enwiki, General Ization, Tau'olunga, Nick Wilson, Palaeologos, Casliber, WillMak050389, Merbabu, Heroeswithmetaphors, PhiLiP, Deflective, OhanaUnited, Magioladitis, KaElin, Craigsapp, Lenticel, Ylangylang, Xlboy~enwiki, Acaramoy~enwiki, Peter coxhead, Hdt83, Deonwilliams, Rochelimit, Eric in SF, Dior.babii, Idioma-bot, BierHerr, Respiritu, VolkovBot, Matahari Pagi, Austriacus, SieBot, Macy, Msrasnw, Hippo99, Alexbot, SchreiberBike, DerBorg, Erodium, Drhealthnutty, JocelyneStager, Addbot, Cuaxdon, Myheartinchile, Luckas-bot, AnomieBOT, Xufanc, João Xavier, Obersachsebot, Gigemag76, Almabot, GrouchoBot, Itineranttrader, FrescoBot, Rrcs law, Pinethicket, RedBot, Jero Smith Ju, TobeBot, Lotje, Theoregonconnection, EmausBot, WTM, WikitanvirBot, Wikipelli, Donner60, Dineshkumar Ponnusamy, Infiniteprojects, ClueBot NG, Skoot13, The Old Trout, Helpful Pixie Bot, KLBot2, Plantdrew, BG19bot, Shhhhwwww!!, Jergees, Bamckean, PeterFox59, P. S. Sena, Poornikannan and Anonymous: 61

- **Cannabis flower essential oil** *Source:* https://en.wikipedia.org/wiki/Cannabis_flower_essential_oil?oldid=682423704 *Contributors:* Alan Liefting, RichardWeiss, BD2412, Ian Pitchford, WriterHound, Anomalocaris, El Cazangero, THB, DAJF, SmackBot, Edgar181, JonHarder, Dreadstar, Wafulz, ToneLeMoan, Karlhahn, Cannabis, CommonsDelinker, Funandtrvl, AllOtherNamesTaken, Miniapolis, Yonskii, Addbot, Yobot, Custoo, ZéroBot, Widr, Addihockey10 (automated), Glharris2011, Mangokeylime, Goonsquad LCpl Mulvaney, P. S. Sena and Anonymous: 11

- **Carrot seed oil** *Source:* https://en.wikipedia.org/wiki/Carrot_seed_oil?oldid=653764477 *Contributors:* Rjwilmsi, Waitak, Pigman, DAJF, SmackBot, Herostratus, Betacommand, Cajolingwilhelm, Fabrictramp, RichMac, Douglasalancole, Tomer T, GlassFET, Patdreams DumZiBoT, Addbot, SpBot, Kevinwells, Itineranttrader, RjwilmsiBot, P. S. Sena and Anonymous: 11

- **Cedar oil** *Source:* https://en.wikipedia.org/wiki/Cedar_oil?oldid=662994386 *Contributors:* Rmhermen, SimonP, Lir, Tim Starling, Starfarmer, Antandrus, Zombiejesus, Melaen, SidP, Drbreznjev, Ghirlandajo, Kazvorpal, Woohookitty, Sparkit, BD2412, WriterHound, Joellbughead, DAJF, 何何何 robot, Huhnra, Bluebot, Nakon, Childzy, Rigurat, Alaibot, Nick Number, Goldenrowley, Malcolm, Jgover, Avicennasis, Birczanin, VolkovBot, Lexington50, AngelOfSadness, Mild Bill Hiccup, WikHead, Steff2, Addbot, Jacopo Werther, AdRem, AnomieBOT, Sthigpen, FrescoBot, BenzolBot, Dinamik-bot, EmBOTellado, TYelliot, ChrisGualtieri, Southwesterncedaroil, Thepasta, Junkyardsparkle, Galahn, P. S Sena and Anonymous: 17

- **Citron** *Source:* https://en.wikipedia.org/wiki/Citron?oldid=683552302 *Contributors:* Danny, Llywrch, Ahoerstemeier, Ugen64, Lou Sander, Tpbradbury, Taxman, Bevo, Wetman, Shafei, Auric, MPF, Gilgamesh~enwiki, Chowbok, Kaldari, Secfan, Oknazevad, Adashiel, DanielCD, Hesperian, Stillnotelf, Kevinskogg, Recury, Kazvorpal, Forteblast, Japanese Searobin, Tournesol, Stemonitis, Jaimetout, Woohookitty, RHaworth, Fbriere, Chochopk, Palica, BD2412, Rjwilmsi, Ricardo Carneiro Pires, Franzeska, Eubot, Ground Zero, Gdrbot, WriterHound, Yur kBot, RussBot, Hede2000, MosheA, Badagnani, Dogcow, Apokryltaros, DAJF, Asarelah, Blacksand, Open2universe, SMcCandlish, Ordinary Person, HereToHelp, Eog1916, SmackBot, Rjmunro, Imz, Brya, Kintetsubuffalo, Oli Filth, Afasmit, Hongooi, Aaron Solomon Adelman, Yidisheryid, Cybercobra, Mgiganteus1, A. Parrot, NYL, Shirahadasha, DeLarge, Neelix, Cydebot, Soureraa, Anshelm '77, Luna Santin, Nipisiqui, Awien, TheEditrix2, Ataltane, BilCat, Bellemichelle, Peter coxhead, Ebizur, Ariel., R'n'B, The Sanity Inspector, MacAuslan, Neutron Jack, Skumarlabot, Acalamari, Skier Dude, Stambouliote, 83d40m, Taosein, Psygnet, Idioma-bot, Philip Trueman, TXiKiBoT, Wikidemon, JhsBot, Alborz Fallah, VidGa, Finnrind, Nick Denkens, SieBot, Pawebster, Rosiestep, Captainfergus, Kloth~enwiki, Wwheaton, Johnbrewe, Moshe Yakob, Yakov shalom, Hafspajen, Niceguyedc, Arunsingh16 Cedro~enwiki, Jason526, SchreiberBike, PAROH, Shoteh, Critisizer, Wikiuser100, Ost316, Vojtěch Dostál, Wikiplantjud, BriefError, Good Olfactory, CitricAsset, Addbot, IOLJeff, Luckas-bot, Yobot, Peter Phillipson, AnomieBOT, Royote, LilHelpa, Gigemag76, Tomdo08, RibotBOT, FrescoBot, Hasiru, Krish Dulal, SpacemanSpiff, Wendolpho, FoxBot, TobeBot, Jonkerz, Lotje, EmausBot, John of Reading, Look2See1, צבי אהרונוב, ZéroBot, Anir1uph, Erianna, Mjbmrbot, ClueBot NG, Justlettersandnumbers, Snotbot, Frietjes, Yshemtovyshemtov, Curb Chain, BG19bot, Bmusician, MKar, Suchetaav, JoshuSasori, Wikiman897, JYBot, Sminthopsis84, Mogism, Corinne, Dineshkumar86, Jordan valdiviez1, Rasayana informatics, Cathcart55, Krutonki, SkateTier, BethNaught, AwesoMar 3000, EsrogHunt, CitriCulture, Riversid, P. S. Sena, Etaoinspiffy, Denniscabrams and Anonymous: 145

- **Citronella oil** *Source:* https://en.wikipedia.org/wiki/Citronella_oil?oldid=663024975 *Contributors:* Jengod, Texture, Loganberry, Selphie, StoatBringer, Walkerma, Gpvos, Shoefly, Gene Nygaard, Kazvorpal, Ceyockey, V8rik, Rjwilmsi, Ground Zero, RussBot, Chris Capoccia, Bovineone, DAJF, TDogg310, Epipelagic, BorgQueen, SmackBot, Edgar181, Armeria Smalltowngirl, Soap, John, A. Parrot, RyJones, BrOnXbOmBr21, IronChris, Longwalkshortpier, Nick Number, Sikkema, Rees11, Seaphoto, John Moss, Magioladitis, STBot, R'n'B, Tgeairn, J.delanoy, Nfette, Skier Dude, Ja 62, Calliopejen1, Superbeecat, Sensonet, Germancapi, Acdbot, Legobot, Yobot, Legobot II, AnomieBOT, Citation bot, FrescoBot, GreenZmiy, Citation bot 4, Jonesey95, Andrew69., Trappist the monk, Phyrexian, Theoregonconnection, Pantherslair, Phlegat, T3dkjn89q00vl02Cxp1kqs3x7, Siden, ClueBot NG, Troglopedetes, Hans Frörum, Fuckthisilledit, Jeanloujustine, AndyTheMonster, Vanamonde93, EvergreenFir, Adderkleet, P. S Sena, Rlread52 and Anonymous: 52

- **Copaiba** *Source:* https://en.wikipedia.org/wiki/Copaiba?oldid=669607336 *Contributors:* Peter Ellis, Discospinster, Oeuftete88, Rjwilmsi, Waitak, Dysmorodrepanis~enwiki, DAJF, BorgQueen, SmackBot, Abrahami, DRyan, Tim Vickers, Robertjohnsonrj, Beagel, Tevcnic, Falcon8765, Emesee, Parkwells, Alexbot, Dthomsen8, Addbot, TutterMouse, Luckas-bot, KamikazeBot, D.antonia, Itineranttrader, H3llBot, Plantdrew, Italstudio, Chiefinesse, P. S. Sena and Anonymous: 11

- **Cymbopogon martinii** *Source:* https://en.wikipedia.org/wiki/Cymbopogon_martinii?oldid=666832030 *Contributors:* Alan Liefting, Hesperian, Rjwilmsi, DAJF, IceCreamAntisocial, Nick Number, Waacstats, TXiKiBoT, Addbot, Flakinho, Luckas-bot, Citation bot, MaurtsBot, Gigemag76, Itineranttrader, Claudio Pistilli, John of Reading, Manytexts, Tchaliburton, ChrisGualtieri, Joseph Laferriere, P. S. Sena and Anonymous: 2

- **Cyperus scariosus** *Source:* https://en.wikipedia.org/wiki/Cyperus_scariosus?oldid=685919560 *Contributors:* Hesperian, Stemonitis, Rjwilmsi, Anomalocaris, DAJF, Asarelah, HeartofaDog, Rkitko, Delink, Shivaexportsindia, Waacstats, VolkovBot, Addbot, Cuaxdon, Flakinho, Yobot, LucienBOT, Trappist the monk, EmausBot, Michael Bailes, Frietjes, Erikoo152, BattyBot, Whitehousee, Khazar2, P. S. Sena and Anonymous: 6

- **Dill oil** *Source:* https://en.wikipedia.org/wiki/Dill_oil?oldid=682603443 *Contributors:* Finlay McWalter, Waitak, RussBot, Alynna Kasmira, DAJF, Asarelah, J. Van Meter, SmackBot, Lord Roghen, KyraVixen, Fabrib, MarshBot, DMR5713, Pharillon, Uncle Dick, Maralia, Cewvero, Cuaxdon, Itineranttrader, Erik9bot, ClueBot NG, FlyinFijian, P. S. Sena and Anonymous: 12

- **Enfleurage** *Source:* https://en.wikipedia.org/wiki/Enfleurage?oldid=680032455 *Contributors:* The Anome, Jengod, Astronautics~enwiki, RupertB, Poccil, Pedant, Polarscribe, Sjschen, Eater~enwiki, Roboto de Ajvol, Curpsbot-unicodify, SmackBot, Quatloo, Clicketyclack, Meng.benjamin, Thijs!bot, AS, Bobsodium, Fcastem, Sensonet, Addbot, Some jerk on the Internet, Oculus42, Luckas-bot, Dancy Sephy, Jim1138, Citation bot, Alexandru Stanoi, ClueBot NG, Curb Chain, DaltonCastle, Lagoset, Monkbot and Anonymous: 16

- **Eucalyptus oil** *Source:* https://en.wikipedia.org/wiki/Eucalyptus_oil?oldid=678133500 *Contributors:* Fubar Obfusco, Jpatokal, PFHLai, Rich Farmbrough, Bender235, Axl, Rjwilmsi, Waitak, JarrahTree, RussBot, Hydrargyrum, DAJF, Zagalejo, Asarelah, Rathfelder, Groyolo, Smack-Bot, Melchoir, Chris the speller, JDCMAN, Stepho-wrs, Zearin, Liam Skoda, CmdrObot, I.M.S., John Moss, DuncanHill, RebelRobot, Prestonmcconkie, WhatamIdoing, Enquire, Th84, DASonnenfeld, VolkovBot, Ktalon, Una Smith, Petteri Aimonen, Logan, Roo1812, Hordaland, Neznanec, Mild Bill Hiccup, SchreiberBike, GKantaris, Dthomsen8, Doug butler, Addbot, Colibri37, Luckas-bot, Bunnyhop11, Evilyoshimax, EryZ, Obersachsebot, Borys bond, FrescoBot, LucienBOT, Citation bot 4, Aareo, Zzzomg2, Tea with toast, Trappist the monk, TjBot, MrFawwaz, GoingBatty, Klbrain, John Cline, AManWithNoPlan, ClueBot NG, Ehrjej, TwoTwoHello, Binko100, SantiLak, P. S. Sena and Anonymous: 45

- **Fragrance extraction** *Source:* https://en.wikipedia.org/wiki/Fragrance_extraction?oldid=680032783 *Contributors:* Brainsik, Monsterinabox, Sjschen, Marudubshinki, BD2412, Dar-Ape, TheMoog, Hairy Dude, Foolestroupe, SmackBot, Edgar181, Chris the speller, A. B., Clicketyclack, Hikaridranz, Seasicksarah, Jay32183, Fabykot, R'n'B, Wrfrancis, Mattchess, Calliopejen1, Sensonet, Razorflame, Anna Frodesiak, ClueBot NG, PrincessWortheverything, Lagoset and Anonymous: 23

- **Fragrance oil** *Source:* https://en.wikipedia.org/wiki/Fragrance_oil?oldid=687800448 *Contributors:* Quarl, Cacycle, Sjschen, Walkerma, Shoefly, Physchim62, DAJF, The Famous Movie Director, Acdx, Christian75, Herbjunkie, Dekimasu, Dusti, Calliopejen1, Addbot, RichFragrance, ZéroBot, Jelly1066, BG19bot, KateWishing, Lagoset, P. S. Sena, Anonimeco, HimanshuDholakia and Anonymous: 9

- **Herbal distillate** *Source:* https://en.wikipedia.org/wiki/Herbal_distillate?oldid=680360636 *Contributors:* Pigsonthewing, Sjschen, Rjwilmsi, DAJF, SmackBot, Ohnoitsjamie, Chris the speller, Deli nk, Kupirijo, Rifleman 82, Mojo Hand, Husond, WhatamIdoing, Ariel., Cindy Jones1, Skier Dude, Calliopejen1, Jkomatsu, Ottawahitech, Sensonet, Ngebendi, Addbot, Cblack2, Xqbot, DKong27, Anna Frodesiak, Look2See1, H3llBot, Theopolisme, Helpful Pixie Bot, Yoyoma101, Sagescript, Lagoset, P. S. Sena and Anonymous: 19

- **Hydnocarpus wightiana seed oil** *Source:* https://en.wikipedia.org/wiki/Hydnocarpus_wightiana_seed_oil?oldid=662491115 *Contributors:* Rjwilmsi, Bgwhite, Malcolma, DAJF, Edgar181, Deli nk, Derek R Bullamore, DASonnenfeld, Dthomsen8, Yobot, AnomieBOT, LilHelpa, Plantdrew, BattyBot, Hmainsbot1, Palagiri and P. S. Sena

- **Jasmine** *Source:* https://en.wikipedia.org/wiki/Jasmine?oldid=687614720 *Contributors:* WojPob, Tarquin, KF, Hephaestos, Infrogmation, Boud, Ahoerstemeier, Mihai~enwiki, Imc, Jetwhiz, Wetman, Jni, Robbot, Academic Challenger, UtherSRG, DocWatson42, MPF, Netoholic, Jackol, Antandrus, MarkSweep, OwenBlacker, Asbestos, Muijz, Liberlogos, Discospinster, Rhobite, Cacycle, Autiger, Mani1, Kbh3rd, CanisRufus, Dara, Kwamikagami, Adambro, Bastique, Ruszewski, Acjelen, Hesperian, MPerel, Nsaa, Alansohn, Rd232, Lightdarkness, Roy-Smith, Idont Havaname, Wtmitchell, BlastOButter42, Kazvorpal, Megan1967, George Hernandez, Sandover, Vanniar, Woohookitty, Camw, LOL, MONGO, Miss Madeline, Isnow, Wayward, Btyner, Eirikr, Mtcurado, Raguks, BorgHunter, Rjwilmsi, Vary, Ligulem, Ghepeu, Eubot, RexNL, Gurch, Chobot, Stormbear, Gdrbot, Cactus.man, Teleolurian, Kummi, Cjs56, YurikBot, Sceptre, SkyCaptain~enwiki, X42bn6, RussBot, Groogle, Stephenb, Polluxian, Gaius Cornelius, Alexgoodell, Draeco, Cquan, Mardochaios, Justin Eiler, DAJF, Matticus78, TDogg310, DeadEyeArrow, Everyguy, IceCreamAntisocial, VederJuda, Tigershrike, Ke6jjj, FF2010, Codrinb, Digfarenough, Peter, Paul Erik, NickelShoe, Luk, SmackBot, WilliamThweatt, C.Fred, Hecktor, Anastrophe, Delldot, Eskimbot, Gilliam, Skizzik, Carl.bunderson, Shoniko, Smt52, Rkitko, Ron E, Dr bab, Hafrul, Lilengine, Melburnian, Droll, Deli nk, Enfantsduparadis, Octahedron80, Frap, KevM, Mhym, VMS Mosaic, Addshore, BostonMA, Hateless, Luc., Mitsuki152, Magialuna, Madeleine Price Ball, Nishkid64, Murdocke, Ergative rlt, SilkTork, Linnell, Green Giant, NongBot~enwiki, IronGargoyle, Paradox11, Smommss, Hu12, Phase4, R~enwiki, Courcelles, Tawkerbot2, Fuddiphat, Artificial Silence, JForget, Tanthalas39, Ale jrb, W guice, Yarnalgo, ShelfSkewed, Cydebot, Mercator, Corpx, Chrislk02, Smiteri, Thijs!bot, Epbr123, Bezking, Whomeam, Enimsaj, Keraunos, N5iln, Marek69, Thevortexofsuck, Rajaramraok, Amjaabc, Big Bird, Tiamut, Mentifisto, Ialsoagree, AntiVandalBot, Widefox, Seaphoto, NeilEvans, Quintote, Paste, Mountolive, Jj137, Ianare, Shivaexportsindia, Res2216firestar, JAnDbot, Deflective, Mvanr, Barek, Geneisner, MER-C, OhanaUnited, Andonic, Roleplayer, Jimmy, PhilKnight, .anacondabot, Bencherlite, Bongwarrior, VoABot II, Firebladed, JNW, Careless hx, Michael Goodyear, Southernwood, WhatamIdoing, Brister28, Mtl1969, Bluemin, Taamu, Adrian J. Hunter, Aziz1005, DerHexer, JaGa, Pyrochem, Khalid Mahmood, Ylangylang, Peter coxhead, Mmustafa~enwiki, MartinBot, Jonathanchad, Gunkarta, Ash, Tgeairn, J.delanoy, Pharaoh of the Wizards, Pimadude, Fowler&fowler, Uncle Dick, Darth Mike, Mzx, Balthazarduju, Joeyrockyhorror, SmilesALot, Ahuskay, Kloisiie, Nadiatalent, Sunderland06, Cometstyles, Jonberry, S, Mochamomma15, CardinalDan, Idioma-bot, 28bytes, VolkovBot, Jeff G., Kyriosity, Barneca, Philip Trueman, Zidonuke, Technopat, Rei-bot, F1090864, WazzaMan, Clarince63, Princessjasmine, Tsteinbach4, McM.bot, Pachyderm13, Billinghurst, Thewords, Jdamianm, Why Not A Duck, Treyw, EJF, SieBot, Coffee, Ethel Aardvark, Euryalus, Jauerback, Caltas, Matthew Yeager, Nate818, Triwbe, Yintan, Santyshyam, Happysailor, Vonsche, Flyer22 Reborn, Jacksonli0210, Orangeyellow1, Moriah Drinkard, AlexWaelde, Neo Zeus, Jfizzz, Angielaj, StaticGull, Cyfal, Slamazzar, Escape Orbit, Angelo De La Paz, Grunthos, Smashville, ClueBot, CarolSpears, Jmgarg1, The Thing That Should Not Be, Cygnis insignis, FeygeleGoy, DigitalNinja, Harland1, Jaza182, Seanwal111111, Excirial, Jusdafax, Lartoven, Philosophist705, Jazmin.mf, Rosabella83, SpectacledDaruma, The Red, Aravindan Shanmugasundaram, Puppyakitty, BarretB, XLinkBot, Ost316, PeterFisk, Luwilt, Addbot, DOI bot, Zozo2kx, Yolgnu, Friginator, Binary TSO, Ronhjones, Mrtwata, Blackbody, CarsracBot, Koolaidohyea, Ahmad2099, Scientiae, AtheWeatherman, GoTheBombers38, Bacoleño, Peti610botH, Jasmineforden, Jjkrbff, Numbo3-bot, Anilbharadwaj125, Tide rolls, Mjquinn id, Nguyễn Thanh Quang, Luckas-bot, Yobot, TaBOT-zerem, Washburnmav, THEN WHO WAS PHONE?, SwisterTwister, IW.HG, Garcon under tree, AnomieBOT, Jkangel4eva, IRP, Xufanc, RandomAct, Materialscientist, Mutzee, Citation bot, OllieFury, Thelittlegreyman, Maxis ftw, Quebec99, Parthian Scribe, TinucherianBot II, Ali944rana, Lolinder, Hikili, Almabot, Fashionquean, Fixthissh1t, J04n, GrouchoBot, Itineranttrader, Amaury, Cakegurl1721, Dodder0, Hamamelis, Empayton, MG1968, FrescoBot, Katrina133113, Mikestevo, Girlwithgreeneyes, Jasmineroxs11, Teinesavaii, Lilaac, Citation bot 1, Kous2v, Kiki maka, Pinethicket, I dream of horses, Samjas1, Calmer Waters, Moonraker, Merlion444, December21st2012Freak, Dave Oceano, FoxBot, Kalaivanan S, Mono, Kandaswamy07, Miracle Pen, Jazzybabyx96x, SadaoGhost, TRYPPN, David Hedlund, Harrisonrh, Mizz.butta, Cjohnweb, Flwr petal fairy, Satdeep Gill, Reach Out to the Truth, Scribble225, This is just some random name, Obsidian Soul, Jazzy1011, TjBot, Noommos, DrJGMD, Max5600, EmausBot, Sophie, Look2See1, Mordgier, RA0808, Larrymacphail, Eman5195, Wikipelli, Mistafire247, Thecheesykid, ZéroBot, Bollyjeff, Abu Shawka, Antmega, Wikfr, Wayne Slam, Lexusuns, Shrigley, Shaamala, Jasmeg, Indiankid96, Sunshine4921, ClueBot NG, Chester Markel, Wikiusername7795, Amr.rs, Asukite, Rezabot, Widr, Rr7, Mcmad358, Helpful Pixie Bot, Curb Chain, Mark Marathon, BG19bot, Neeya The Great, PhnomPencil, ElphiBot, Mark Arsten, Saba rathnam, CitationCleanerBot, Tu7uh, Jason1918, Magentic Manifestations, Mogism, Kahanaknight, Healtia, Akshay.paramatmuni1987, Faizan, Eyesnore, Durga Destroyer, DavidLeighEllis, Gen2255, Ugog Nizdast, عزالدين السبيني‎, CarmineRed, Bjcurrie56, JaconaFrere, Monkbot, Toonrobbierocks, Someanonymoususer12, PotatoNinja, P. S. Sena, Jazzzzzy cx, Orduin, TaqPol, XxxJesus103Xxx, Cpriyad3, CAPTAIN RAJU, JasmineS081903 and Anonymous: 541

- **Juniper berry** *Source:* https://en.wikipedia.org/wiki/Juniper_berry?oldid=667614412 *Contributors:* Enchanter, Ixfd64, Ebruchez, Wetman, HaeB, MPF, ComaVN, Jason Quinn, OldakQuill, RetiredUser2, Rich Farmbrough, Bobo192, Circeus, Alansohn, Keenan Pepper, Ish ishwar, Walshga, Sandover, Bunchofgrapes, Ttwaring, WriterHound Noclador, Wavelength, SkyCapta n~enwiki, Pigman, Calicore, Curtis Clark, Astral, Veledan, DAJF, Lockesdonkey, Asarelah, Smaines, BorgQueen, DVD R W, SmackBot, Melchoir, Kintetsubuffalo, Here.it.comes.again, Nakon, BullRangifer, MrDarwin, Iridescent, Pukkie, ShelfSkewed, Cydebot, Kozuch, JorgonQ, Antique Rose, JAnDbot, Jdcook, Natureguy1980, Fradlin, VoABot II, Rarian rakista, McSly, DASonnenfeld, Salvar, Lamro, BotanyBot, Mr.Sourcebook, Radon210, ClueBot, Justin W Smith, Takeaway, Sun Creator, Addbot, Cuaxdon, Tide rolls, Lightbot, Kenraiz, Mattchow, AnomieBOT, AmritasyaPutra, Citation bot, Cheryenwen, Nasnema, Trdsf, Iceyisawesome, Emredjan, Maxgilead, Chickadee1999, Charles sk, Sp33dyphil, Slightsmile, Tommy2010, K6ka, Erianna, ClueBot NG, What?7652134, HippieflowsBZ, Noyster, P. S. Sena and Anonymous: 60

- **Lavender oil** *Source:* https://en.wikipedia.org/wiki/Lavender_oil?oldid=684256944 *Contributors:* Wm, Docu, Poor Yorick, Dysprosia, Imc, Merovingian, Texture, Bobo192, Remuel, Walkerma, BDD, Ceyockey, Rjwilmsi, Ctdunstan, Jivecat, AED, WriterHound, Dforest, Badagnani, Tearlach, DAJF, Elkman, 2over0, Kradak, 김개 robot, SmackBot, Steven Kippel, Edgar181, Ohnoitsjamie, Mairibot, Smalltowngirl, Deli nk, Sadads, Stedder, Disavian, Joelmills, Interlingua, Ale jrb, Rhiom, Johner, Master son, On5deu, JustAGal, Hvw, Luna Santin, Julia Rossi, Herbjunkie, Epeefleche, Kyleberk, Alberto Enriquez, Magiolacitis, Puellanivis, EagleFan, Dr algorythm, Welshleprechaun, ChemNerd, Feanutry, IrisWings, Siraj88, STBotD, Equazcion, DorganBot, Tourbillon, Philip Trueman, Kumorifox, Optigan13, Slagell, Alexbrn, Zentomologist, Tanvir Ahmmed, Lianiwidjaja, Jytdog, Dthomsen8, Addbot, Grayfell, Jacopo Werther, Serrac, Yobot, Anypodetos, Honey badger 08, AnomieBOT, KentigernEnnis, Citation bot, Xqbot, Erron3000, Itineranttrader, Doc1arid, HJ Mitchell, Un Mundo, Konradov, WikitanvirBot, ZéroBot, Chris-pastonBot, Michael Bailes, ClueBot NG, Widr, Helpful Pixie Bot, Plantdrew, Gatheringwithin, Haslantis, TylerDurden8823, I am One of Mary, PSUCamson, LeanneKitchin, Tertiaryresources, P. S. Sena, Nordiskk, Bvasilev1 and Anonymous: 55

- **Lemon oil** *Source:* https://en.wikipedia.org/wiki/Lemon?oldid=684671718 *Contributors:* Vicki Rosenzweig, Bryan Derksen, Malcolm Farmer, Dragon Dave, Rmhermen, Toby Bartels, William Avery, SarahEmm, Leandrod, Michael Hardy, BrianHansen~enwiki, DopefishJustin, Liftarn, Mic, Ixfd64, Delirium, (, Shimmin, Mdebets, Ahoerstemeier, Synthetik, Ronz, Jimfbleak, TUF-KAT, Angela, Jebba, Andrewa, Poor Yorick, Mxn, Dwo, Ideyal, Mulad, Agtx, Hollgor, Mpt, Stone, JCarriker, WhisperToMe, Zoicon5, Tpbradbury, Imc, Furrykef, Fvw, Metasquares, Wetman, Pakaran, Pollinator, Francs2000, Shantavira, Robbot, Sensor, Hankwang, Moriori, R3m0t, Naddy, Babbage, Merovingian, Rfc1394, Academic Challenger, Texture, LGagnon, Bkell, Alan De Smet, UtherSRG, Wikibot, Dina, Giftlite, DocWatson42, Bob Palin, MPF, E.f, Wolfkeeper, BenFrantzDale, Everyking, Anville, Moyogo, Gamaliel, Markus Kuhn, Yekrats, Dmmaus, Eequor, Khalid hassani, Jackol, Pre, Bobblewik, Jurema Oliveira, Dyfrgi, Utcursch, Gdr, Dirus, Noe, Antandrus, Bgbot, JoJan, MisfitToys, RichardAmes, Jossi, Rdsmith4, Kesac, DragonflySixtyseven, Bumm13, Mrtrey99, Marcus2, Deandeto, Revised~enwiki, Fanghong~enwiki, Squash, Grunt, Canterbury Tail, Mike Rosoft, Imroy, DanielCD, Discospinster, Helohe, Vsmith, ESkog, Jameschipmunk, Kbh3rd, Steerpike, Jonathanischoice, Aqua008, *drew, Joanjoc~enwiki, Edward Z. Yang, Shanes, Mr. Strong Bad, Femto, Jpgordon, Adambro, Bobo192, Longhair, Fir0002, Olve Utne, Cmdrjameson, Fqsik, Darwinek, Thewayforward, Minghong, Kickstart70, Hesperian, Sam Korn, Haham hanuka, Fox1, Prevert, HasharBot~enwiki, Nemalki, Alansohn, MatthiasKabel, Ibn zareena, Keenan Pepper, Sjschen, Mmmready, Riana, Pdboddy, Mac Davis, Redfarmer, Mysdaao, Snowolf, Jm51, Wtmitchell, Dschwen, Melaen, TaintedMustard, Fledgeling, Sunbun, Aka, Irfanh, Drat, Sciurinæ, Gene Nygaard, Redvers, HerryLi, TShilo12, Feezo, Angr, Vashti, Woohookitty, Melgibson999, LizardWizard, Lydia Pryon, Mindmatrix, Shreevatsa, PoccilScript, WadeSimMiser, JeremyA, MONGO, Jean-Pol Grandmont, Blacknproud92, Kmg90, Cbdorsett, Al E., Sengkang, SDC, Fxer, Ggonnell, Dysepsion, Graham87, Magister Mathematicae, BD2412, Chun-hian, Bunchofgrapes, FreplySpang, Enzo Aquarius, Rjwilmsi, Tizio, Theobromos, Linuxbeak, Seraphimblade, MZMcBride, Nneonneo, XLerate, HappyCamper, Ricardo Carneiro Pires, Brighterorange, The wub, Hermione1980, Yamamoto Ichiro, Fish and karate, Blacknproud992, Eubot, RobertG, Latka, Nihiltres, Nivix, RexNL, Gurch, Bigdottawa, Karrmann, KFP, ViriiK, TeaDrinker, Codex Sinaiticus, EronMain, M7bot, Innnotminkus, King of Hearts, Chobot, Bjwebb, Gdrbot, Cactus.man, Tone, Debivort, YurikBot, Wavelength, Sortan, RobotE, Rob T Firefly, Hairy Dude, Jimp, RussBot, Serinde, Maxistheman, Lar, Stephenb, Manop, Lovesick, Rsrikanth05, Pseudomonas, Wimt, Friday, NawlinWiki, Anomie, EWS23, Wiki alf, Bachrach44, Grafen, Badagnani, Cquan, RealWingus, Justin Eiler, Chunky Rice, Robchurch, Davfoster88, Yoninah, CHBlogger, Cleared as filed, Nick, Deodar~enwiki, Malcolma, Raven4x4x, Synthiss, DeadEyeArrow, Someones life, .marc., DRosenbach, Csobankai Aladar, Trainra, Haemo, Wknight94, Orioane, Zzuuzz, StuRat, Lt-wik -bot, Joethegirl, Closedmouth, SMcCandlish, BorgQueen, GraemeL, TBadger, Davidals, CWenger, Chrishmt0423, Natgoo, Ajuk, Katieh5584, EtherealPurple, GrinBot~enwiki, SkerHawx, DVD R W, Mynabull, AndrewWTaylor, Hiddekel, SmackBot, MattieTK, Ratarsed, Unschool, Brya, Herostratus, KnowledgeOfSelf, Hydrogen Iodide, McGeddon, Unyoyega, Huhnra, C.Fred, Skooky, Vald, Kilo-Lima, Pkirlin, Jrockley, Delldot, Peloneous, Jab843, Hardyplants, Jlahorn, ZS, Edgar181, HalfShadow, BustlinSlug, Gilliam, Donama, Hmains, Oscarthecat, Angelbo, Cowman109, Hugo-cs, Anwar saadat, Smalltowngirl, Quinsareth, Persian Poet Gal, Ksenon, Sirex98, Aro888, Bonesiii, Etcher, SchfiftyThree, Jeff5102, Darth Panda, Gracenotes, Poobarb, Scwlong, Zsinj, Kotra, Can't sleep, clown will eat me, Nick Levine, Brimba, Furby100, Nixeagle, TheKMan, Rrburke, Worland102688, Krsont, VMS Mosaic, Japeo, Jezpuh, Mr.Z-man, Arab Hafez, Jmlk17, Cybercobra, Khukri, Nakon, TedE, Blake-, AdeMiami, Richard001, -Ozone-, DMacks, Jitterro, Wombat1138, Zeamays, Vina-iwbot~enwiki, Kukini, Will Beback, Thejerm, L337p4wn, Natpowning, HighwayCello, Thesmothete, Rory096, Ser Amantio di Nicolao, Howdoesthiswo, Valfontis, Kuru, John, Fremte, Kipala, Heimstern, Soumyasch, Denimcat, Chodorkovskiy, Evan Robidoux, Jevit, Onlyme2007, Joshua Scott, CoolKoon, Ckatz, Alfadark, MarkSutton, Andypandy.UK, Slakr, Munita Prasad, Murrian, Yvesnimmo, SQGibbon, Mr Stephen, SirFozzie, Vandin, Samm, Fangfufu, Waggers, Doczilla, Nwwaew, Tuspm, LaMenta3, Onionmon, Caiaffa, Darry2385, Hu12, Pejman47, SimonD, BranStark, HisSpaceResearch, Iridescent, Zmmz, Creeknet, Green Bay, J Di, CapitalR, Majora4, Ewulp, Courcelles, Gilabrand, Sabb0ur, Frank Lofaro Jr., Matangkad, Tau'olunga, Tawkerbot2, Dlohcierekim, Dani415247, Amartinez, ChrisCork, Paulistano, JForget, FleetCommand, Chyran, CR-Greathouse, Dkazdan, Phillip J, CmdrObot, Tanthalas39, Ale jrb, Sid Carter, The Font, Ilikefood, Radihh, Binky The WonderSkull, Runningonbrains, CWY2190, Abbzzieee, Schlampeamber, Dgw, OMGsplosion, MarsRover, Phatom87, Sopoforic, CumbiaDude, Cydebot, Stebbins, Fl, Alfirin, Goldfritha, Gogo Dodo, Bridgecross, JFreeman, Flowerpotman, Indeterminate, Corpx, Edmund1989, Wikipediarules2221, Wildnox, Dancter, Dave10115, Crab230, Roberta F., DumbBOT, Optimist on the run, Slinking ferret, Nsaum75, Wikiwikiwild, Omicronpersei8, EvocativeIntrigue, FrancoGG, Devl2666, Thijs!bot, Epbr123, Qwyrxian, GentlemanGhost, Mojo Hand, Purple Paint, Marek69, Calahäst, John254, Tapir Terrific, Doyley, X201, Tellyaddict, Benqish, Dfrg.msc, Brahmaputra, Farrtj, Sturm55, Philippe, Zachary, Tim1988 2, Big blue veiner, Mike.blitz, Escarbot, Rothefyre, Pie Man 360, ReallyMale, CerealBabyMilk, Ialsoagree, AntiVandalBot, Glegoo, Baggyeyescar, Nickle pickle, Majorly, Luna Santin, Seaphoto, Emeraldcityserendipity, QuiteUnusual, 17Drew, TimVickers, Lordmetroid, PhJ, Bata 43, Spencer, PTWC, David Shankbone, John Moss, Lonestar662p3, Canadian-Bacon, BeefRendang, Sluzzelin, JAnDbot, DuncanHill, Barek, MER-C, Kiwi Tiwi6969, Instinct, Fetchcomms, Db099221, Andonic, YK Times, TAnthony, TheEditrix2, LittleOldMe, Steveprutz, Acroterion, Bencherlite,

Connormah, Bongwarrior, VoABot II, AuburnPilot, MJD86, Maxwellversion2, Yandman, Shmuelakam, JamesBWatson, Aznguy93, Faizhaider, Froid, SparrowsWing, Avicennasis, BrianGV, Catgut, Hipatian, Indon, Animum, Cyktsui, 28421u2232nfenfcenc, Allstarecho, DerHexer, Khalid Mahmood, Nevit, Tarcus, WLU, TheRanger, Patstuart, Charitwo, Kables, Oroso, Gjd001, Hdt83, MartinBot, CliffC, Matt03777, Bfesser, Ron2, Vamooom, TomSmith123, Robnsamm, Tholly, Roastytoast, Juansidious, FruitLover, AlexiusHoratius, Bobdaman11, PrestonH, Proabivouac, LedgendGamer, Tgeairn, J.delanoy, 031586, Captain panda, Pharaoh of the Wizards, Trusilver, Bogey97, Mthibault, Uncle Dick, Ashcraft, Jerry, Skumarlabot, Exit47motel, Gzkn, Acalamari, Onlyhelp onlyhope, Katalaveno, Smeira, Ncmvocalist, McSly, Watermelonlover123, Skier Dude, Psyklic, AntiSpamBot, (jarbarf), The clyde, Colchicum, Belovedfreak, ReHaNCaN, Richard D. LeCour, NewEnglandYankee, Avocado122, Bobber0001, Bobianite, Toon05, ThinkBlue, Unflavoured, JohnnyRush10, Tanaats, Shoessss, Avocados11, Brancron, Wavemaster447, Ionescuac, Cometstyles, Equazcion, Lukeolivertomben, Zxcvbnmioupailfs, Chachacha123, Manga-Me, HighKing, TheNewPhobia, Mas Ahmad, Abigirl164, Catluver101, SoCalSuperEagle, Xiahou, Zertly14, Idioma-bot, Funandtrvl, Spellcast, Xnuala, Wikieditor06, Lights, X!, Deor, VolkovBot, TreasuryTag, CWii, Thedjatclubrock, Murderbike, DSRH, Leebo, Indubitably, Nburden, Pizzaluver910, Chango369w, Gambito~enwiki, Soliloquial, TheOtherJesse, Dreddmoto, Chitrapa, Barneca, Philip Trueman, Dadude123, Llamasmoker, TXiKiBoT, Mercurywoodrose, Steve Wise, Who wants to knows, Lottiotta, Mathwiz3141, GDonato, NPrice, Z.E.R.O., Anonymous Dissident, Midlandstoday, AlysTarr, Qxz, Alistairrivers, Hglickman, Oxfordwang, Anna Lincoln, Cheez freak777, Una Smith, H. Carver, Onyx the hero, VogueLovesU2, DSWebb, Corvus cornix, Man united321, Ferretremover, LeaveSleaves, Seb az86556, Sbrandle, Benhead 07, Bearian, PaladinWhite, Maxim, ACEOREVIVED, Jasz, Jebman, Stephanie herman, Alborz Fallah, Greswik, Lerdthenerd, Ultafulta, Cantiorix, Evilratboy64iscool, The Endis-Near1994, Dan0411, Rossdaboss11492, Michaelhogard, Falcon8765, Enviroboy, Insanity Incarnate, Hytham123, Litsdakewlest, Why Not A Duck, Ceranthor, Op kutiee1115, Bluedenim, Lando5, Logan, Atlantabravz, Science148, Kmalino, Newbyguesses, EJF, Jimboneyjonelby, SieBot, Zenlax, WOW Teeandbee77, Dr.b&t, Jmg2493, Ethel Aardvark, Tresiden, Tiddly Tom, Moonriddengirl, Scarian, Euryalus, Fabullus, DestroyerOfWiki, Dawn Bard, User217, Caltas, Connor1000, RJaguar3, Triwbe, Peter cohen, Lesyemm, Keilana, Happysailor, Tiptoety, Oysterguitarist, JD554, Oda Mari, Cheeseyj, Bananastalktome, Bob98133, Oxymoron83, Antonio Lopez, Faradayplank, Avnjay, Nuttycoconut, Harry~enwiki, Targeman, AnonGuy, Steven Crossin, Life in a shoe, Tombomp, Poindexter Propellerhead, Alex.muller, Wonderpet, Mikecraig003, Samster 93, Jamarimutt, Oooliamooo, Purpleicefairy, Rocksanddirt, Georgette2, Spazure, Meowist, Mygerardromance, Hamiltondaniel, BoomBoomBoomlol, Mr. Stradivarius, Dabomb87, Nn123645, Pinkadelica, DRTllbrg, Vilnisr, Escape Orbit, Jordan 1972, Explicit, Angel caboodle, Missing Ace, DirtyDisco, Elassint, ClueBot, CarolSpears, Fyyer, Foxj, The Thing That Should Not Be, Alhuth, Lalafface, Rodhullandemu, Jadamatta, Kafka Liz, Felixclaw, Techdawg667, MikeVitale, Anondeliversssslolcat, StatfordUponLexington, Arakunem, Niruja1, Meekywiki, Mini greek, Pyroen21, Camp6ell, Yamakiri, Regibox, CounterVandalismBot, StigBot, Infolepsy, Giuseppema, Egglemoncheese, Lemonpwr, Winchesterlemon, Pras, Auntof6, PMDrive1061, Maccy69, Starcraft88, Snaxalotl, Pumpmeup, Edo 555, Jusdafax, Benjamizal13uk, Maxinelunn, Gtstricky, Lartoven, Elliottbrooks, NuclearWarfare, Ice Cold Beer, Morel, Razorflame, Redthoreau, Dekisugi, Gnormashingday, Kilsss, Thehelpfulone, Stepheng3, Bapithakur, RachieBabez91, C628, Audionaut, Wardleisfat, Thingg, Redrocketboy, Marsbarz, Hohohomerrychristmasy, Baggiesfan2k7, Aitias, Littleteddy, Jamaicanbobsledteam, Berean Hunter, TheProf07, Apparition11, Shoteh, Roozbeh.a, Crazy Boris with a red beard, Skunkboy74, TED, Stickee, Tscooter11, Wikiuser100, Feinoha, Little Mountain 5, BriefError, Pyros550, IngerAlHaosului, Mrvagtastic, Alexius08, Noctibus, JinJian, Mrmooseman, Airplaneman, Kbkirby, Thatguyflint, Samkino, Starwarz24, Cameronlofgren, Nylad tuck, Passportguy, Bookbrad, Addbot, Wildplum69, AMB03, Orac7, Willking1979, Shneebly, C6541, Manuel Trujillo Berges, AVand, Tcncv, Captain-tucker, OldSpot61, Pjc jrtl, Akajiff, Dizzee09, Mww113, Jncraton, Fieldday-sunday, CanadianLinuxUser, Fluffernutter, Tigerange1, Corrie108, Cst17, Zeeshan.rahim, Mjr162006, Glane23, Bassbonerocks, Brassmonky25000, Paris 16, Debresser, Favonian, Doniago, 5 albert square, Thetomcruise, CuteHappyBrute, Peridon, Abc12345689, DeusExBarba, HazelRawr, Tide rolls, Kakashi-poo, Lemons332, James-f-doherty, Jan eissfeldt, Squidinater88, Pietrow, સત્યશિલ્રે, Teles, Bob the Beaner, Luckas-bot, ZX81, TheSuave, Ashleygrint, Andersishere, Orac29, TaBOT-zerem, Cflm001, Legobot II, Ethanco, Gobbleswoggler, Washburnmav, Mmxx, THEN WHO WAS PHONE?, Kumslee, Brougham96, Рес「эм Нур̌ьев, 33Peterpan, Alexkin, Backtothemacman32, MassimoAr, MacTire02, Gustavoreyeslican, Haylemarie, Synchronism, Fudge984, Juliancolton Alternative, AnomieBOT, Rubinbot, Götz, Daniele Pugliesi, Jim1138, IRP, Teamnumberawesome, Ipatrol, AdjustShift, Fahadsadah, KRLS, Shadow majora, Kingpin13, Law, Lemongirl23, Csigabi, Flewis, Furfur111, Giants27, Materialscientist, Emobutpsyco, GreenLight7, The High Fin Sperm Whale, Citation bot, Donutman555, 666maggot666, Owlindaylight, RevelationDirect, Maxis ftw, Xapo, GB fan, Shasta6, T-applesauce, Xqbot, Mrs.Ripken Jr, Bmx776688, Strikerforce, Jassybaby100029, TinucherianBot II, Dognuts33, Gigemag76, B&B1992, Jeffrey Mall, Upum, Yodog456789, Sellyme, Dr54gtr51t5er1, DSisyphBot, Lemonhead111, Dmausser19, Midnightsun65, Maddie!, Hydrodd, Dontfeedmyfrog, Feistybtch, GrouchoBot, Abce2, Michaelfol0, Mario777Zelda, Itineranttrader, Frankie0607, Zefr, Saalstin, L THExONE l, Mayor mt, Master Meow, AntiAbuseBot, Itami-chan, Alfred lover, IcedNut, B claudia13, Gummybear2009, Florencegregory, JayJay, Noder4, Hooberbloob, A.amitkumar, RightCowLeftCoast, Firewire95, Uusijani, Liderek, Sky Attacker, 天下第一, Trikki Motiv, EricLaporteEn, D'ohBot, Mfwitten, Craig Pemberton, Jamesooders, Arcendet, Glamourgalpl, Assassinsblade, Flint McRae, Pinethicket, Metricmike, 95j, Baz2bad, Batman n' robin, Imgonnacry, RedBot, Agong1, Samtomjess, Fridgegunk, Egoorefiesh, Theenglishway88, FoxBot, Lando Calrissian, Ox Loveless xo, اكشف عقیل12345drbob, Liztanp, Jonkerz, Lotje, Sexist banana, Divhead, Vrenator, Goglin30, Henso au, Extra999, Chaching2323, Steelcity398, Bluefist, Robboisfunky, Ahmed saade, Wizardboyniga, TRYPPN, Petar43, Diannaa, Weedwhacker128, Vera.tetrix, Satdeep Gill, Alexanderbielby, Bobby122, MornMore, Mean as custard, Nwgeorge98, ArwinJ, RjwilmsiBot, Ncerlan, Shoehornian, NInTeNdO, Skamecrazy123, DASHBot, Elmodude5, EmausBot, John of Reading, Orphan Wiki, Immunize, Sophie, Deanbird98753154, Katherine, AJona1992, RoflWaffleCopter, Joeywallace9, Osmangulsen, Tommy2010, Historygeek222, Wikipelli, Djembayz, William Hung for President, Linzey999, Fæ, Traxs7, Shuipzv3, Herrogurlll123, Jcpurleigh, Jaydiem, AIRWaLkersiLLysmile, Willgrulich, Bryce Carmony, Aamto24, Bahudhara, Brettburcham, Francesca Sandys, Wiooiw, Ryugeist, Orlando2345, Fossilized77777, Wayne Slam, 11colsor, OnePt618, Crazyhug, Mitchell9812, Lemon00000, Squidyy, Esimon221, Venom789456123, SupercatsGizzle, L Kensington, Mayur, Ciaran10, Grooveboy102, Puffin, ShatteredAnon, Evan-Amos, Pooo123, LikeLakers2, Lil'meowmeow14, Cjlemon, Autodidact1, Est.r, ClueBot NG, Spike-TorontoRCP, Mechanical digger, MattyMerrt, Michaelmas1957, Minerv, Sportsrob31, Poiui, ReroFlow, Hon-3s-T, Supermonnom, Ilikeorangesido, O.Koslowski, ScottSteiner, Crazymonkey1123, Fugyoo, Helpful Pixie Bot, Reanimatedgif, Limdog333lemon, Sabbbyy, Doctorwho1234, Chang101LOL, Cleo, Gauravjuvekar, Lowercase sigmabot, Northamerica1000, ProjectManhattan, Sailing to Byzantium, Jogi don, Jahnavisatyan, Jeancey, Snow Blizzard, Maurice Flesier, H4X0R626, Tenoukii, Glacialfox, Kfcdesuland, Amindayo2, Llamallamaz, Klilidiplomus, Skifer92108, RichmanT, FreeRogue, IWannaPeterPumpkinEaterPeterParker, Xoyellowgirl, BattyBot, N64dude, StipeST, Walruslemon, Darorcilmir, Several Pending, BADGIRLSCLUBLUVVER, Anaximander01, Popizzamanjoe, JoshuSasori, MangoMania69, Abblo321la, Katiejordahl, Jacktoots, Spencer Asral, Paxman155, Surferjamjill, Lishageb, Khazar2, H2NCH2COOH, AutomaticStrikeout, BrightStarSky, Dexbot, Sminthopsis84, Webclient101, ColonelHenry, Lugia2453, SFK2, Corn cheese, Laddo, Tim Alberdingk Thijm, Jacisjoe, Dominikretro, Ray Lightyear, Omgwtf321, Mahmoud naseem, Me1482, Blissbliss101, General534, Kind Tennis Fan, HalfGig, Raymond37, Ladyblackmetal,

AwesoMan3000, Swidran, Ochilov, Riversid, P. S. Sena, Sarr Cat, Yellow Dingo, KasparBot, Anjali das gupta and Anonymous: 1370

- **Monoi oil** *Source:* https://en.wikipedia.org/wiki/Monoi_oil?oldid=675198552 *Contributors:* Robbot, D6, RussBot, Malcolma, DAJF, Frap, Stephenjh, Daodonnell, Fabrictramp, Jimmilu Katharineamy, Squids and Chips, Jackfork, Jennifergaglione, Dawn Bard, Lightmouse, JL-Bot, Niceguyedc, Good Olfactory, Addbot, FreeRangeFrog, Xqbot, FrescoBot, John of Reading, ZéroBot, AvicAWB, ZoschH, ClueBot NG, Monoitiare, Monoitiki, KLBot2, MusikAnimal, AK456, Bylanre, Maururu~enwiki, Bammbii, Sarasedgewick, P. S. Sena and Anonymous: 20

- **Mustard oil** *Source:* https://en.wikipedia.org/wiki/Mustard_oil?oldid=678976711 *Contributors:* AxelBoldt, Scott, Antandrus, Burschik, Klemen Kocjancic, Acsenray, Rich Farmbrough, Kwamikagami, Kjkolb, Lightdarkness, Mindmatrix, Jpramas, Etan Wexler, Rjwilmsi, Ground Zero, YurikBot, Waitak, Badagnani, Inhighspeed, DAJF, Alexandrov, SmackBot, Timotheus Canens, Edgar181, TRosenbaum, ERcheck, Jishnua, Hgrosser, RandomP, Andrew c, Ian Spackman, Dl2000, DabMachine, Radiant chains, WeggeBot, AdamRoach, Cacahuate, Robzz, Mr. G. Williams, ChemNerd, Pharaoh of the Wizards, Maproom, Acalamari, LittleHow, Yespriminister, MartinBotIII, Leopart, TXiKiBoT, Hcb, Rajuonline, SieBot, Rajantak, Newsingh, Seuraza, DrippingGoofball, Alexbot, Eeekster, RPSM, BobKawanaka, Amlanray, NJGW, Ryckmans thomas, Jytdog, Alicecullengirl, Addbot, Michaelm 22, Glane23, Luckas-bot, Yobot, AnomieBOT, ThaddeusB, Hatmaskin, Feowren Hwaerthgeld, Citation bot 1, Preetsingh13, RjwilmsiBot, ZéroBot, Trinanjon, Erianna, Khaydock, ClueBot NG, الأغذية الزاوية, Helpful Pixie Bot, Curb Chain, Hans Frörum, Lpupkiewicz, Northamerica1000, AhMedRMaaty, Jahnavisatyan, Gyanvigyan1, Sparkie82, Luckydhaliwal, Faizan, Monkbot, P. S. Sena and Anonymous: 79

- **Myrrh** *Source:* https://en.wikipedia.org/wiki/Myrrh?oldid=687393861 *Contributors:* Bryan Derksen, Malcolm Farmer, SimonP, Leandrod, Llywrch, Lexor, Liftarn, Ihcoyc, Mkweise, Ellywa, Rossami, Tkinias, Evercat, [212], RodC, Fvw, JorgeGG, Peak, Xyzzyva, MPF, Philwelch, Herbee, Gus Polly, Rpyle731, ZeroJanvier, Tagishsimon, Andycjp, JoJan, Mike Rosoft, Rich Farmbrough, Dbachmann, Bender235, JamesR1701E, Minghong, Hesperian, Polylerus, Musiphil, Anthony Appleyard, Supine, Sjschen, Linmhall, Ringbang, WojciechSwiderski~enwiki, HenryLi, Kazvorpal, Stemonitis, Sandover, -Ril-, John Hill, BD2412, DiamonDie, Search4Lancer, Koavf, SMC, FlaBot, Naraht, Eubot, Avalyn, Maustrauser, Travis.Thurston, VolatileChemical, WriterHound, Therefore, YurikBot, Wavelength, Whoisjohngalt, SkyCaptain~enwiki, RussBot, Gaius Cornelius, El Cazangero, DAJF, Merosonox, Asarelah, SmackBot, Dweller, Elonka, McGeddon, AnOddName, Khepidjemwa'atnefru, Ohnoitsjamie, So hungry, The Invisible Hand, Rkitko, Muggwort17, Mladifilozof, SheeEttin, Flyguy649, Bdiscoe, Wombat1138, Andrew Dalby, Will Beback, Polihale, SilkTork, Gorosaurus, Feterlewis, LuYiSi, Smenjas, PaulGS, NEMT, Orangutan, Covalent, Dia^, Iuio, Greg.loutsenko, Karenjc, ObiterDicta, Ph0kin, Cydebot, Byronreese, Lugnuts, Mycroft.Holmes, Gonzo fan2007, Dyanega, Epbr123, Mojo Hand, Sturm55, Therequiembellishere, Heroeswithmetaphors, Mitkat, Seaphoto, KP Botany, Pollira, Penjr, Danny lost, Huttarl, JAnDbot, Deflective, Joshryre, Wasell, Bencherlite, Emperorgrey, Vssun, Ksvaughan2, SquidSK, Mylabrie, R'n'B, CommonsDelinker, Lax4mike, Zeragito, Maproom, Chiswick Chap, BrettAllen, Gr8white, MishaPan, Ogranut, DASonnenfeld, Spellcast, Meiskam, AlnoktaBOT, Ravhovel, Philip Trueman, Raymondwinn, Rovingrover, AlleborgoBot, SieBot, YonaBot, Jojalozzo, Jtrainier80, Grim-Gym, Calatayudboy, Torchwoodwho, CultureDrone, Raasgat, TheCatalyst31, ClueBot, Icarusgeek, Ottawahitech, Rotational, PFRSC87, PixelBot, Estirabot, Stretchcat, Whaddawinna, F0110w3r, Kayjay76, HawaiiHangin10, ZooFari, Addbot, Grayfell, Jdevola, Tcncv, Jncraton, Cuaxdon, Leszek Jańczuk, TNA64, Millwonder, Ahmad2099, Flappychappy, Zorrobot, Legobot, Middayexpress, Luckas-bot, Yobot, Maxí, AnomieBOT, Aargian, AdjustShift, Xqbot, Capricorn42, Gigemag76, Lewbly, Itineranttrader, RibotBOT, Reginald.pipecleaner, Basharh, Sophus Bie, Schekinov Alexey Victorovich, Kierkkadon, Frozenevolution, Custoo, FrescoBot, Citation bot 1, DKMell, Pinethicket, Meaghan, Tedency, PrinceRegentLuitpold, Koakhtzvigad, Corinne68, Trappist the monk, Veron, Pubfac, EmausBot, Ashdavies46, John of Reading, Orphan Wiki, Lipsio, Black Yoshi, Paul Bedson, Josve05a, Cobaltcigs AManWithNoPlan, Coasterlover1994, Donner60, Odysseus1479, Thefalseprofit, Matthew L. Green, ClueBot NG, Magneticfield123, Afcpakistan, Jacopo188, Greenknight dv, Glacialfox, Cyberbot II, ChrisGualtieri, YFdyh-bot, Ahpavel, Sminthopsis84, Morfusmax, Robski57, Shangri-La-la-land, WineMyrrh, Nixon333, P. S. Sena, Sarr Cat, Alchavers21, Savir and Anonymous: 201

- **Myrtol standardized** *Source:* https://en.wikipedia.org/wiki/Myrtol_standardized?oldid=653764092 *Contributors:* Bearcat, Malcolma, DAJF, Jahibadkaret, PixelBot, Addbot, Citation bot, Martijnd, FrescoBot, P. S. Sena and Anonymous: 3

- **Neroli** *Source:* https://en.wikipedia.org/wiki/Neroli?oldid=686675569 *Contributors:* Brainsik, Zoicon5, Texture, Jeroboambramblejam, TonyW, Corti, Brianhe, Srkingdavy, Physicistjedi, MPerel, Keenan Pepper, Woohookitty, FlaBot, DAJF, BOT-Superzerocool, Dddstone, Rcharman, SmackBot, Edgar181, Chris the speller, Smalltowngir-, A. B., PamD, Nipisiquit, Dombett, Schmloof, CommonsDelinker, ChrisNickson, Winecellar, Funandtrvl, Grammarmonger, Andy Dingley, SieBot, Calliopejen1, Timothy Cooper, Procrastinatrix, Keraunoscopia, Sensonet, Eeekster, Ladygrey21, Addbot, Glane23, Lightbot, Ytiugbma, AnomieBOT, Shootbamboo Gigemag76, Itineranttrader, Abductive, Sprout House, ZéroBot, Cjsunbird, Alyssa Janney, Tgvornado, ClueBot NG, Elizaacd, Wh1teChocolatte, Kai Ojima, Oscardeklan, Thrub, Riversid, P. S. Sena, MadameAnglaise and Anonymous: 36

- **Nutmeg oil** *Source:* https://en.wikipedia.org/wiki/Nutmeg_oil?oldid=664377036 *Contributors:* Walkerma, Heah, Waitak, DAJF, Feng Aili, Alexandrov, SmackBot, The Famous Movie Director, Cygnus78, Ewulp, Sensonet, HawaiiHangin10, Addbot, Walrus heart, Gigemag76, Itineranttrader, Erik9bot, Minimac, Cjsunbird, P. S. Sena and Anonymous: 6

- **Oil of clove** *Source:* https://en.wikipedia.org/wiki/Oil_of_clove?oldid=653764506 *Contributors:* William Avery, Ehn, WhisperToMe, YpsilantiBruin, DMG413, Thorwald, Rich Farmbrough, Gene Nygaard, Technochocolate, Rjwilmsi, Ground Zero, WriterHound, Cliffb, Kyorcsuke, Sanguinity, EgbertW, DAJF, Alpha 4615, Preczewski, Alexandrov, SmackBot, Setanta747 (locked), Geoff B, Gilliam, Deli nk, Bouncingmolar, Pgr94, Rifleman 82, Dom0803, John Moss, Shivaexportsindia, Appraiser, Bwhack, Sixit, ChemNerd, McSly, Alnokta, IceDragon64, ReefkprZ, Saber girl08, Natek2142, GustavoJoseph, CMBJ, Badvibes101, Bpeps, ClueBot, Celiakozlowski, Ronaldcmarks, Djneufville, Buggia, NellieBly, Addbot, DOI bot, Calartifex, Fu ran, Tassedethe, MuZemike, EnochBethany, AnomieBOT, Citation bot, LilHelpa, Ragityman, Itineranttrader, Masterbowker, Citation bot 1, Felis domestica, Vrenator, Fanfardon, RjwilmsiBot, Ajsanch, CopperSquare, Helpful Pixie Bot, Darorcilmir, Linguisticphilo, Ritika3339, YiFeiBot, Onuphriate, Monkbot, Honeybeesweettree, P. S. Sena and Anonymous: 65

- **Oil of guaiac** *Source:* https://en.wikipedia.org/wiki/Oil_of_guaiac?oldid=687321559 *Contributors:* Infrogmation, Gjbloom, Naddy, Fabloflores, Flyhighplato, Brim, Prime Entelechy, DAJF, Edgar181, Adrigon, Clicketyclack, Aspern, Rg998, Daniel Olsen, Rosarinagazo, Belovedfreak, Calliopejen1, Sensonet, Addbot, THEN WHO WAS PHONE?, Plantdrew, P. S. Sena and Anonymous: 4

- **Olbas Oil** *Source:* https://en.wikipedia.org/wiki/Olbas_Oil?oldid=659507393 *Contributors:* DAJF, Mike hayes, Geach, AdamRoach, CrossHouses, Editor510, Xqbot, BG19bot, BattyBot, Deveron28, P. S. Sena, Teacher was here and Anonymous: 1

- **Orange oil** *Source:* https://en.wikipedia.org/wiki/Orange_oil?oldid=658256551 *Contributors:* Stone, Dusik, Quarl, Icairns, Klemen Kocjancic, Discospinster, 1-is-blue, Rd232, DrGaellon, V8rik, Rjwilmsi, Jweiss11, YurikBot, Waitak, Shaddack, DAJF, NHSavage, SmackBot, Peloneous,

Mister Magotchi, Rilr, Thumperward, Valenciano, Smokefoot, Bejnar, Rockpocket, Ohconfucius, Piramidon, Gogo Dodo, Brewsum, Ccrrccrr, Magioladitis, Rklecka, NReitzel, Acalamari, Buxley Hall, Signalhead, VolkovBot, Calliopejen1, OKBot, Mild Bill Hiccup, Niceguyedc, Sensonet, PixelBot, Eeekster, Slidinandridin06, Daviejoe77, XLinkBot, Addbot, Jacopo Werther, DOI bot, Cinicalknowledge, Ginosbot, Luckasbot, AnomieBOT, Rubinbot, Eoilco, MichaelSterlingSF, Saehrimnir, Girlwithgreeneyes, Citation bot 1, Charlielacosta, Termiteguy, Trappist the monk, Jonkerz, Oktanyum, Mean as custard, Look2See1, GoingBatty, ZéroBot, Erianna, ClueBot NG, Helpful Pixie Bot, Furyofnasa, MusikAnimal, Badon, Christinareese7, Stvhwl, Artfully69, CliffordBanes, Devxnregan, Awesomebala, INDIATAXINFOPRIVATELIMITED, Tiradlover101, Chronomaster5779, Asds34fox, Riversid, P. S. Sena, Kate jonson, Fresshh and Anonymous: 34

- **Orris oil** *Source:* https://en.wikipedia.org/wiki/Orris_oil?oldid=669043794 *Contributors:* Avriette, I9Q79oL78KiL0QTFHgyc, Malcolma, DAJF, SmackBot, Deli nk, Addshore, WhatamIdoing, Erik9bot, Snotbot, Northamerica1000, Flashy1010, BattyBot, Deputydog7781, Chris-Gualtieri, MrNiceGuy1113, Leecanham18, P. S. Sena and Anonymous: 3

- **Palmarosa Oil** *Source:* https://en.wikipedia.org/wiki/Palmarosa_Oil?oldid=667904065 *Contributors:* Ewen, Rjwilmsi, DAJF, Cesium 133, Billinghurst, Yobot, Josve05a, Plantdrew, Tchaliburton, P. S. Sena and Aconne01

- **Patchouli** *Source:* https://en.wikipedia.org/wiki/Patchouli?oldid=682284436 *Contributors:* PierreAbbat, Booyabazooka, Kwertii, Dante Alighieri, Bogdangiusca, Tkinias, RickK, Eugene van der Pijll, Texture, Garrett Albright, NeoThe1, Varlaam, Cantus, Neutrality, Jimaginator, Rich Farmbrough, Zombiejesus, Bender235, ESkog, Dennis Brown, Tigerente, Bobo192, Circeus, Seanturvey, Hesperian, Jhfrontz, Alansohn, Supine, Sjschen, Snachodog, Beakerboy, Versageek, Kazvorpal, Richwales, Dismas, SDC, Liface, V8rik, BD2412, Island, Rjwilmsi, Vary, Nandesuka, FlaBot, Seinfreak37, Gdrbot, WriterHound, Cassius987, YurikBot, Umlaut, The Hokkaido Crow, Dppowell, Fleet Pete, Lucasreddinger, Kadaniel~enwiki, TastyCakes, Vaisnavi, Nikki88, 21655, Esprit15d, Fram, EtherealPurple, Groyolo, SmackBot, Fueled~enwiki, Gilliam, The Famous Movie Director, Keegan, Smalltowngirl, Thumperward, Jax184, Deli nk, Mooterj, Aldaron, BostonMA, Vprajkumar, SnappingTurtle, Nrcprm2026, NaySay, ABoerma, Kendrick7, Harryboyles, SilkTork, Gobonobo, NewTestLeper79, Meco, Wwagner, Iridescent, Kaarel, DavidOaks, Cherryeater987, Van helsing, Cydebot, Meeprophone, Faigl.ladislav, Marek69, James086, Mule Man, Heroeswithmetaphors, AntiVandalBot, Dekkanar, Goldenband, Davewho2, Shinola, Swpb, Adavies42, Rarian rakista, Cecilkorik, The ninjalectual, AlexiusHoratius, Lifebonzza, J.delanoy, Katalaveno, Carolfrog, DarwinPeacock, Balajijagadesh, Jeff G., Amikake3, TXiKiBoT, Noopinonada, Yilloslime, UnitedStatesian, Chuck02, Dirkbb, SieBot, Euryalus, Hippybobb, Steven Crossin, Sharac, ClueBot, Rayne-goodechilde, Lobotomoy, Penguin6635, EoGuy, Dgp2, LarryMorseDCOhio, Hollyroseeva, Mfrench518, Canuckin, Wikiuser100, Ost316, Jht4060, Dchristofi, MystBot, Sgpsaros, Wyatt915, Addbot, LatitudeBot, Scrdcow, Cuaxdon, Lightbot, Tanár, Luckas-bot, KamikazeBot, AnomieBOT, Daniele Pugliesi, Chuckiesdad, Tiggsy, Steve8394, Sledgeas, Itineranttrader, Prunesqualer, Rosomak~enwiki, U336, FrescoBot, Citation bot 1, Redrose64, Pinethicket, HRoestBot, Impala2009, Miriote, Herbie.stafford, Goanaut, RjwilmsiBot, Solmique, Slon02, EmausBot, Sliceofmiami, WikitanvirBot, Helium4, Racerx11, Wikipelli, Spawnish, Tednightingale, Esandaas, Mjbmrbot, ClueBot NG, MelbourneStar, Helpful Pixie Bot, Jamie Tubers, Plantdrew, Iansha, KClarky, YFdyh-bot, Cerabot~enwiki, Monkbot, BethNaught, Ryan Kearns and Anonymous: 235

- **Pelargonium graveolens** *Source:* https://en.wikipedia.org/wiki/Pelargonium_graveolens?oldid=682048606 *Contributors:* Brainsik, Stan Shebs, Rich Farmbrough, Sjschen, Stemonitis, Bfigura, FlaBot, Eubot, WriterHound, SkyCaptain~enwiki, DAJF, SmackBot, The Famous Movie Director, Rkitko, Init~enwiki, Mgiganteus1, Benqish, Akhonji, DerHexer, Peter coxhead, MoiraMoira, Edgeweyes, Agyle, Jaguarlaser, Atubeileh, SieBot, Calliopejen1, Laitche, Tlustulimu, DragonBot, Skunkboy74, Jovianeye, HexaChord, Openevan, Addbot, C6541, Cuaxdon, Debresser, Flakinho, רוד55, Yobot, AnomieBOT, Yachtsman1, LilHelpa, Xqbot, Gigemag76, Itineranttrader, Citation bot 1, EmausBot, ChuispastonBot, Sierra Shaver, ClueBot NG, Dietitian3, Bernolákovčina, Plantdrew, BG19bot, NotWith, Xprofj, P. S. Sena, TMcB23 and Anonymous: 32

- **Petitgrain** *Source:* https://en.wikipedia.org/wiki/Petitgrain?oldid=653763905 *Contributors:* Sjschen, FlaBot, DAJF, Alexandrov, SmackBot, PamD, Auntof6, Brewcrewer, WikHead, Addbot, SpBot, PoizonMyst, Itineranttrader, SassoBot, Cjsunbird, NotWith, P. S. Sena and Anonymous: 5

- **Pine oil** *Source:* https://en.wikipedia.org/wiki/Pine_oil?oldid=667302251 *Contributors:* Auric, Timrollpickering, I9Q79oL78KiL0QTFHgyc, Great Scott, Garrisonroo, Gene Nygaard, DePiep, Fish and karate, Eubot, Gurch, Waitak, Bhny, MadMax, Stephanos Georgios John, Chem-Gardener, SmackBot, Edgar181, Deli nk, Ken Gallager, Gogo Dodo, ChemNerd, Boghog, VolkovBot, TXiKiBoT, Una Smith, Ravanacker, Chem-awb, ClueBot, Inver471ness, Addbot, 超级猪哥, Ronhjones, TaBOT-zerem, CheMoBot, Xqbot, Itineranttrader, Zefr, GreenZmiy, DrilBot, Pinethicket, RedBot, Bgpaulus, BogBot, EmausBot, Heymid, ZéroBot, The chemistds, Dan653, P. S. Sena, Anonimeco and Anonymous: 31

- **Rose oil** *Source:* https://en.wikipedia.org/wiki/Rose_oil?oldid=687510979 *Contributors:* Ixfd64, Texture, DocWatson42, CanisRufus, Shenme, Hooperbloob, Sjschen, Gene Nygaard, Feline1, Marudubshinki, Dar-Ape, Hairy Dude, Waitak, Family Guy Guy, TodorBozhinov, Reo On, Curtis Clark, Adamrush, Igiffin, Modify, John Broughton, Alexandrov, SmackBot, Melchoir, EncycloPetey, Hardyplants, Edgar181, Xaosflux, Gilliam, Chris the speller, Smalltowngirl, Deli nk, Clicketyclack, Pinktulip, White Ash, CmdrObot, Rifleman 82, Palaeologos, B, EvocativeIntrigue, Thijs!bot, Headbomb, Shivaexportsindia, Prestonmcconkie, Kyle824, LordAnubisBOT, Manager00104~enwiki, AndreasJSbot, Tourbillon, Mehdizare, David Condrey, Mattchess, Denisarona, Hanter, Mild Bill Hiccup, Sensonet, Vulgarian, SchreiberBike, Addbot, Jacopo Werther, Jim10701, SamatBot, Luckas-bot, Tempodivalse, AnomieBOT, ArthurBot, Capricorn42, Anna Frodesiak, Francescobianchi, Itineranttrader, Zefr, Andromeas, FrescoBot, Nojan, EmausBot, Klbrain, Ph111P20079, ChuispastonBot, Socialservice, ClueBot NG, JasminSullivan, Bceduval, Lagoset, Neatsfoot, P. S. Sena and Anonymous: 50

- **Rosewood oil** *Source:* https://en.wikipedia.org/wiki/Rosewood_oil?oldid=680728737 *Contributors:* Waitak, RussBot, Dweller, Melchoir, EncycloPetey, Grahamec, AnomieBOT, Itineranttrader, Ericreid57 and Lagoset

- **Sage oil** *Source:* https://en.wikipedia.org/wiki/Sage_oil?oldid=676406548 *Contributors:* Berek, Greydream, Ari x, Rjwilmsi, Waitak, Kafziel, DAJF, Edgar181, Dr Don, Ckatz, Dugwiki, Lupusrex, Acalamari, Unbuttered Parsnip, Sensonet, Addbot, DOI bot, AnomieBOT, Gigemag76, Mean as custard, Iamaveronica, P. S. Sena, Kate jonson and Anonymous: 10

- **Salvia sclarea** *Source:* https://en.wikipedia.org/wiki/Salvia_sclarea?oldid=676952310 *Contributors:* Tarquin, Olivier, Stan Shebs, Imc, Eugene van der Pijll, WormRunner, MPF, Mike Rosoft, DanielCD, Rich Farmbrough, Mwng, Circeus, Elipongo, Hesperian, Stemonitis, SP-KP, Ricardo Carneiro Pires, FlaBot, Eubot, Gdrbot, SkyCaptain~enwiki, RussBot, Rada, Dtrebbien, DAJF, SMcCandlish, SmackBot, Edgar181, DabMachine, Iridescent, Paul venter, Cydebot, Thijs!bot, Epbr123, Hydro, Apsley, Sweetshana3, Taotriad, TXiKiBoT, SieBot, Elie plus, Sjwells53, Fratrep, Alexbot, BOTarate, Addbot, Cuaxdon, First Light, Luckas-bot, Yobot, AnomieBOT, LilHelpa, Xqbot, Skrod, Itineranttrader, FrescoBot, GreenZmiy, RedBot, EmausBot, Ancient Gardener, Ecochicagoland, موشلك بن ورمع, Hectonichus, Helpful Pixie Bot, Xenxax, P. S. Sena and Anonymous: 17

- **Sandalwood oil** *Source:* https://en.wikipedia.org/wiki/Sandalwood_oil?oldid=679043227 *Contributors:* Pol098, DAJF, Melchoir, Edgar181, Hgrosser, Leyo, DASonnenfeld, DumZiBoT, WikHead, Addbot, AnomieBOT, Rubinbot, Citation bot, Itineranttrader, Theoregonconnection, WikitanvirBot, ZéroBot, ClueBot NG, CopperSquare, Monkbot, P. S. Sena and Anonymous: 6

- **Santalum album** *Source:* https://en.wikipedia.org/wiki/Santalum_album?oldid=686441109 *Contributors:* Shyamal, Pengo, Alan Liefting, Everyking, Ary29, Mike Rosoft, Hesperian, Stemonitis, Woohookitty, BD2412, Rjwilmsi, Ricardo Carneiro Pires, Eubot, RussBot, Chris Capoccia, DAJF, TDogg310, Epipelagic, SmackBot, Bidgee, Rkitko, MalafayaBot, Tripledot, Snowgrouse, KarlM, DangerousPanda, AdamMorton, Calvero JP, Barticus88, Phoe, J. Patrick Fischer, JAnDbot, CommonsDelinker, Fred.e, Clocktower, DorganBot, Balajijagadesh, Idioma-bot, Xnuala, Sam Blacketer, Sankalpdravid, Jaguarlaser, SieBot, Meinpng, Jmgarg1, Wwheaton, Cygnis insignis, Alexbot, DumZiBoT, Addbot, VASANTH S.N., 丁丁丁, Yobot, Viking59, Soaringhawk21, AnomieBOT, Materialscientist, Citation bot, Krish Dulal, Full-date unlinking bot, MegaSloth, John of Reading, Prabinepali, Snotbot, Helpful Pixie Bot, YVSREDDY, ChrisGualtieri, SantoshBot, Biswapriya123, Soham, Buffbills7701, Filedelinkerbot, P. S. Sena and Anonymous: 21

- **Santalum spicatum** *Source:* https://en.wikipedia.org/wiki/Santalum_spicatum?oldid=653763416 *Contributors:* Alan Liefting, PDH, Kevyn, Rich Farmbrough, Peter Greenwell, Brim, Hesperian, Sjschen, Eubot, JarrahTree, DAJF, TDogg310, SmackBot, Brya, Rkitko, Xyzzyplugn, Iridescent, Xtrappl8, Cydebot, Fred.e, Plasticup, Berichard, Jaguarlaser, Moonriddengirl, Editore99, Cygnis insignis, DumZiBoT, Addbot, Lil-Helpa, Jenks24, Rcsprinter123, Monkbot, P. S. Sena and Anonymous: 3

- **Sfumatura** *Source:* https://en.wikipedia.org/wiki/Sfumatura?oldid=653763388 *Contributors:* DAJF, Melchoir, Jon186, H. Carver, Schreiber-Bike, Addbot, Jacopo Werther, Yobot, Citation bot and P. S. Sena

- **Spearmint** *Source:* https://en.wikipedia.org/wiki/Spearmint?oldid=671260067 *Contributors:* Hephaestos, Zanimum, Snoyes, Kragen, Johnwhite79, Andrewman327, Silvonen, Pedant17, Tpbradbury, Eugene van der Pijll, Robbot, Rfc1394, MPF, Mintleaf~enwiki, Sunny256, Espetkov, Yath, Williamb, JoJan, Quarl, Manny551~enwiki, Burschik, Mormegil, DanielCD, Moverton, Jaberwocky6669, C1k3, Bobo192, Circeus, Hesperian, Jonathunder, Msh210, Oleg Alexandrov, Stemonitis, Oliphaunt, Graham87, Rjwilmsi, Oo64eva, Mikecron, Catsmeat, Jrtayloriv, Gdrbot, YurikBot, SkyCaptain~enwiki, Chris Capoccia, Dysmorodrepanis~enwiki, Inhighspeed, Zwobot, Morgan Leigh, DeadEyeArrow, BorgQueen, Nekura, SmackBot, Slashme, Rebollo fr~enwiki, Rojomoke, Cazort, Durova, SaltyWater, Mensch, Perlmonger42, RedHillian, Abrahami, Kingdon, Andrew Dalby, SilkTork, Mgiganteus1, Libertyblues, Shoeofdeath, Rm1854, Philiptdotcom, InspiredLight, Karenjc, Rifleman 82, Synergy, Nick Number, Dezidor, Keeganspeck, Peacefool, Autumnko, Michael Goodyear, CommonsDelinker, Victor Blacus, Athaenara, Igno2, Idioma-bot, Philip Trueman, Watercat04, Nefabit, NHStormie, SieBot, Scarian, Elie plus, Arda Xi, Poissonrouge, IvanTortuga, ClueBot, Jan1nad, Jusdafax, Ravenna1961, Iohannes Animosus, Amaltheus, Canihaveacookie, HawaiiHangin10, Addbot, DOI bot, Laaknor-Bot, Tassedethe, Luckas-bot, Yobot, KamikazeBot, AnomieBOT, Citation bot, Xqbot, Janet Davis, Ani medjool, Zefr, Andromeas, FrescoBot, LucienBOT, XLR808, Citation bot 1, Pinethicket, AmphBot, TobeBot, Dinamik-bot, Theoregonconnection, Erianna, Will Beback Auto, ClueBot NG, Pika32141, Xenophonix, Plantdrew, Vagobot, Supernerd11, Tu7uh, Shisha-Tom, Qskb, Corn cheese, Clr324, AfadsBad, NutrientGirl, Joseph Laferriere, Coltsman12 and Anonymous: 100

- **Styrax balsam** *Source:* https://en.wikipedia.org/wiki/Styrax_balsam?oldid=684446086 *Contributors:* Jake Nelson, Eugene van der Pijll, MPF, LHOON, Mindmatrix, Hydrargyrum, El Cazangero, Black-Velvet, SmackBot, Maxima m, EncycloPetey, Can't sleep, clown will eat me, SilkTork, Minisarm, Nick Number, Hoffmeier, Magioladitis, EscapingLife, Nadiatalent, Penarc, Calliopejen1, Flyer22 Reborn, LarryMorseDCChio, Addbot, Peridon, WuBot, Gilo1969, Berylcloud, Mad4Linux, Plantdrew, Rileybk, Grumpir.hard, Lemnaminor and Anonymous: 17

- **Tea tree oil** *Source:* https://en.wikipedia.org/wiki/Tea_tree_oil?oldid=687570354 *Contributors:* AxelBoldt, GTBacchus, Egil, Kragen, Cherkash, Stone, Maximus Rex, Texture, Hadal, Mandel, MPF, Wolfkeeper, Niteowlneils, Jfdwolff, Mckaysalisbury, Trilobite, Briar-Willoughby, Perey, Rich Farmbrough, Cacycle, Mummymonkey, Mwanner, Davidruben, Viriditas, ZayZayEM, Arcadian, Maebmij, Mpulier, Abstraktn, Alansohn, Oasisbob, Walkerma, Bobrayner, Love3child, Rjwilmsi, Darguz Parsilvan, Dudegalea, Musical Linguist, Jrtayloriv, Yurik-Bot, Chris Capoccia, Gaius Cornelius, Brec, Shaddack, The Hokkaido Crow, Keithonearth, DAJF, Asarelah, 2over0, Mike Dillon, Jacklee, Foolestroupe, SmackBot, Rayward, Kintetsubuffalo, Edgar181, Gilliam, The Famous Movie Director, Gene Thomas, Durova, Chris the speller, Smalltowngirl, RDBrown, JoeAustralia, Oatmea. batman, Frap, Cybercobra, BullRangifer, Bejnar, John, Sbmehta, Cubefrenzy, Joelmills, Gregorydavid, Dodo bird, Simon12, Paul venter, Yhager, FabioLb, Tawkerbot2, Shkirenko, Bubbha, Switchercat, JJiggssaw, Linuxerist, CmdrObot, Green caterpillar, Rhode Island Red, Dr.enh, DumbBOT, TheJC, Catawba, Thijs!bot, Barticus88, Qwyrxian, Headbomb, Sean7phil, Uses2, Second Quantization, Benqish, Nick Number, Tean91, Tjmayerinsf, John Moss, JAnDbot, MER-C, Aekbal, Freedomlinux, Lex Kitten Indon, Buddhadev1, Hdt83, Gandydancer, DBlomgren, Bmrbarre, Manticore, Dicotyledon, Trusilver, MistyMorn, LesWeller, Hippi ippi, Naniwako, HiLo48, Molly-in-md, Siraj88, Siraj555, Atooms, DASonnenfeld, Lights, My Core Competency is Competency, Ryan032, Wikidemor, Galialuna, Piperh, Leafyplant, TempeBrennan, Moses shepard, Ziounclesi, Henryodell, Stephanie herman, Roxya, Stvfetterly, SkyViewOrphanage, Cactus26, Mohansen11, Djayjp, Imaginenow, Alexbrn, Darladeer, Rhesusmonkeyboy, ClueBot, Lianiwidjaja, Hutcher, Litmaerle, Unbuttered Parsnip, Plankwalking, WDM27, Csonnenf, Gtstricky, Slidinandridin06, Wnt, Jewelchild, DumZiBoT, TimTay, Roxy the dog, Drhealthnutty, HawaiiHangin10, Randominity14, Leoniana, Vdeck, Addbot, Deepmath, DOI bot, Cssiitcic, The last slice of pizza, Samat-Bot, West.andrew.g, Numbo3-bot, Tide rolls, Legobot, Luckas-bot, Yobot, EnochBethany, AnomieBOT, Jim1138, Citation bot, Mejohn7779, ArthurBot, FreeRangeFrog, Solace1, Gigemag76, JWBE, Itineranttrader, Taka76, Froggysocks, GliderMaven, Surv1v4l1st, NSH002, Adamsintime, Citation bot 1, Front Runner 8, Un Mundo, Hoo man, Aareo, GabrielGL, Kgrad, Trappist the monk, Medical Studies, Vrenator, RjwilmsiBot, Steve03Mills, EmausBot, T3dkjn89q00vl02Cxp1kqs3x7, HiMyNameIsFrancesca, Philippe (WMF), Dewritech, Frglz, ZéroBot, Cogiati, Csunbird, Bazzel, Netha Hussain, Arbowmd, JoeSperrazza, FloGreen, Teapeat, DASHBotAV, Rememberway, ClueBot NG, Uzma Gamal, This lousy T-shirt, AerobicFox, Ramillav, GlassLadyBug, Theonesean, Helpful Pixie Bot, Valimets, Mark Marathon, BG19bot, Gurt Posh, Jamespenn1234, PhnomPencil, Luceth, NotWith, Shisha-Tom, Rytyho usa, BattyBot, Biosthmors, Cclehnen, Ajithrocksca, Tyler-Durden8823, TheAnonymousRabbit, EncycloCritique, FriendlyParasprite, Clr324, Dough34, Mogs03, RYasmeen (WMF), Anamikagioiaxo, Monkbot, ACathe-Leigh, Apkurnia1, Markie1992, P. S. Sena, Requiem for a Daydream, Blascelle, שמעוני and Anonymous: 250

- **Volatility (chemistry)** *Source:* https://en.wikipedia.org/wiki/Volatility_(chemistry)?oldid=642101313 *Contributors:* Ellywa, Giftlite, Discospinster, Vsmith, Alansohn, Walkerma, Commander Keane, JRHorse, KKramer~enwiki, Carrionluggage, Erik4, YurikBot, Buster79, Trovatore, Dhollm, Poppy, Infinity0, Itub, FocalPoint, Victor M. Vicente Selvas, GregRM, Nbarth, Colonies Chris, Mbeychok, GetsEclectic, LouisBB, Rifleman 82, Christian75, Epbr123, Headbomb, Marek69, Pfranson, Txomin, WilfriedC, Comrade Tux, Kbrose, PlanetStar, Faradayplank,

Simkiss3, JL-Bot, Leighwaldon, ClueBot, Goodvac, Addbot, Tide rolls, Yobot, Aboalbiss, Daniele Pugliesi, Citation bot, زادگان قلی, Jonesey95, Double sharp, Sumone10154, Vekov, Katherine, ה הריא., Wikipelli, RaymondSutanto, Δ, ClueBot NG, MerlIwBot, Prouder Mary, YiFeiBot, CogitoErgoSum14, Monkbot, Crossark and Anonymous: 46

- **Wintergreen** *Source:* https://en.wikipedia.org/wiki/Wintergreen?oldid=680739206 *Contributors:* Heron, Glenn, Ike9898, Dogface, MPF, Daibhid C, Andycjp, Elektron, Ukexpat, Zaslav, Hesperian, Velella, Captainsquare, Kazvorpal, BlueCanoe, Woohookitty, Spettro9, Carmeld1, Choess, Srleffler, The Rambling Man, Bullzeye, Awiseman, Gadget850, Mike Serfas, Akrabbim, Veinor, SmackBot, Oceanbourne, Kintetsubuffalo, Edgar181, Rkitko, Thumperward, Melburnian, Lesnail, IronGargoyle, Dionysia, Bridesmill, CWY2190, WeggeBot, LaFoiblesse, Chris CII, Mojo Hand, Just Chilling, Gabbyhayes, Soulbot, Hdt83, Belovedfreak, Nadiatalent, Jamesontai, Richard New Forest, Flyer22 Reborn, Cthunter44, DumZiBoT, SMP0328., Drhealthnutty, Addbot, Cuaxdon, NjardarBot, Teles, Jarble, Ben Ben, Yobot, AnomieBOT, Harne, Coolsgain, Kingpin13, Bcw142, Capricorn42, J04n, Itineranttrader, Hamamelis, DrilBot, Funnykid777, Hollyjean380, ClueBot NG, Cwinstanley, Helpful Pixie Bot, Plantdrew, Tfbybyhf, Kellarcarnes, Lagoset and Anonymous: 62

- **Yarrow oil** *Source:* https://en.wikipedia.org/wiki/Yarrow_oil?oldid=647710158 *Contributors:* J3ff, Grutness, Walkerma, SmackBot, Beetstra, Hdt83, Murderbike, Drhealthnutty, Dthomsen8, Dawynn, Yobot, Erik9bot, Btilm, SunnyInHouston, Rubbish computer and Anonymous: 1

- **List of essential oils** *Source:* https://en.wikipedia.org/wiki/List_of_essential_oils?oldid=687817346 *Contributors:* Michael T. Richter, Jason Quinn, Ryanaxp, Cacycle, Oolong, Sjschen, Beakerboy, Versageek, Woohookitty, Miss Madeline, BD2412, Rjwilmsi, MZMcBride, Bgwhite, WriterHound, Waitak, RussBot, Tearlach, CLW, Open2universe, ViperSnake151, SmackBot, McGeddon, Hardyplants, Edgar181, Ohnoitsjamie, Balin42632003, J306, Geqo, Nehrams2020, Iepeulas, Eastlaw, CmdrObot, Requestion, Johner, Cydebot, Mccojr02, Barticus88, Shivaexportsindia, Epeefleche, Robina Fox, Cannabis, WhatamIdoing, Nips, R'n'B, Reedy Bot, Rod57, Belovedfreak, Siraj88, Pghosh428, Una Smith, January2007, Alexbrn, Darladeer, JL-Bot, Lianiwidjaja, Robbiemuffin, Egogordo, Niceguyedc, No such user, Mirlanda92, XLinkBot, Addbot, Jacopo Werther, Cblack2, AnomieBOT, Anna Frodesiak, Taka76, Nagualdesign, GoingBatty, A Scents Worth, H3llBot, Mueka238, DavidAnstiss, Plantdrew, Sminthopsis84, SFK2, World of vetiver, Lagoset, O4organics, Ecosumit and Anonymous: 36

- **List of vegetable oils** *Source:* https://en.wikipedia.org/wiki/List_of_vegetable_oils?oldid=663595556 *Contributors:* Rmhermen, Mac, Ronz, Ike9898, CBDunkerson, Donarreiskoffer, Academic Challenger, Alan Liefting, RetiredUser2, Neutrality, Rich Farmbrough, Vsmith, Arthena, Sjschen, Lkinkade, Stemonitis, Soultaco, Kam Solusar, Prashanthns, Rjwilmsi, Quiddity, Vegaswikian, Ricardo Carneiro Pires, Choess, OpenToppedBus, Wavelength, Waitak, Jimp, Peter G Werner, RussBot, Sarranduin, Chris Capoccia, C777, Tavilis, Sanguinity, Curtis Clark, Grafen, Badagnani, BorgQueen, Fram, Anthony717, SmackBot, Victor M. Vicente Selvas, Alex Ex, AndreasJS, Commander Keane bot, Bluebot, Stevage, Deli nk, TheFeds, CSWarren, Frap, JonHarder, ClairSamoht, Sei Shonagon~enwiki, Monotonehell, G716, BullRangifer, J306, Bonzi, Cmh, Hu12, B7T, Colonel Warden, RekishiEJ, CmdrObot, KyraVixen, Neelix, Pro bug catcher, Cydebot, Rifleman 82, Trident13, Narayanese, Trev M, Itsmejudith, KP Botany, Mattgow, Oleochemist, Catgut, WLU, Peter coxhead, ChemNerd, Beechnut, Masebrock, Angela C, 83d40m, Juliancolton, DASonnenfeld, Funandtrvl, Johnfos, Jmrowland, Davehi1, Gueneverey, UnitedStatesian, Alex.muller, Anchor Link Bot, ClueBot, Phytotrade, Piledhigheranddeeper, Auntof6, Dagordon01, DOHill, NuclearWarfare, Arjayay, NJGW, Nepenthes, Olaffpomona, Freetrashbox, Basilicofresco, DOI bot, Giants2008, Download, LinkFA-Bot, HAmpzter, The Earwig, Aboalbiss, AnomieBOT, Citation bot, GB fan, Quebec99, Gilo1969, Amada44, FrescoBot, Citation bot 1, Killian441, Emyil, WaitingForConnection, RjwilmsiBot, WildBot, Skamecrazy123, Cogiati, H3llBot, SporkBot, Brandmeister, Jacobponnose, ClueBot NG, Widr, Helpful Pixie Bot, Plantdrew, ELNO Checking, Northamerica1000, Mark Arsten, CitationCleanerBot, 86.** IP, BattyBot, Dexbot, Joeinwiki, Habibibibalani, Daniel Gadsby, Noyster, Monkbot, سيسىراي and Anonymous: 56

3.2   Images

- **File:2012lemon_and_lime.png** *Source:* https://upload.wikimedia.org/wikipedia/commons/e/ea/2012lemon_and_lime.png *License:* CC BY-SA 4.0 *Contributors:* Own work *Original artist:* Swidran

- **File:3-Caren.svg** *Source:* https://upload.wikimedia.org/wikipedia/commons/8/87/3-Caren.svg *License:* Public domain *Contributors:* ? *Original artist:* ?

- **File:3_etrog.JPG** *Source:* https://upload.wikimedia.org/wikipedia/commons/0/0b/3_etrog.JPG *License:* Public domain *Contributors:* Own work *Original artist:* Yankelowitz

- **File:4628_-_Bacche_di_ginepro_al_mercato_di_Ortigia,_Siracusa_-_Foto_Giovanni_Dall'Orto,_20_marzo_2014.jpg** *Source:* https://upload.wikimedia.org/wikipedia/commons/f/fa/4628_-_Bacche_di_ginepro_al_mercato_di_Ortigia%2C_Siracusa_-_Foto_Giovanni_Dall%27Orto%2C_20_marzo_2014.jpg *License:* Attribution *Contributors:* Self-photographed *Original artist:* Giovanni Dall'Orto

- **File:4_color_mix_of_peppercorns.jpg** *Source:* https://upload.wikimedia.org/wikipedia/commons/f/f6/4_color_mix_of_peppercorns.jpg *License:* CC BY-SA 3.0 *Contributors:* Own work *Original artist:* Ragesoss

- **File:A_species_of_citrus_fruit_(Citrus_sarcodactylis_Hort._Bog.);_Wellcome_V0042687.jpg** *Source:* https://upload.wikimedia.org/wikipedia/commons/1/1d/A_species_of_citrus_fruit_%28Citrus_sarcodactylis_Hort._Bog.%29%3B_Wellcome_V0042687.jpg *License:* CC BY 4.0 *Contributors:*
http://wellcomeimages.org/indexplus/obf_images/48/0b/44970f4fb13df266e26819437638.jpg
Original artist: ?

- **File:AdhesiveBandage.png** *Source:* https://upload.wikimedia.org/wikipedia/commons/5/5c/AdhesiveBandage.png *License:* CeCILL *Contributors:* ? *Original artist:* ?

- **File:Alice_par_John_Tenniel_21.png** *Source:* https://upload.wikimedia.org/wikipedia/commons/a/a4/Alice_par_John_Tenniel_21.png *License:* Public domain *Contributors:* Scanned from "The collected verse of Lewis Carroll". New York, The Macmillan Co., 1933. ([1]) *Original artist:* Sir John Tenniel

- **File:Alpha-pinen.svg** *Source:* https://upload.wikimedia.org/wikipedia/commons/6/69/Alpha-pinen.svg *License:* CC-BY-SA-3.0 *Contributors:* Own work *Original artist:* J.delanoy

- **File:Cryptone.svg** *Source:* https://upload.wikimedia.org/wikipedia/commons/f/f1/Cryptone.svg *License:* CC BY-SA 3.0 *Contributors:* Own work *Original artist:* Nuklear

- **File:Davana-Dried.jpg** *Source:* https://upload.wikimedia.org/wikipedia/commons/6/69/Davana-Dried.jpg *License:* CC BY-SA 3.0 *Contributors:* Own work *Original artist:* Sahyadri

- **File:DavanaEssOil.png** *Source:* https://upload.wikimedia.org/wikipedia/commons/b/b7/DavanaEssOil.png *License:* Public domain *Contributors:* Own work *Original artist:* Itineranttrader

- **File:Dentistry_stub.svg** *Source:* https://upload.wikimedia.org/wikipedia/commons/5/51/Dentistry_stub.svg *License:* GFDL *Contributors:* Based upon tooth section shown in Image:ToothSection.jpg *Original artist:* Ch1902 vectorized, Asbestos raster

- **File:DillEssOil.png** *Source:* https://upload.wikimedia.org/wikipedia/commons/5/5b/DillEssOil.png *License:* Public domain *Contributors:* Own work *Original artist:* Itineranttrader

- **File:Dried_Peppercorns.jpg** *Source:* https://upload.wikimedia.org/wikipedia/commons/a/a8/Dried_Peppercorns.jpg *License:* CC-BY-SA-3.0 *Contributors:* en:Image:Dried Peppercorns.jpg *Original artist:* en:User:Bunchofgrapes

- **File:Duftlampen.jpg** *Source:* https://upload.wikimedia.org/wikipedia/commons/2/29/Duftlampen.jpg *License:* CC BY-SA 3.0 *Contributors:* Own work *Original artist:* Micha L. Rieser

- **File:Emoji_u1f33f.svg** *Source:* https://upload.wikimedia.org/wikipedia/commons/e/eb/Emoji_u1f33f.svg *License:* Apache License 2.0 *Contributors:* https://code.google.com/p/noto/ *Original artist:* Google

- **File:Epikutanni-test.jpg** *Source:* https://upload.wikimedia.org/wikipedia/commons/4/4c/Epikutanni-test.jpg *License:* CC BY-SA 3.0 *Contributors:* Own work *Original artist:* Jan Polák

- **File:Eterično_ulje.jpg** *Source:* https://upload.wikimedia.org/wikipedia/commons/a/a4/Eter.%C4%8Dno_ulje.jpg *License:* CC BY-SA 3.0 *Contributors:* Own work *Original artist:* SpeedyGonsales

- **File:Eucalyptol.png** *Source:* https://upload.wikimedia.org/wikipedia/commons/3/31/Eucalyptol.png *License:* Public domain *Contributors:* en: Image:Eucalyptol.png *Original artist:* Edgar181

- **File:EucalyptusGlobulusEssOil.png** *Source:* https://upload.wikimedia.org/wikipedia/commons/f/fa/EucalyptusGlobulusEssOil.png *License:* Public domain *Contributors:* Own work *Original artist:* Itineranttrader

- **File:Eucalyptus_polybractea_leaf.JPG** *Source:* https://upload.wikimedia.org/wikipedia/commons/4/45/Eucalyptus_polybractea_leaf.JPG *License:* Public domain *Contributors:* Own work *Original artist:* John Moss

- **File:Flag_of_Argentina.svg** *Source:* https://upload.wikimedia.org/wikipedia/commons/1/1a/Flag_of_Argentina.svg *License:* Public domain *Contributors:* Based on: http://manuelbelgrano.gov.ar/bandera/creacion-de-la-bandera-nacional/ *Original artist:* (Vector graphics by Dbenbenn)

- **File:Flag_of_Brazil.svg** *Source:* https://upload.wikimedia.org/wikipedia/en/0/05/Flag_of_Brazil.svg *License:* PD *Contributors:* ? *Original artist:* ?

- **File:Flag_of_India.svg** *Source:* https://upload.wikimedia.org/wikipedia/en/4/41/Flag_of_India.svg *License:* Public domain *Contributors:* ? *Original artist:* ?

- **File:Flag_of_Iran.svg** *Source:* https://upload.wikimedia.org/wikipedia/commons/c/ca/Flag_of_Iran.svg *License:* Public domain *Contributors:* URL http://www.isiri.org/portal/files/std/1.htm and an English translation / interpretation at URL http://flagspot.net/flags/ir'.html *Original artist:* Various

- **File:Flag_of_Italy.svg** *Source:* https://upload.wikimedia.org/wikipedia/en/0/03/Flag_of_Italy.svg *License:* PD *Contributors:* ? *Original artist:* ?

- **File:Flag_of_Mexico.svg** *Source:* https://upload.wikimedia.org/wikipedia/commons/f/fc/Flag_of_Mexico.svg *License:* Public domain *Contributors:* This vector image was created with Inkscape. *Original artist:* **Alex Covarrubias**, 9 April 2006

- **File:Flag_of_Spain.svg** *Source:* https://upload.wikimedia.org/wikipedia/en/9/9a/Flag_of_Spain.svg *License:* PD *Contributors:* ? *Original artist:* ?

- **File:Flag_of_Turkey.svg** *Source:* https://upload.wikimedia.org/wikipedia/commons/b/b4/Flag_of_Turkey.svg *License:* Public domain *Contributors:* Turkish Flag Law (Türk Bayrağı Kanunu), Law nr. 2893 of 22 September 1983. Text (in Turkish) at the website of the Turkish Historical Society (Türk Tarih Kurumu) *Original artist:* David Benbennick (original author)

- **File:Flag_of_the_People'{}s_Republic_of_China.svg** *Source:* https://upload.wikimedia.org/wikipedia/commons/f/fa/Flag_of_the_People%27s_Republic_of_China.svg *License:* Public domain *Contributors:* Own work, http://www.protocol.gov.hk/flags/eng/n_flag/design.html *Original artist:* Drawn by User:SKopp, redrawn by User:Denelson83 and User:Zscout370

- **File:Flag_of_the_United_States.svg** *Source:* https://upload.wikimedia.org/wikipedia/en/a/a4/Flag_of_the_United_States.svg *License:* PD *Contributors:* ? *Original artist:* ?

- **File:Folder_Hexagonal_Icon.svg** *Source:* https://upload.wikimedia.org/wikipedia/en/4/48/Folder_Hexagonal_Icon.svg *License:* Cc-by-sa-3.0 *Contributors:* ? *Original artist:* ?

- **File:Foodlogo2.svg** *Source:* https://upload.wikimedia.org/wikipedia/commons/d/d6/Foodlogo2.svg *License:* CC-BY-SA-3.0 *Contributors:* Original *Original artist:* Seahen

- **File:FountainSpringsWintergreen.png** *Source:* https://upload.wikimedia.org/wikipedia/commons/0/0b/FountainSpringsWintergreen.png *License:* Public domain *Contributors:* Own work *Original artist:* Mike Serfas

- **File:Fragonard_small_perfume_distillery.JPG** *Source:* https://upload.wikimedia.org/wikipedia/commons/9/95/Fragonard_small_perfume_distillery.JPG *License:* CC-BY-SA-3.0 *Contributors:* Own work *Original artist:* BrokenSphere

- **File:Macchina_calabrese.jpg** *Source:* https //upload.wikimedia.org/wikipedia/commons/e/ec/Macchina_calabrese.jpg *License:* Public domain *Contributors:* SSEA - Experimental Station of Essential Oil and Citrus Products - Reggio Calabria *Original artist:* Unknown

- **File:Marotti.jpg** *Source:* https://upload.wikimedia.org/wikipedia/commons/7/75/Marotti.jpg *License:* CC BY-SA 3.0 *Contributors:* Own work *Original artist:* Anoopmail

- **File:Meenakshi_Sundareswarar.jpg** *Source:* https://upload.wikimedia.org/wikipedia/commons/d/dd/Meenakshi_Sundareswarar.jpg *License:* CC BY-SA 3.0 *Contributors:* Own work *Original artist:* Saba rathnam

- **File:Melaleuca_alternifolia_(Maria_Serena).jpg** *Source:* https://upload.wikimedia.org/wikipedia/commons/3/34/Melaleuca_alternifolia_%28Maria_Serena%29.jpg *License:* Public domain *Contributors:* Own work *Original artist:* Tangopaso

- **File:Merge-arrow.svg** *Source:* https://upload.wikimedia.org/wikipedia/commons/a/aa/Merge-arrow.svg *License:* Public domain *Contributors:* ? *Original artist:* ?

- **File:Mergefrom.svg** *Source:* https://upload.wikimedia.org/wikipedia/commons/0/0f/Mergefrom.svg *License:* Public domain *Contributors:* ? *Original artist:* ?

- **File:Monoi_Fakarava.JPG** *Source:* https://upload.wikimedia.org/wikipedia/commons/6/61/Monoi_Fakarava.JPG *License:* GFDL *Contributors:* Own work *Original artist:* Verodemortillet

- **File:Mustard_oil.JPG** *Source:* https://upload.wikimedia.org/wikipedia/en/4/47/Mustard_oil.JPG *License:* Fair use *Contributors:*
  Own work by uploader; I release the photo under cc-by-sa-3.0 and GFDL
  Original artist: ?

- **File:Myrcen.svg** *Source:* https://upload.wikimedia.org/wikipedia/commons/8/8c/Myrcen.svg *License:* Public domain *Contributors:* Own work *Original artist:* Yikrazuul

- **File:MyrrhEssentialOil.png** *Source:* https://upload.wikimedia.org/wikipedia/commons/1/14/MyrrhEssentialOil.png *License:* Public domain *Contributors:* Own work *Original artist:* Itineranttrader

- **File:Neroli.png** *Source:* https://upload.wikimedia.org/wikipedia/commons/c/c0/Neroli.png *License:* Public domain *Contributors:* Own work *Original artist:* Itineranttrader

- **File:NutmegEssentialOil.png** *Source:* https://upload.wikimedia.org/wikipedia/commons/0/08/NutmegEssentialOil.png *License:* Public domain *Contributors:* Own work *Original artist:* Itineranttrader

- **File:Ocimene.png** *Source:* https://upload.wikimedia.org/wikipedia/commons/8/89/Ocimene.png *License:* Public domain *Contributors:* Own work *Original artist:* Edgar181

- **File:Ocimene_-_cis.png** *Source:* https://upload.wikimedia.org/wikipedia/commons/3/3c/Ocimene_-_cis.png *License:* Public domain *Contributors:* Own work *Original artist:* Edgar181

- **File:Olive_oil_from_Oneglia.jpg** *Source:* https://upload.wikimedia.org/wikipedia/commons/4/49/Olive_oil_from_Oneglia.jpg *License:* GFDL *Contributors:* Own work *Original artist:* Lemone

- **File:P2101990,lemon.jpg** *Source:* https://upload.wikimedia.org/wikipedia/commons/5/59/P2101990%2Clemon.jpg *License:* CC BY 3.0 *Contributors:* Own work (????) *Original artist:* Kiyochan50

- **File:PLoS_Mu_transposon_in_maize.jpg** *Source:* https://upload.wikimedia.org/wikipedia/commons/f/fe/PLoS_Mu_transposon_in_maize.jpg *License:* CC BY 2.5 *Contributors:* Transposon Silencing Keeps Jumping Genes in Their Place; Liza Gross PLoS Biology *Original artist:* Damon Lisch

- **File:PatchouliEssentialOil.png** *Source:* https://upload.wikimedia.org/wikipedia/commons/7/72/PatchouliEssentialOil.png *License:* Public domain *Contributors:* Own work *Original artist:* Itineranttrader

- **File:People_icon.svg** *Source:* https://upload.wikimedia.org/wikipedia/commons/3/37/People_icon.svg *License:* CC0 *Contributors:* OpenClipart *Original artist:* OpenClipart

- **File:Pepper091.jpg** *Source:* https://upload.wikimedia.org/wikipedia/commons/9/9c/Pepper091.jpg *License:* CC BY 3.0 *Contributors:* Transfered from en.wikipedia *Original artist:* Original uploader was Devadaskrishnan at en.wikipedia

- **File:Pepper_tree_in_Kolli_Hills.JPG** *Source:* https://upload.wikimedia.org/wikipedia/commons/9/9b/Pepper_tree_in_Kolli_Hills.JPG *License:* CC BY-SA 3.0 *Contributors:* Own work *Original artist:* Docku

- **File:PetitgrainEssentialOil.png** *Source:* https://upload.wikimedia.org/wikipedia/commons/3/36/PetitgrainEssentialOil.png *License:* Public domain *Contributors:* Own work *Original artist:* Itineranttrader

- **File:Pfeffermuehlen_S7301812.jpg** *Source:* https://upload.wikimedia.org/wikipedia/commons/b/b0/Pfeffermuehlen_S7301812.jpg *License:* FAL *Contributors:* Own work *Original artist:* smial

- **File:Phase_change_-_en.svg** *Source:* https://upload.wikimedia.org/wikipedia/commons/0/0b/Phase_change_-_en.svg *License:* Public domain *Contributors:* Own work *Original artist:* F l a n k e r, penubag

- **File:Phellodendron_amurense2.jpg** *Source:* https://upload.wikimedia.org/wikipedia/commons/5/50/Phellodendron_amurense2.jpg *License:* CC-BY-SA-3.0 *Contributors:* caliban.mpiz-koeln.mpg.de/mavica/index.html part of www.biolib.de *Original artist:* Kurt Stüber [1]

- **File:PineEssentialOil.png** *Source:* https://upload.wikimedia.org/wikipedia/commons/3/39/PineEssentialOil.png *License:* Public domain *Contributors:* Own work *Original artist:* Itineranttrader

- **File:Pine_forest_in_Sweden.jpg** *Source:* https://upload.wikimedia.org/wikipedia/commons/4/42/Pine_forest_in_Sweden.jpg *License:* CC BY-SA 2.0 *Contributors:* http://www.flickr.com/photos/tetrapak/5956902891/sizes/m/in/set-72157628342553177/ *Original artist:* AB Tetra Pak

- **File:StarAnise.jpg** *Source:* https://upload.wikimedia.org/wikipedia/commons/b/be/StarAnise.jpg *License:* CC-BY-SA-3.0 *Contributors:* ? *Original artist:* ?
- **File:Starr_010309-0546_Calophyllum_inophyllum.jpg** *Source:* https://upload.wikimedia.org/wikipedia/commons/5/5c/Starr_010309-0546_Calophyllum_inophyllum.jpg *License:* CC BY 3.0 *Contributors:* Plants of Hawaii, Image 010309-0546 from http://www.hear.org/starr/plants/images/image/?q=010309-0546 *Original artist:* Forest & Kim Starr
- **File:Starr_061224-2876_Cananga_odorata.jpg** *Source:* https://upload.wikimedia.org/wikipedia/commons/9/91/Starr_061224-2376_Cananga_odorata.jpg *License:* CC BY 3.0 *Contributors:* Plants of Hawaii, Image 061224-2876 from http://www.hear.org/starr/plants/images/image/?q=061224-2876 *Original artist:* Forest & Kim Starr
- **File:Sunflowers.jpg** *Source:* https://upload.wikimedia.org/wikipedia/commons/d/d5/Sunflowers.jpg *License:* Public domain *Contributors:* This image was released by the Agricultural Research Service, the research agency of the United States Department of Agriculture, with the ID K5751-1 <a class='external text' href='//commons.wikimedia.org/w/index.php?title=Category:Media_created_by_the_United_States_Agricultural_Research_Service_with_known_IDs,<span>,&,</span>,filefrom=K5751-1#mw-category-media'>(next)</a>. *Original artist:* Bruce Fritz
- **File:Symbol_book_class2.svg** *Source:* https://upload.wikimedia.org/wikipedia/commons/8/89/Symbol_book_class2.svg *License:* CC BY-SA 2.5 *Contributors:* Mad by Lokal_Profil by combining: *Original artist:* Lokal_Profil
- **File:TVM_Pepper.JPG** *Source:* https://upload.wikimedia.org/wikipedia/commons/f/f2/TVM_Pepper.JPG *License:* CC BY-SA 3.0 *Contributors:* Transferred from ml.wikipedia; transferred to Commons by User:binoyjsdk. *Original artist:* Aruna at ml.wikipedia
- **File:Tea_tree_plantation.JPG** *Source:* https://upload.wikimedia.org/wikipedia/commons/1/1b/Tea_tree_plantation.JPG *License:* Public domain *Contributors:* Own work *Original artist:* John Moss
- **File:Terpinolene.svg** *Source:* https://upload.wikimedia.org/wikipedia/commons/1/19/Terpinolene.svg *License:* Public domain *Contributors:* Own work *Original artist:* Ed (Edgar181)
- **File:Tiaré_tahiti.jpg** *Source:* https://upload.wikimedia.org/wikipedia/commons/2/2f/Tiar%C3%A9_tahiti.jpg *License:* CC-BY-SA-3.0 *Contributors:* ? *Original artist:* ?
- **File:Tree_template.svg** *Source:* https://upload.wikimedia.org/wikipedia/commons/9/98/Tree_template.svg *License:* CC BY-SA 3.0 *Contributors:*
  - File:Tango icon nature.svg
  - File:Blank_template.svg

Original artist:

  - DarKobra
  - Urutseg
  - Ain92

- **File:Treestub.jpg** *Source:* https://upload.wikimedia.org/wikipedia/commons/1/1b/Treestub.jpg *License:* CC-BY-SA-3.0 *Contributors:* Transferred from en.wikipedia; transfer was stated to be made by User:Rockfang. *Original artist:* Original uploader was MPF at en.wikipedia
- **File:Tucuma-oleo-frut4.JPG** *Source:* https://upload.wikimedia.org/wikipedia/commons/e/ed/Tucuma-oleo-frut4.JPG *License:* CC BY-SA 4.0 *Contributors:* Own work *Original artist:* P. S. Sena
- **File:Vapor_Pressure_Chart.png** *Source:* https://upload.wikimedia.org/wikipedia/commons/9/96/Vapor_Pressure_Chart.png *License:* Public domain *Contributors:* Own work *Original artist:* Mbeychok
- **File:Variants_of_Pepper.jpg** *Source:* https://upload.wikimedia.org/wikipedia/commons/0/0a/Variants_of_Pepper.jpg *License:* CC BY-SA 3.0 *Contributors:* Own work *Original artist:* Chirdukulkarni
- **File:Vitellaria_paradoxa_MS4195.JPG** *Source:* https://upload.wikimedia.org/wikipedia/commons/7/7f/Vitellaria_paradoxa_MS4195.JPG *License:* CC BY-SA 2.5 *Contributors:* Own work (own foto) *Original artist:* Marco Schmidt
- **File:White_Pepper_Grains.jpeg** *Source:* https://upload.wikimedia.org/wikipedia/commons/2/21/White_Pepper_Grains.jpeg *License:* CC BY-SA 3.0 *Contributors:* Own work *Original artist:* OttawaAC
- **File:Wiki_letter_w.svg** *Source:* https://upload.wikimedia.org/wikipedia/en/6/6c/Wiki_letter_w.svg *License:* Cc-by-sa-3.0 *Contributors:* ? *Original artist:* ?
- **File:Wikibooks-logo-en-noslogan.svg** *Source:* https://upload.wikimedia.org/wikipedia/commons/d/df/Wikibooks-logo-en-noslogan.svg *License:* CC BY-SA 3.0 *Contributors:* Own work *Original artist:* User:Bastique, User:Ramac et al
- **File:Wikispecies-logo.svg** *Source:* https://upload.wikimedia.org/wikipedia/commons/d/df/Wikispecies-logo.svg *License:* CC BY-SA 3.0 *Contributors:* Image:Wikispecies-logo.jpg *Original artist:* (of code) cs:User:-xfi-
- **File:Wiktionary-logo-en.svg** *Source:* https://upload.wikimedia.org/wikipedia/commons/f/f8/Wiktionary-logo-en.svg *License:* Public domain *Contributors:* Vector version of Image:Wiktionary-logo-en.png. *Original artist:* Vectorized by Fvasconcellos (talk · contribs), based on original logo tossed together by Brion Vibber
- **File:Wiktionary-logo.svg** *Source:* https://upload.wikimedia.org/wikipedia/commons/e/ec/Wiktionary-logo.svg *License:* CC BY-SA 3.0 *Contributors:* ? *Original artist:* ?
- **File:Wild_Almond.jpg** *Source:* https://upload.wikimedia.org/wikipedia/commons/3/39/Wild_Almond.jpg *License:* CC BY 2.0 *Contributors:* http://www.flickr.com/photos/75380256@N06/6925170900/ *Original artist:* jayeshpatil912

3.3 Content license